T0332816

# Essential Physics for Manual Medicine

To my former pupils, a promise fulfilled . . . .

. . . and to Lisa, for helping me fulfill it.

For Elsevier

*Commissioning Editor:* Claire Wilson
*Development Editors:* Ailsa Laing and Sally Davies
*Project Managers:* Anne Dickie and Srikumar Narayanan
*Designer:* Kirsteen Wright
*Illustration Manager:* Gillian Richards

# Essential Physics for Manual Medicine

**Martin Young** BSc(Hons) DC FCC
Private Practice,
Yeovil, Somerset, UK

Illustrations by

**Simon Venn**
Technical Illustrator
Simon Venn Graphic
Shaftesbury, Dorset, UK

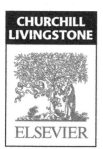

CHURCHILL
LIVINGSTONE

ELSEVIER

Edinburgh  London  New York  Oxford  Philadelphia  St Louis  Sydney  Toronto  2010

CHURCHILL
LIVINGSTONE
ELSEVIER

ISBN 978-0-443-10342-1

**British Library Cataloguing in Publication Data**
A catalogue record for this book is available from the British Library

**Library of Congress Cataloging in Publication Data**
A catalog record for this book is available from the Library of Congress

**Notice**
Neither the Publisher nor the Author assume any responsibility for any loss or injury and/or damage to persons or property arising out of or related to any use of the material contained in this book. It is the responsibility of the treating practitioner, relying on independent expertise and knowledge of the patient, to determine the best treatment and method of application for the patient.

*The Publisher*

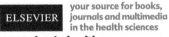

your source for books,
journals and multimedia
in the health sciences
**www.elsevierhealth.com**

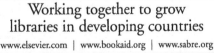

Working together to grow
libraries in developing countries
www.elsevier.com | www.bookaid.org | www.sabre.org

ELSEVIER    BOOK AID International    Sabre Foundation

The
Publisher's
policy is to use
paper manufactured
from sustainable forests

Printed in China

# Contents

Preface . . . . . . . . . . . . . . . . . . . . . . . . . . . . . . . . . . . . ix

How to use this book . . . . . . . . . . . . . . . . . . . . . . . . . . . . xi

**Chapter 1    The tools of the trade** . . . . . . . . . . . . . . . 1

Check your existing knowledge . . . . . . . . . . . . . . . . . . . . . 1
Weights and measures . . . . . . . . . . . . . . . . . . . . . . . . . . 2
Vectors and scalars . . . . . . . . . . . . . . . . . . . . . . . . . . . . 7
Algebra . . . . . . . . . . . . . . . . . . . . . . . . . . . . . . . . . . . 9
Trigonometry . . . . . . . . . . . . . . . . . . . . . . . . . . . . . . . 12
Vectors and scalars (continued) . . . . . . . . . . . . . . . . . . . . 15
Coordinates and planes . . . . . . . . . . . . . . . . . . . . . . . . . 16
Learning outcomes . . . . . . . . . . . . . . . . . . . . . . . . . . . . 24
Check your existing knowledge: answers . . . . . . . . . . . . . . . 24
Bibliography . . . . . . . . . . . . . . . . . . . . . . . . . . . . . . . . 25

**Chapter 2    Natural philosophy** . . . . . . . . . . . . . . . . . 27

Check your existing knowledge . . . . . . . . . . . . . . . . . . . . . 27
Introduction . . . . . . . . . . . . . . . . . . . . . . . . . . . . . . . . 28
Velocity, angular velocity and acceleration . . . . . . . . . . . . . . 30
Mass and momentum . . . . . . . . . . . . . . . . . . . . . . . . . . . 31
Force . . . . . . . . . . . . . . . . . . . . . . . . . . . . . . . . . . . . 32
Newton's laws and equations of motion . . . . . . . . . . . . . . . . 33
Workshop . . . . . . . . . . . . . . . . . . . . . . . . . . . . . . . . . . 36
Gravity . . . . . . . . . . . . . . . . . . . . . . . . . . . . . . . . . . . 36
Energy and work . . . . . . . . . . . . . . . . . . . . . . . . . . . . . 37
Learning outcomes . . . . . . . . . . . . . . . . . . . . . . . . . . . . 46
Check your existing knowledge: answers . . . . . . . . . . . . . . . 46
Workshop: answers . . . . . . . . . . . . . . . . . . . . . . . . . . . . 47
Bibliography . . . . . . . . . . . . . . . . . . . . . . . . . . . . . . . . 47

**Chapter 3    Applied physics** . . . . . . . . . . . . . . . . . . . 49

Check your existing knowledge . . . . . . . . . . . . . . . . . . . . . 49
Levers, beams and moments . . . . . . . . . . . . . . . . . . . . . . 50
Workshop . . . . . . . . . . . . . . . . . . . . . . . . . . . . . . . . . . 57
Bending moments and torsion . . . . . . . . . . . . . . . . . . . . . 58
Second moment of area . . . . . . . . . . . . . . . . . . . . . . . . . 60

Polar moment of inertia . . . . . . . . . . . . . . . . . . . . . . . . . 62
Centre of gravity . . . . . . . . . . . . . . . . . . . . . . . . . . . . . . 63
Instantaneous axis of rotation . . . . . . . . . . . . . . . . . . . . . 64
Property of materials . . . . . . . . . . . . . . . . . . . . . . . . . . . 65
Stress and strain . . . . . . . . . . . . . . . . . . . . . . . . . . . . . . 66
Moduli of elasticity . . . . . . . . . . . . . . . . . . . . . . . . . . . . 66
Learning outcomes . . . . . . . . . . . . . . . . . . . . . . . . . . . . 68
Check your existing knowledge: answers . . . . . . . . . . . . . . 68
Workshop: answers . . . . . . . . . . . . . . . . . . . . . . . . . . . . 68
Bibliography . . . . . . . . . . . . . . . . . . . . . . . . . . . . . . . . . 69

Chapter 4    The anatomy of physics . . . . . . . . . . . . . . . . . . . . . . 71
Check your existing knowledge . . . . . . . . . . . . . . . . . . . . . 71
The classification of joints . . . . . . . . . . . . . . . . . . . . . . . 72
Fibrous joints . . . . . . . . . . . . . . . . . . . . . . . . . . . . . . . . 74
Cartilaginous joints . . . . . . . . . . . . . . . . . . . . . . . . . . . . 76
Synovial joints . . . . . . . . . . . . . . . . . . . . . . . . . . . . . . . 77
Structural classification . . . . . . . . . . . . . . . . . . . . . . . . . 83
Ligaments . . . . . . . . . . . . . . . . . . . . . . . . . . . . . . . . . . 83
The classification of muscle . . . . . . . . . . . . . . . . . . . . . . 84
Learning outcomes . . . . . . . . . . . . . . . . . . . . . . . . . . . . 97
Check your existing knowledge: answers . . . . . . . . . . . . . . 97
Bibliography . . . . . . . . . . . . . . . . . . . . . . . . . . . . . . . . . 98

Chapter 5    The physics of anatomy . . . . . . . . . . . . . . . . . . . . . . 99
Check your existing knowledge . . . . . . . . . . . . . . . . . . . . . 99
Joint movement . . . . . . . . . . . . . . . . . . . . . . . . . . . . . . 99
Arthrokinematics . . . . . . . . . . . . . . . . . . . . . . . . . . . . . 102
Joint features . . . . . . . . . . . . . . . . . . . . . . . . . . . . . . . 105
Posture . . . . . . . . . . . . . . . . . . . . . . . . . . . . . . . . . . . 116
Gait . . . . . . . . . . . . . . . . . . . . . . . . . . . . . . . . . . . . . 120
Learning outcomes . . . . . . . . . . . . . . . . . . . . . . . . . . . 121
Bibliography . . . . . . . . . . . . . . . . . . . . . . . . . . . . . . . . 122

Chapter 6    Atomic structure . . . . . . . . . . . . . . . . . . . . . . . . . 125
Check your existing knowledge . . . . . . . . . . . . . . . . . . . . 125
Atomic theory . . . . . . . . . . . . . . . . . . . . . . . . . . . . . . . 126
Electrons and electron shells . . . . . . . . . . . . . . . . . . . . . 136
Intramolecular bonding . . . . . . . . . . . . . . . . . . . . . . . . . 143
Intermolecular bonding . . . . . . . . . . . . . . . . . . . . . . . . . 147
Learning outcomes . . . . . . . . . . . . . . . . . . . . . . . . . . . 148

Check your existing knowledge: answers . . . . . . . . . . . . . . . . 148
Bibliography . . . . . . . . . . . . . . . . . . . . . . . . . . . . . . . . 149

Chapter 7    Electricity and magnetism . . . . . . . . . . . . . . . . . . . . 151

Check your existing knowledge . . . . . . . . . . . . . . . . . . . . 151
Introduction . . . . . . . . . . . . . . . . . . . . . . . . . . . . . . . 152
Electromagnetism . . . . . . . . . . . . . . . . . . . . . . . . . . . . 153
Electrostatics . . . . . . . . . . . . . . . . . . . . . . . . . . . . . . 154
Electric potential . . . . . . . . . . . . . . . . . . . . . . . . . . . . . 155
Conductors and insulators . . . . . . . . . . . . . . . . . . . . . . . 156
Electrodynamics . . . . . . . . . . . . . . . . . . . . . . . . . . . . . 158
Electronics . . . . . . . . . . . . . . . . . . . . . . . . . . . . . . . . 161
Systems . . . . . . . . . . . . . . . . . . . . . . . . . . . . . . . . . 165
Magnetism . . . . . . . . . . . . . . . . . . . . . . . . . . . . . . . . 168
Electromagnetic induction . . . . . . . . . . . . . . . . . . . . . . . 168
The transformer . . . . . . . . . . . . . . . . . . . . . . . . . . . . . 169
Electricity in the home and clinic . . . . . . . . . . . . . . . . . . . 171
Learning outcomes . . . . . . . . . . . . . . . . . . . . . . . . . . . 175
Check your existing knowledge: answers . . . . . . . . . . . . . . . 175
Bibliography . . . . . . . . . . . . . . . . . . . . . . . . . . . . . . . 177

Chapter 8    Electromagnetic radiation and radioactivity . . . . . . . . . . . 179

Check your existing knowledge . . . . . . . . . . . . . . . . . . . . 179
Introduction . . . . . . . . . . . . . . . . . . . . . . . . . . . . . . . 180
The electromagnetic spectrum . . . . . . . . . . . . . . . . . . . . . 182
Radioactivity . . . . . . . . . . . . . . . . . . . . . . . . . . . . . . . 187
Visible light . . . . . . . . . . . . . . . . . . . . . . . . . . . . . . . . 192
X-rays . . . . . . . . . . . . . . . . . . . . . . . . . . . . . . . . . . 194
Learning outcomes . . . . . . . . . . . . . . . . . . . . . . . . . . . 199
Check your existing knowledge: answers . . . . . . . . . . . . . . . 199
Bibliography . . . . . . . . . . . . . . . . . . . . . . . . . . . . . . . 199

Chapter 9    Diagnostic imaging . . . . . . . . . . . . . . . . . . . . . . . . 203

Introduction . . . . . . . . . . . . . . . . . . . . . . . . . . . . . . . 203
The x-ray machine . . . . . . . . . . . . . . . . . . . . . . . . . . . 204
Computed tomography . . . . . . . . . . . . . . . . . . . . . . . . . 218
Magnetic resonance imaging . . . . . . . . . . . . . . . . . . . . . 221
Positron emission tomography (PET) . . . . . . . . . . . . . . . . . 226
Diagnostic ultrasonography . . . . . . . . . . . . . . . . . . . . . . 227
Learning outcomes . . . . . . . . . . . . . . . . . . . . . . . . . . . 231
Bibliography . . . . . . . . . . . . . . . . . . . . . . . . . . . . . . . 231

Chapter 10  Making it better . . . . . . . . . . . . . . . . . . . . . . 235

Check your existing knowledge . . . . . . . . . . . . . . . . . . . . . 235
Introduction . . . . . . . . . . . . . . . . . . . . . . . . . . . . . . . 235
Ultrasound . . . . . . . . . . . . . . . . . . . . . . . . . . . . . . . . 235
Cryotherapy . . . . . . . . . . . . . . . . . . . . . . . . . . . . . . . 238
Electromagnetic field therapies . . . . . . . . . . . . . . . . . . . . . 238
Magnetic field therapy . . . . . . . . . . . . . . . . . . . . . . . . . . 239
TENS . . . . . . . . . . . . . . . . . . . . . . . . . . . . . . . . . . 240
Interferential . . . . . . . . . . . . . . . . . . . . . . . . . . . . . . . 240
Electrical muscle stimulation . . . . . . . . . . . . . . . . . . . . . . . 241
Learning outcomes . . . . . . . . . . . . . . . . . . . . . . . . . . . . 241
Bibliography . . . . . . . . . . . . . . . . . . . . . . . . . . . . . . . 242

Index . . . . . . . . . . . . . . . . . . . . . . . . . . . . . . . . . . . 245

Almost everything that students of manual medicine study at College is physics, even though lecturers in some subjects occasionally try to disguise this. Take, for example, the core subject of biochemistry. Far from being a discipline in its own right, biochemistry is nothing more than the physics of the outer electron shells of a rather narrow range of elements. Physiology is simply what happens when you get a lot of biochemistry going on; anatomy merely describes where the physiology is taking place and pathology is just an overview of what can happen when the physiology stops working properly.

Then there's neurology, the study of changing electron potentials and capacitance effects, and radiography, which is what happens when you put together nuclear physics and quantum mechanics with sufficient electrical power. Radiology, meanwhile, is no more than the interpretation of a rather clever bit of physical chemistry; biomechanics speaks for itself and orthopaedics is merely biomechanics going wrong. Learning to manipulate is the intuitive application of moments of inertia to third order levers whilst modalities, such as ultra-sound, infra red, interferential and the like, are classic examples of applied physics. In fact, there is really not much that you're going to do that *isn't* physics – even relativity comes into it, as anyone who has sat through histology on a Friday afternoon, and wondered how a one-hour lecture can seem to last several days, will testify!

I know of many colleagues who regarded learning physics as a nightmare but, if they thought that learning it was tough, they should have tried teaching the subject! I can still remember my first class, sitting with mixed expressions of fear, boredom and resentment. I already knew from the admissions office that I would be teaching a class with mixed abilities; however, try to imagine my dismay when I discovered that this had been taken – as it would be in subsequent years – to ridiculous extremes. Within one body of students were several who had quit physics aged 14; a fair number who had rote-learned sufficiently to pass basic examinations, albeit with little or no actual understanding; a majority who had given up at 16 to concentrate on Biology and Chemistry; several high flyers who did well enough at 18 to have taken their studies further; and, for good measure, a couple of engineering graduates.

So, where to pitch the level of the course, without either losing the bottom end or boring the top end? The seemingly impossible answer to that question forms the basis of this textbook. Contained within these pages is stuff that you (probably) already know like the back of your hand – unless of course you quit physics aged 14, in which case I would highly recommend starting at page 1. Then there will be the stuff that you think you know but in fact don't. There is a world of difference between knowing enough about a subject to pass an examination and actually understanding it well enough to put it into practice: ask any teacher. If you are going to be treating patients, it is never enough to try to get away with the former: you will, sooner or later, be found out.

Read the following section on how to use this book to its best advantage and you'll quickly discover which areas need either to be revised or even learnt afresh as well as discovering the stuff that you don't know. It doesn't matter if you're an honours physics graduate or finished *summa cum laude* in your mechanical engineering degree course, there WILL be stuff in this book that you don't know and, what's really great, is that by reading the next section, you can easily find out what these bits are and know which chapters and sections you can skip with impunity. So yield not to the temptation to skip the stuff at the beginning and get stuck in to Chapter 1; this next bit is the instruction manual for the mobile phone of life – you will probably be able to make metaphorical calls without reading it, but to achieve full 3G multi-media functionality, it will require a further five minutes of your time.

Once done, you will hopefully find this a physics text like no other. I had the good fortune to be a not very good physicist (academically, not morally). That means that, unlike many of the brilliant minds that tried to teach me, I can understand why students have problems understanding certain concepts, what those problems are and how they can best be addressed. Some of the approaches may be unorthodox – but if you want orthodox, there are plenty of those books out there already, although you may have to shell out a fair amount: I believe this is the only book that caters to the unique requirements of the manual physician. I have tried to encapsulate all the requirements of learning basic science, diagnostic imaging, treatment modalities, clinical applications and biomechanics in simple, understandable language: a trick that I picked up and, hopefully, perfected in a previous existence as a freelance writer composing technical articles for lay audiences (well, nobody would employ me as a physicist).

I also remain, at heart, a clinician who prefers treating patients to physics. I fully appreciate that it can be a dry, difficult subject and have tried, wherever possible, to spice it up with anecdotes and clinical facts that will put the material into context for the student of manual medicine.

In writing this book I have also fulfilled a promise made to my fellow students who struggled through our biophysics syllabus in bored bewilderment, longing for a single textbook, written in clear English that would explain what it was we needed to know. To the three-quarters of my *alma mater* who failed biophysics for want of such a book, I offer this volume as evidence of a promise fulfilled.

Martin F. Young
Yeovil, England

# How to use this book

One of the best bits of advice I was ever given was, in a previous existence, by a training officer for a firm of English wine merchants who was teaching me how to tutor new recruits to be able to run their own branches. 'Check existing knowledge,' he would drum into me once or twice a day. 'Do nothing until you have checked their existing level of knowledge.'

Unless you did this, he explained, you would either patronize the person to whom you were explaining (by telling them, in detail, things that they had known for years) or bore them (by losing them completely within the first sentence or two). This, as I was to later discover, applies as much to communicating with your patient as to teaching students or professionals. As an undergraduate student, I rapidly discovered the same dictum applies to textbooks. Too many academic books seemed to have been written so that the author could prove to his professorial colleagues his intellectual brilliance by dint of terrorizing undergraduates (completely unnecessarily, we already *knew* that they were geniuses; that, presumably, is why they were made professors and asked to write books in the first place).

The problem with genius, however, is that it has difficulty in dealing with and understanding the mundane. One of the professors who taught – or tried to teach – me physics was regarded as one on the top five researchers in his field in the whole world. You might think it a privilege to be taught by such a man; it may well be, but I and 95% of my classmates never got a chance to find out – his lectures were so bad that, in time-honoured undergraduate fashion, we decided we could learn more easily from books (no matter how daunting) and voted with our feet. Why were his lectures so abysmal? Some thought it was because his mind wasn't on the job (he often would stop and stare into space for several minutes at a time; once, he concluded this hiatus by rushing out mid-lecture not to return); some thought he was ill-prepared because his heart only had room for his true passion, research, from which teaching undergraduates was an unwanted distraction. My own theory was that he was just too clever for the job: an IQ of 180+ and he struggled to understand why anybody wouldn't find quantum mechanics a bit of a doddle (in much the same way he struggled to find two matching socks or to couple buttons with button-holes).

Most physics texts have the same problem. They are written (for the most part) by people who achieved their first-class honours with effortless ease and thereafter soared into the stratosphere of *n*-dimensional space-time to ponder at length on the particle path of the Higgs' boson. If they ever did struggle with a basic concept, it was so long ago that they have forgotten it.

As an undergraduate, I liked books that had the reassuring words 'Basic', 'Elementary' or 'Essential' in their title. One somehow thought (often erroneously) that the author would not be making the assumption that you already knew the subject and had purchased the book as a little light night-time read. So, as with any class, how do you reach all levels at once? The answer is to aim at the lowest common denominator but to give the high-fliers and the previously informed a fast-track through to the information they require.

At the start of every chapter, there is either a quick quiz or an explanation of the knowledge the user should already have before they proceed. Answers to the quizzes can be found at the end of the chapter, along with a rough scale indicating whether you can skip the chapter completely; skim through it in order to patch up any leakages in your grasp of the subject area; or work though it in detail to learn new material.

This also gives you the chance to go back and retest yourself at the end of the chapter to ensure you have mastery before deciding whether it is appropriate to move on – the crucial thing is to build on firm foundations. That is why the basic

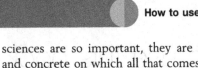

sciences are so important, they are the hard core and concrete on which all that comes after is built. You are going to learn so much during the course of your studies that, in many ways, it matters little what you learned in the past – that represents a mere drop in the ocean to what is to come. The only important thing is to make sure you access the information in a logical order so that it makes sense, rather than try to learn facts in isolation. That way the examiners will be testing your knowledge rather than your memory, and your future patients will benefit from treatment by a rounded clinician rather than a therapist hoping their areas of ignorance won't be exposed.

# Chapter One

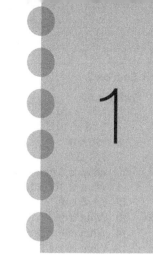

# The tools of the trade

## CHAPTER CONTENTS

Check your existing knowledge . . . . . . .  1
Weights and measures  . . . . . . . . . . . .  2
   Numbers  . . . . . . . . . . . . . . . . . . . . . .  2
   Scientific notation  . . . . . . . . . . . . . . .  3
   Units  . . . . . . . . . . . . . . . . . . . . . . . . .  4
Vectors and scalars  . . . . . . . . . . . . . .  7
Algebra  . . . . . . . . . . . . . . . . . . . . . . . .  9
Trigonometry . . . . . . . . . . . . . . . . . . . .  12
   Conclusion . . . . . . . . . . . . . . . . . . . . .  14
Vectors and scalars (continued)  . . . . . . .  15

Resolving vectors  . . . . . . . . . . . . . . . .  15
Addition of vectors  . . . . . . . . . . . . . . .  16
Coordinates and planes . . . . . . . . . . . . .  16
   The anatomical system  . . . . . . . . . . . .  16
   The orthogonal system  . . . . . . . . . . . .  19
   Three-dimensional movement  . . . . . . . .  21
Learning outcomes . . . . . . . . . . . . . . . .  24
Check your existing knowledge:
answers  . . . . . . . . . . . . . . . . . . . . . . . .  24
Bibliography  . . . . . . . . . . . . . . . . . . . . .  25

## CHECK YOUR EXISTING KNOWLEDGE

### Section 1

1 If $4x + 4y - 12z = 32$, derive an expression for $x$.
2 Expand $(x - y)(2x + y)$

In the diagram below:

3 What is $x$?
4 What is $\theta$?
5 What is $\gamma$?

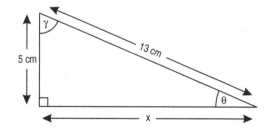

## Section 2

Write in full:
6  $1.67 \times 10^{12}$
7  $1.76 \times 10^{-9}$
8  716 km
9  671 GJ
10  What is 3 mm + 4 μm?
11  What is $10^0 \times 10^1 \times 10^2 \times 10^3$?
12  What is $9^{\frac{1}{2}}$?
13  What is $9^{-1}$?
14  What is the SI unit of temperature?
15  What is the SI unit of electrical resistance?
16  What is a scalar?
17  An object is acted upon by two forces. One, from the south, acts with a force of 4 newtons; the other, of equal magnitude, acts from the west.
   a  In which direction does the object move?
   b  What is the magnitude of the resultant force?
18  The YZ orthogonal plane is the equivalent to which anatomical plane?
19  If a person's body undergoes $-\theta_y$ rotation, what action are they performing?

# Weights and measures

In order to measure something, you need two elements: a quantity and a unit. If you enquire as to the distance to the nearest town and got the reply, 'miles' (as can often be the case in certain rural parts), it is of limited use. Of course, you can infer that the distance is one that you would be inclined to measure using miles rather than, say, inches or parsecs and that it is, by the use of the plural, more than a single mile; however, knowing whether it was 2 miles or 200 miles would be useful. Units require numbers to quantify them.

In a similar fashion, an answer of '17' is even more unhelpful. Seventeen what? Miles? Kilometres? Leagues? Furlongs? So numbers, when used for measuring things, need units to quantify them.

 **DICTIONARY DEFINITION**

### PARSEC

An astronomical measure equivalent to the distance travelled by light in 3.26 years (30 700 000 000 000 km), a distance that would take you three-quarters of the way to alpha centauri proxima, the nearest star (other than the sun) to earth.

### LEAGUE

An archaic measure of distance equal to about three miles, now only remembered from the fairy tale of the *Seven league boots* and Tennyson's 'Half a league, half a league, half a league onward' from *The charge of the light brigade*.

### FURLONG

Originally the length of a furrow in mediaeval strip farming; now an eighth of a mile and only commonly used in horse racing.

# Numbers

The problem with numbers is that there are an awful lot of them. In fact, there are an infinite number of them – they continue, quite literally, forever: take the largest number you can imagine ... and then add one! With smaller numbers, it is often easier to write the numeral than the number itself: '8' is quicker to write (and spell) than 'eight'; '1327' requires seven pen-strokes, 'one-thousand, three-hundred-and-twenty-seven' needs 78.

Numbers are also much more useful for mathematics than words. Organizing them into representations of units, tens, hundreds, thousands and having a 'zero' allows us to manipulate them arithmetically – see how easy you find the following sums:

    a   Twenty-six plus forty-eight plus nineteen equals?

    b   XXVI + XLVIII + XIX =

    c    26
       +48
       +19

(The answers are: a) ninety-three; b) XCIII and c) 93.)

The decimal (base ten) numeral system that we use is certainly more convenient on an everyday basis, and having a 'zero' enables us to perform mental calculations that were unavailable to the Romans – which is why the Greeks and the Arabs, from whom we obtained our digits (including the zero), were far more advanced in mathematics than the speakers of Latin, including the mediaeval scholars of Western Europe.

However, left to themselves, numbers become cumbersome for physicists, who must be able to measure everything from the size of a sub-atomic particle to the number of such particles in the universe. There are three ways of doing this: you can put up with writing down very long numbers, you can adapt the units you are using or you can find a short-hand way of recording very large (and very small) numbers.

The first of these options is impractical. Whereas the diameter of an atomic nucleus is approximately 0.000 000 000 000 01 metres – a number that is tedious to write on a regular basis – the number of particles in the universe is estimated as being somewhere in the region of 1 followed by eighty zeros, a number so big that it would fill several lines, take several minutes to write and even longer to read, painstakingly counting out the zeros in groups of three without losing track of one's place.

It wasn't long before people began adapting units to suit their needs, as has always been the case (an inch is the width of a thumb, a foot the length of a foot, a pace is a yard, and a fathom the arm span of a man). So, carpenters, in this metric age, use millimetres; engineers, microns (a thousandth of a millimetre); molecular scientists, Angstrøms (a ten-millionth of a millimetre). Although this is convenient if all your measurements are conducted in the same way and for discussions or recording

of data, it does not allow for easy manipulation of data. It is important to know and remember that you can only add, subtract, multiply and divide quantities if they are in the same units. You can't add millimetres directly to Angstrøms any more than you can directly add a distance measured in miles to one measured in kilometres.

## Scientific notation

There is, however, a way of recording all numbers in a convenient way using **scientific notation**, a universally agreed system for expressing any number in terms of its power of ten. You will already be familiar with certain powers of ten:

$10^2$ = **ten squared = 100**
$10^3$ = **ten cubed = 1000**

The digit to the top right is the number of times the main figure is multiplied together:

$2^4 = 2 \times 2 \times 2 \times 2 = 16$

The number ten is useful in that multiplying by ten simply involves adding a nought to the end of the number you are multiplying (e.g. $10 \times 10\,000 = 100\,000$); therefore, the power to which ten is raised is *also* equal to the number of noughts:

$10^6$   = **1 000 000**
$10^{10}$ = **10 000 000 000**

Suddenly, the number of particles in the universe becomes a much more manageable $10^{80}$ (estimates actually range from $10^{72}$ to $10^{87}$)!

This convention also skirts around another problematical area, that of nomenclature. Although people are generally agreed as to the meanings of 'hundred', 'thousand' and 'million', thereafter American English diverges from its mother tongue and works in increments of a thousand rather than a million so, on one side of the Atlantic, a billion is a *thousand* million ($10^9$) and, on the other, it has traditionally been a *million* million ($10^{12}$), except in some European countries, such as France, who have adopted the American convention. As the numbers get larger, so does the confusion: a British trillion ($10^{18}$) is an American quintillion whilst an American trillion is a British billion. Because international finance uses the American convention, the trend is increasingly to follow this, even in the UK, but the use of scientific convention removes all ambiguity ... as well as doing away with the need to remember how many noughts there are in a septillion! (For the record, in the US, 24; in the UK, 42.)

For numbers that aren't exact multiples of ten, scientific notation uses multiplication so:

$$2 \times 10^6 = 2\,000\,000$$

and

$$2.64 \times 10^6 = 2\,640\,000$$

For numbers between 0 and 1000, it is usual to write them in full but, just so you know, any number raised to the power of one is itself ($x^1$ is $x$; $10^1$ is 10) and any number raised to the power of zero is 1 ($x^0$ is 1; $10^0$ is also 1). It is also worth pointing out at this stage that multiplying powers is quite simple – you just add them together:

$$10^6 \times 10^2 = 10^{6+2} = 10^8$$

or

$$1\,000\,000 \times 100 = 100\,000\,000$$

It is also, at this stage, worth quickly dealing with **fractional powers**: if a number is raised to the power of a $\frac{1}{2}$, it is the number's square root; raised to $\frac{1}{3}$, it is the number's cube root and so on:

$$100^{\frac{1}{2}} = \sqrt{100} = 10$$

$$1000^{\frac{1}{3}} = \sqrt[3]{1000} = 10$$

Having dealt with the very big, it is a relatively easy matter to deal with the very small. If a number is raised to a **negative power**, it is the *inverse* of the positive power:

$$x^{-y} = \frac{1}{x^y}$$

or

$$\frac{1}{10^6} = \frac{1}{1\,000\,000} = 0.000\,001$$

so

$$\frac{1}{2.64 \times 10^6} = \frac{1}{2\,640\,000} = 0.000\,002\,64$$

Now we have a way of representing any number, large or small, in a concise, consistent and comprehensible manner. This can take us from the unimaginably small to the incomprehensibly large (Fig. 1.1); however, bear in mind that the scale in this figure is not linear but **logarithmic**; that is, it rises in powers of ten: $10^6$ is not *twice* as big as $10^3$, it is *one thousand* times bigger. If we used a normal, linear scale, it wouldn't just be a case being hard to fit Figure 1.1 on the page – it would be hard to fit into the known universe!

## Units

Since the dawn of time, humans have been measuring things. Thousands of years ago, the ancient Egyptians and Chinese had discovered sophisticated ways of measuring distances (for building purposes – walls, pyramids and the like) and time (the cyclical passage of astronomical bodies; clocks would come later). Thousands – possibly tens of thousands – of years before that, early man had almost certainly found ways of describing to their friends how far it was to the mammoth hunting grounds, and to their womenfolk the enormous size of the mammoth they had so nearly managed to kill.

The problem with ancient measuring systems was that they were either comparative (my club is bigger than your club) or local to one tribe or one area. On a day-to-day basis, this was not a problem but, as civilization became more international, the need for uniformity became more pronounced. One only has to look at the story of the cubit to get an idea of size of the problem.

Originally, a cubit was the distance from one's fingertips to one's elbow. Quite obviously, this varies from one individual to the next but will suffice if the measurement is a personal one (I want to cut a piece of wood as long as the measurement I just made) or if there's only one carpenter in town and he's willing to make house calls in order to measure up for jobs.

As soon as commerce was invented, this definition lost its usefulness – as anyone familiar with the story of *The King's New Bed* will know (a king kept having problems ordering a bed that he had

| Power | Description |
|---|---|
| | Distance (in metres) to the edge of the visible universe |
| $10^{24}$ | |
| | Mass of the Earth (kg) |
| $10^{21}$ | Diameter (in metres) of the Milky Way galaxy |
| $10^{18}$ | Mass of free water on the Earth (kg) |
| | Number of metres in a light year |
| $10^{15}$ | Age of the Universe (in seconds) |
| $10^{12}$ | |
| | Distance (in metres) to the sun |
| $10^{9}$ | Average human lifespan (in seconds) |
| | Speed (in metres per second) of light in a vacuum |
| | Temperature (in Kelvin) of Sun's core |
| $10^{6}$ | |
| | Frequency (in Hertz) of bat's squeak |
| $10^{3}$ | Speed (in metres per second) of sound at sea level |
| | Height (in metres) of Mount Everest |
| | Gravitational force (in Newtons) on Earth's surface |
| $10^{0}$ | Number of atoms in a square metre of outer space |
| | Wavelength of microwaves (metres) |
| $10^{-3}$ | |
| | Wavelength of infra-red radiation (metres) |
| $10^{-6}$ | |
| | Wavelength of visible light (metres) |
| | Lowest artificially obtained temperature (Kelvin) |
| $10^{-9}$ | |
| | Separation of atoms in a solid (metres) |
| | Wavelength of x-rays (metres) |
| $10^{-12}$ | |
| | Binding energy of helium nucleus (Joules) |
| | Diameter (in metres) of atomic nuclei |
| $10^{-15}$ | |
| | Energy of an ultra-violet photon (Joules) |
| $10^{-18}$ | |
| | Charge (in coulombs) on an electron |

**Figure 1.1** • From the very small to the very large.

measured as 6 feet long by 4 feet wide until he found a carpenter with feet the same size as his own; thereafter, he made models of his foot for his citizens to use for measurements throughout his realm and so everyone lived happily ever after … except for a couple of carpenters who had had their heads removed for failing to make a bed that came up to royal requirements).

A number of non-fictional rulers tried to standardize the cubit; the trouble was – much like the eponymous king – they presumably used their own personal cubit as the standard. This means that the biblical cubit (as used to lay down Noah's Ark, God presumably having Noah's arm measurements down pat when issuing his omnipotent blueprints) at 56 cm was different from that of the Egyptians (53 cm), which, in turn, was different from that of the Romans (44 cm), which was slightly shorter than that of the British (46 cm).

Where trade failed to agree communal weights and measures, empires enforced them. The Romans at one time ruled almost half the population of the known world and, even if they failed in the long-term standardization of the cubit, from them, we get the *mille* or mile, a thousand (double) paces … even if the statute mile is approximately 140 yards longer than the Roman one … and, for various technical reasons, 265 yards less than a nautical mile.

## Fact File

### THE MILE

The Roman foot measured 11.68 modern inches, divided, as is its modern day successor, into 12 parts (uniciae). Five feet made for one passus (from pace, meaning 'double step') and the mille passus (Roman mile) was 1000 paces or 5000 feet long – for the record, the cubit was one and a half feet long.

The statute mile of 5280 feet is so-called as it was formalized in a Parliamentary statute in 1592 by Elizabeth I, having been in usage since the 13th century. Different countries (including the US) had slight variations on this distance (the US Survey mile is longer by $\frac{1}{10}$ inch) and it was not until 1959 that a standard length was agreed.

The nautical mile of 2025 yards bears only a coincidental relationship to the statute mile, being a measure of 1' (one minute = one-sixtieth of a degree) of latitude.

## The Imperial system

The British Empire, being predominantly a vehicle for trade, had a little more success at imposing its weights and measures upon the world ... indeed, that is why the system of feet and inches; ounces and pounds; pints and gallons is called the Imperial system (of, or pertaining to, an empire). Even then, different towns often had differing ideas as to what constituted a pound and what qualified as short measure and, even today, there is a difference between the amount – and spelling – of units: a US gallon is 3.79 *liters* and a UK gallon, 4.55 *litres*.

If you think this haphazard, bear in mind that, until the need for conformity was driven by railway timetabling in the mid-19th century, different towns not only could have different weights and measures but even their clocks were set differently, not just by seconds but by minutes!

## The MKS system

Whilst science was still limited to the leisurely pursuit of gentleman amateurs, such variations mattered little as long as there was internal consistency; however, as the pace of scientific and technical advance started to snowball in the early 19th century, scientists began to seek a means of developing international conformity. The first international system devised was called the metre-kilogram-second (MKS) system whereby scientists agreed to use metres for measuring all distances, kilograms for mass and seconds for time. There was, of course, a schism almost straight away with some scientists championing centimetres, grammes and seconds (CGS system), which, as you will see later, explains some of the derived units with which we have been historically endowed.

Importantly though, there was also, for the first time, international agreement as to what the exact definition of these quantities should be.

A metre had already been defined by the French Academy of Science in the post-revolution fervour for change as $^1/_{10\ 000\ 000}$ of the quadrant of the Earth's circumference running from the North Pole through Paris to the equator. The kilogram was defined as the mass of 1000 cubic centimetres of water, the second as $^1/_{86\ 400}$ of the average period of rotation of the Earth on its axis relative to the Sun. Unfortunately, as measurements became ever more precise, the definitions were no longer accurate enough: the Earth's crust is a dynamic, moving structure subject to alteration at short notice; its

rotation is also (very) gradually slowing. The density of water changes according to temperature and pressure (not to mention to regional fluctuations in the Earth's gravitational field).

The problem was temporarily solved by relating the definitions of mass and length to the parameters of two lumps of platinum and iridium (and thus highly inert and resistant to oxidation) that were kept locked in a Parisian vault ... which was fine if you were a Parisian scientist but was a bit tough on anyone else who wanted to calibrate their instruments.

Today, wherever possible, we use highly precise definitions based on constant phenomena that are observable by any scientist working anywhere in the world or, indeed, off it. A metre is now defined as the distance travelled by light in a vacuum in $^1/_{299\ 792\ 458}$ of a second; a second is 9 192 631 770 cycles of radiation associated with the transition between the two hyperfine levels of the ground state of the caesium-133 atom (a statement that will be understandable by the end of Ch. 8). A kilogram, however, remains as the mass of a cylinder of French platinum-iridium until somebody can think of anything better.

## The SI system

By this time, three new units had been added, all named after eminent scientists: a unit of force (the **newton**, N), defined as that force which gives to a mass of one kilogram an acceleration of one metre per second per second; a unit of energy (the **joule**, J), defined as the work done when the point of application of a newton is displaced one metre in the direction of the force; and a unit of power (the **watt**, W), which is the power that, in one second, gives rise to energy of one joule.

These additional units, which built upon the MKS system, were called the *Système International D'unités*, known as the **SI system**. Since its formal adoption in 1960, many more units have been added. There are now seven basic units (Table 1.1): in addition to the metre, the kilogram and the second, we now have the **ampere**, A, for electric current; for luminous intensity, the **candela**, cd; for temperature, **kelvin**, K; and for quantity of substance, the **mole**, mol.

The three original derived units have also been built upon considerably; however, *all* these other SI units can – as Tables 1.2, 1.3 and 1.4 show – be defined in terms of these seven basic units, either directly or indirectly. Many of these units have their

**Table 1.1** The seven base SI units

| Unit | Symbol | Definition |
|---|---|---|
| Metre | m | The distance travelled by light in a vacuum in $^1/_{299\ 792\ 458}$ second |
| Kilogram | kg | Defined by the international prototype kilogram of platinum-iridium in the keeping of the International Bureau of Weights and Measures in Sèvres, France |
| Second | s | The duration of 9 192 631 770 periods of radiation associated with a specified transition of the cesium-133 atom |
| Ampere | A | The current that, if maintained in two wires placed one metre apart in a vacuum, would produce a force of $2 \times 10^{-7}$ newton per metre of length |
| Kelvin | K | $^1/_{273.16}$ of the triple point of pure water (corresponding to $-273.15°$ on the Celsius scale and to $-459.67°$ on the Fahrenheit scale). It is calculated by extrapolating the point at which an ideal gas and constant pressure would reach zero volume |
| Mole | mol | The amount of a given substance that contains as many elementary entities as there are atoms in 0.012 kilogram of carbon-12 |
| Candela | cd | The intensity in a given direction of a source emitting radiation of frequency $540 \times 10^{12}$ hertz and that has a radiant intensity in that direction of $^1/_{683}$ watt per steradian |

own special names (such as the newton and joule). At this stage, there may appear to be an alarming number of these units with peculiar names that define quantities of which you may never have heard – and the lists given are by no means complete, these are merely the units that a health professional is likely to encounter! However, by the time you have finished the book, all these terms should be like regular acquaintances. Do not try to memorize them all at this stage,

rather familiarize yourself with the names and use the table as a reference so that, when you encounter a new term or an unfamiliar symbol, you can refer back and learn the detail in its correct context.

There is one other trick to know about when it comes to units, which can – and often does – serve as an alternative to scientific nomenclature. In everyday conversation, it becomes a bit tedious to say 'it's six times ten to the three metres to the nearest town' so, instead, we say 'it's six *kilo-metres*', 'kilo' being a prefix meaning 'one thousand'. Scientists do the same in *their* everyday conversation too: there are a stack of these prefixes, some of which – kilo ($10^3$), centi ($10^{-2}$), milli ($10^{-3}$) – you will be familiar with as you will with their common abbreviations: k, c and m respectively. Table 1.5 shows the abbreviations and symbols from $10^{-24}$ to $10^{24}$, which, whilst not exhaustive, is enough for most eventualities that you are likely to encounter. So you are now able to express large and small quantities in two ways, by saying, for example:

**6.5 × 10$^7$ watts or 65 megawatts**
**8.9 × 10$^{-16}$ joules or 890 attojoules**

## Vectors and scalars

Even when you have put together a quantity with its unit, there is one other consideration that may need to be made, that of *direction*. With units such as mass, there is no directional element: 5 kg is 5 kg whether it is heading north or south, upside down or back to front. Such units are known as **scalars**. Quantities such as temperature and time are also scalar.

By contrast, it is easy to appreciate that, for other measures, direction is all-important. Movement of 600 m in a westerly direction is not at all the same thing as movement of 600 m in an easterly direction; the same applies to velocity, force and magnetic field strength. So for these quantities, known as **vectors**, direction must also be specified and, unless the vectors are all acting in the same direction, we need to be able to *resolve* the vectors if we wish to multiply or add them. For this, we need some basic mathematical tools: algebra and trigonometry, which we will also utilize elsewhere in the book. For those who sailed through this section in the test at the start of the chapter, move on to

**Table 1.2** Some derived SI units

| Quantity | Unit | Symbol |
|---|---|---|
| Acceleration ($a$) | Metres per second per second | $m/s^2 = ms^{-2}$ |
| Area ($A$) | Square metre | $m^2$ |
| Current density ($j$) | Ampere per metre | $A/m^2 = Am^{-2}$ |
| Density ($\rho$) | Kilogram per cubic metre | $kg/m^3 = kgm^{-3}$ |
| Luminance ($L_v$) | Candela per square metre | $cd/m^2 = cdm^{-2}$ |
| Magnetic field strength ($H$) | Ampere per metre | $A/m = Am^{-1}$ |
| Substance concentration ($c$) | Mole per cubic metre | $mol/m^3 = mol.m^{-3}$ |
| Volume ($V$) | Cubic metre | $m^3$ |
| Velocity ($v$) | Metres per second | $m/s = ms^{-1}$ |
| Wave number ($\sigma$) | Reciprocal metre | $m^{-1}$ |

**Table 1.3** Some derived SI units with special names and symbols

| Quantity | Unit | Symbol | Derivation |
|---|---|---|---|
| Angle, plane | Radian | rad | $2\pi\,rad = 360°$ |
| Angle, solid ($\Omega$) | Steradian | sr | The angle that, having its vertex in the centre of a sphere, cuts off an area of the surface of the sphere equal to the square of the radius |
| Capacitance ($C$) | Farad | F | $m^{-2}.kg^{-1}.s^4.A^2 \left(= {}^C/_V\right)$ |
| Electric charge ($Q$) | Coulomb | C | $s.A$ |
| Electric conductance ($\sigma$) | Siemens | S | $m^{-2}.kg^{-1}.s^3.A^2 \left(= {}^A/_V\right)$ |
| Electric potential difference ($V$) | Volt | V | $m^2.kg.s^{-3}.A^{-1} \left(= {}^W/_A\right)$ |
| Electrical resistance ($R$) | Ohm | $\Omega$ | $m^2.kg.s^{-3}.A^{-2} \left(= {}^V/_A\right)$ |
| Energy/work ($W$) | Joule | J | $m^2.kg.s^{-2} (= N.m)$ |
| Force ($F$) | Newton | N | $m.kg.s^{-2}$ |
| Frequency ($f,\nu$) | Hertz | Hz | $s^{-1}$ |
| Inductance ($L$) | Henry | H | $m^2.kg.s^{-2}.A^{-2} \left(= {}^{Wb}/_A\right)$ |
| Luminous flux ($\Phi_v$) | Lumen | lm | $cd.sr^{-1}$ |
| Magnetic flux ($\Phi$) | Weber | Wb | $m^2.kg.s^{-2}.A^{-1} (= V.s)$ |
| Magnetic flux density ($\beta$) | Tesla | T | $kg.s^{-2}.A^{-1} \left(= {}^{Wb}/_{m^2}\right)$ |
| Pressure ($p$) | Pascal | Pa | $m^{-1}.kg.s^{-2} \left(= {}^N/_{m^2}\right)$ |
| Radiation, absorbed dose ($\alpha$) | Gray | Gy | $m^2.s^{-2} \left(= {}^J/_{kg}\right)$ |
| Radiation dose equivalence ($D_e$) | Sievert | Sv | $m^2.s^{-2} \left(= {}^J/_{kg}\right)$ |
| Radionuclide activity ($A$) | Becquerel | Bq | $s^{-1}$ |

**Table 1.4** Some SI units with derived unit names

| Quantity | Unit | Derivation |
|---|---|---|
| Absorbed dose rate | Gray per second | $Gy.s^{-1}$ |
| Angular acceleration ($\alpha$) | Radian per second per second | $rad.s^{-2}$ |
| Angular velocity ($\omega$) | Radian per second | $rad.s^{-1}$ |
| Electric charge density ($P$) | Coulomb per cubic metre | $C.m^{-3}$ |
| Electric field strength ($E$) | Volt per metre | $V.m^{-1}$ |
| Exposure, X- & $\gamma$-ray | Coulomb per kilogram | $C.kg^{-1}$ |
| Moment of force ($F_m$) | Newton metre | $N.m$ |
| Thermal conductivity ($\lambda$) | Watts per metre per kelvin | $Wm^{-1}K^{-1}$ |
| Viscosity ($\pi$) | Pascal second | $Pa.s$ |

**Table 1.5** Commonly used prefixes for SI units. Note the use of capital letters for units of $10^6$ and above and lower case for $10^3$ and below

| | | |
|---|---|---|
| $10^{24}$ | Yotta | Y |
| $10^{21}$ | Zetta | Z |
| $10^{18}$ | Exa | E |
| $10^{15}$ | Peta | P |
| $10^{12}$ | Tera | T |
| $10^9$ | Giga | G |
| $10^6$ | Mega | M |
| $10^3$ | Kilo | k |
| $10^2$ | Hecto | h |
| $10^1$ | Deka | da |
| $10^{-1}$ | Deci | d |
| $10^{-2}$ | Centi | c |
| $10^{-3}$ | Milli | m |
| $10^{-6}$ | Micro | $\mu$ |
| $10^{-9}$ | Nano | n |
| $10^{-12}$ | Pico | p |
| $10^{-15}$ | Femto | f |
| $10^{-18}$ | Atto | a |
| $10^{-21}$ | Zepto | z |
| $10^{-24}$ | Yocto | y |

'Coordinates and planes'; for those who did not, there now follows a short crash course in the basic mathematics you will need to become an adequate physicist.

# Algebra

It is surprising that many people, who have no problems with arithmetic, often stumble when it comes to algebra – yet all that has happened is that numbers, which represent specific instances or events, have been replaced with letters to signify general rules. There is a linguistic equivalent: if you say, "I need to drink two litres of water a day", this relates only to you . . . it may be a matter of personal preference, desire, pathology or neurosis. The statement is true and valid but it is not a generality, it applies only and specifically to the person making the statement; however, if you were instead to say, "One needs to drink two litres of water a day", the statement can then apply to any individual and implies that it is necessary for people as a whole to drink that much in order to maintain their health.

Thus, if we say that if bananas cost \$2/kg; the cost of 10 kg is \$20, we are covering only one single

instance – the statement is no longer true if the price of bananas changes. By contrast, if we say that bananas cost \$$a$/kg, therefore the cost of 10 kg is \$10$a$, we have made a statement that is true for all eventualities – you can replace the term $a$ with whatever the current price happens to be and you have means to calculate the cost of 10 kg bananas. It is possible to go even further: what happens if you want a different quantity of bananas? Ten kilograms of bananas is, after all, rather a large quantity for any primate who has actually stopped swinging from branches. Therefore, we can say that, if the cost of bananas is \$$a$/kg, then the cost of $b$ kg is \$$ab$. We can then substitute the appropriate numerical values for $a$ and $b$ and we have a means to calculate our banana expenditure.

There are similar generalized rules for addition, subtraction and division. Until you become comfortably familiar with algebra, it often helps with understanding the statements if you substitute real numbers (of your choice) for the algebraic letters:

- If a boy is $b$ years old and his younger sister is $g$ years old, the boy is $(b - g)$ years older than his sister.

  *(If a boy is 9 years old and his younger sister is 6 years old, the boy is (9 − 6 = 3) years older than his sister.)*

- If 5 lorries carry a load of $l$ kg each and 8 vans carry a load of $v$ kg each, then the total load carried is $(5l + 8v)$ kg.

  *(If 5 lorries carry a load of 1000 kg each and 8 vans carry a load of 350 kg each, then the total load carried is (5 × 1000 + (8 × 350) = 7800 kg).*

- If a syndicate of $s$ people win a prize of $\$p$, then they each get:

$$\$\frac{p}{s}$$

*(If a syndicate of 10 people wins a prize of \$100 000, then they each get:*

$$\$\frac{100\,000}{10} = \$10\,000)$$

There are also rules for simplifying algebraic expressions:

For addition and subtraction (once again, you can check the rules by inserting real numbers of your own, you will find the rules work whatever your choice of number; an example is given in the first instance; thereafter, you can provide your own):

$2a + a = 3a$   {if $a = 6$, then $(2 × 6) + 6 = 3 × 6 = 18$}

$10b - b = 9b$

$5c - 5c = 0$

$6d + e - d - 3e = 5d - 2e$

For multiplication:

$3 × f × g = 3fg$

$h × h = h^2$

$i × i × i = i^3$

For indices:

$$j^2 × j^3 = j^{2+3} = j^5$$
$$k^6 ÷ k^3 = k^{6-3} = k^3$$
$$(l^4)^2 = l^4 × l^4 = l^8$$
$$m^2 + m^2 = 2m^2$$
$$3n^3 × 2n^4 = 6n^7$$
$$9p^3 ÷ 3p = \frac{9p^3}{3p} = 3p^2$$
$$\sqrt{(16q^2)} = 4q$$

And, finally, you will need to know and understand how to use and manipulate *brackets*. Brackets are used to remove ambiguity from mathematical expressions. Take the arithmetical statement $4 × 3 + 2 = ?$

There is no way to tell whether this means 'four-times-three, then add two' $\{(4 × 3) + 2 = 14\}$ or 'four times three-plus-two' $\{4 × (3 + 2) = 20\}$, unless you add brackets. The following rules apply to removing brackets:

$$3(r + 7s) = 3r + 21s$$
$$t(4t - 3u) = 4t^2 + 3ut$$
$$2v(3v + 6w - 2) = 6v^2 + 12vw - 4v$$
$$3(x + 4y) + 4(3x - 2y) = 3x + 12y + 12x - 8y$$
$$= 15x + 4y$$
$$(2z + \alpha) × (3z - 2\alpha) = 6z^2 - 4z\alpha + 3z\alpha - 2\alpha^2$$
$$= 6z^2 - z\alpha - 2\alpha^2$$

(NB Multiply the first term in the left hand bracket, $2z$, by the first and then the second term in the right hand bracket and then do the same for the second term in the left hand bracket.)

By this rule, we should note that:

$$(2x - y)^2 \neq 4x^2 - y^2$$

But rather:

$$(2x - y)^2 = (2x - y) × (2x - y)$$
$$= 4x^2 - 2xy - 2xy + y^2 = 4x^2 - 4xy + y^2$$

(NB: If you were wondering why the $y^2$ term is positive, it is because two negatives multiplied together make a positive – just as they do linguistically: "'I'm *not* saying 'No'" means that you are in fact saying 'Yes'.)

You will most often encounter algebra in formulae, when it is a relatively simple matter of substituting numerical values that relate to the instance with which you are dealing for the algebraic letter. For example, if we take the world's most famous equation:

$$E = mc^2$$

and we wish to know how much energy ($E$) can be gained from 5 kg of mass ($m$) – knowing as we do that the speed of light ($c$) is $3 \times 10^8$ ms$^{-1}$ – then the equation becomes:

$$E = 5 \times (3 \times 10^8)^2 = 4.5 \times 10^{17} \text{ kg.m.s}^{-1} = 450 \text{ PJ}$$

However, equations and formulae aren't always written in the manner that we want to use them. This doesn't matter; any equation contains other equations just itching to get out ... all you have to do to release them is play detective using a few simple rules.

It helps if you think of an equation as a set of balance scales with the equals sign acting as the central fulcrum. An equation states that both sides of the balance are in equilibrium. There are all kinds of things you can do to an equation – add to it, subtract from it, divide it, multiply it, square it, etc. – so long as you *do the same thing to BOTH sides of the equation*, just as you would to keep the scales balanced.

To return to Einstein's classic; it may be that we actually want to calculate the mass we would require to create 1 megajoule of energy. The formula as it is written doesn't tell us this, so we need to use our detective skills to isolate $m$ in order that the equation is written in terms of $m =$ something. If we were to divide BOTH sides of the equation by $c^2$ then we would not be affecting its balance:

$$\frac{E}{c^2} = \frac{mc^2}{c^2}$$

However,

$$c^2 \div c^2 = 1,$$

and

$$1 \times m = m;$$

Therefore:

$$m = \frac{E}{c^2}$$

Therefore $m = 10^6/(3 \times 10^8)^2 = 1.11 \times 10^{-11}$g

A similar trick can be performed using addition or subtraction. If we take one of the equations of motion that you will be meeting in the next chapter:

$$v^2 = u^2 + 2as$$

where $v$ is the object's velocity, $u$ is its initial velocity, $a$ its acceleration and $s$ the distance travelled. You may like to quickly test your skills at substitution by seeing how fast a car is travelling if it accelerated from 10 ms$^{-1}$ at a rate of 20 ms$^{-2}$ over a distance of 20 m.

{The answer is 30 ms$^{-1}$ (don't forget, you will need to take the square root of the product; the formula is for $v^2$ not $v$) and, in case you were wondering, ms$^{-1}$ means m/s or 'metres per second'.}

However, say that you knew the initial and final velocities and the distance travelled, and wanted to work out your acceleration. You would need to manipulate the equation so that it is expressed in terms of $a =$.

This can be done by subtracting $u^2$ from both sides of the equation, which (as $u^2 - u^2 = 0$) eliminates it from the right hand side completely so that:

$$v^2 - u^2 = 2as$$

We can then use the same division technique as before (this time, dividing by $2s$), to arrive at:

$$a = \frac{v^2 - u^2}{2s}$$

## CLINICAL FOCUS

You will get plenty of chance to practise equation transformation during the course of this book – where appropriate, the derivation of equations is given: not because you have to learn them but, by understanding *how* the formulae came to be and what their relationship is to other formulae, it makes them much easier to remember and to understand. So, it is important that, when you come to such a derivation, you don't just skip through it; rather, you should work carefully line by line and then close the book and make sure you can recreate the steps you have just studied independently.

Although you may seldom need to use the formulae you will encounter, you will need to have a deep familiarity with the concepts and relationships that they represent. Whether you are interpreting an x-ray or testing the strength of a leg muscle, you need to understand the physical implications of the relationships involved and the effects of changing the variables therein.

# Trigonometry

The only branch of trigonometry with which we will need to deal in any detail is that relating to a very special sort of triangle, those in which one of the internal angles is a right-angle (90°) as shown in Figure 1.2. As the sum of *all* triangles' internal angles is 180°, this means that the sum of the other two angles must also be 90°.

In a right-angled triangle, all three sides have different names. The only thing about this that can be slightly confusing is that the name of two of the sides can vary as they are named in relation to the angle that one happens to be discussing; however, one side – the longest one – is *always* called the **hypotenuse** (Fig. 1.3). The other two sides are known as the **opposite** (the side opposite the angle under consideration) and the **adjacent** (the side next to the angle).

Before we start studying angles, there is one law relating to the length of the sides that is useful to know: **Pythagoras' theorem**.

This states that the square of the hypotenuse is equal to the sum of the squares of the other two sides. This is represented in Figure 1.4 and can be expressed algebraically as:

$$c^2 = a^2 + b^2 \text{ or } c = \sqrt{(a^2 + b^2)}$$

You can check this yourself by drawing two lines at right angles to each other, one 3 cm long, the other 4 cm long. If you join together their free ends to make a right-angled triangle and measure the hypotenuse, you will find that it is 5 cm long, which is predicted by Pythagoras' theorem:

$$c = \sqrt{(a^2 + b^2)} = \sqrt{(3^2 + 4^2)} = \sqrt{(9 + 16)} = \sqrt{25} = 5 \text{ cm}$$

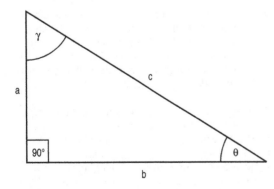

**Figure 1.2** • A right-angled triangle with sides of lengths *a*, *b* and *c*. The internal angles are θ, γ and 90° and total 180°.

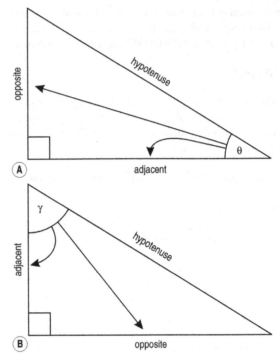

**Figure 1.3** • The nomenclature of a right-angled triangle. Two of the sides – the *opposite* and *adjacent* – are named in relation to the angle that is being studied. The names are therefore interchangeable depending on whether we are referring to the angle θ (A) or γ (B).

Obviously, this theorem can be rearranged in order to be expressed in terms of *a* = ... or *b* = ... (you could try doing this as an exercise), so we now have a method of calculating the length of the third side of a right-angled triangle if we know the other two.

We have also previously seen how to calculate the third angle if we know the other two. We shall now concentrate on finding the value of an angle if two sides are known, or the value of a side if one side and one angle are known.

There are three main relationships of which you need to be aware. Take the right-angled triangle in Figure 1.2.

The **sine** of angle θ is equal to the ratio of the opposite side and the hypotenuse:

$$\sin \theta = a/c$$

The **cosine** of the angle θ is equal to the ratio of the adjacent side and the hypotenuse:

$$\cos \theta = b/c$$

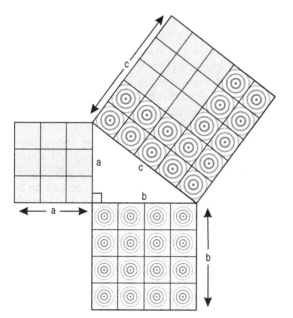

**Figure 1.4** • A graphical representation of Pythagoras' theorem: a square with sides equal to the length of the hypotenuse (*c*) has the same area as squares with sides equal to the length of the other two sides of the triangle (*a* and *b*).

Finally, the **tangent** of the angle θ is equal to the ratio of the opposite side to the adjacent side.

**tan $\theta = a/b$**

To solve problems using these formulae, you will need either a calculator that has trig functions (make sure that it is set to work in degrees [deg] rather than radians [rad] or gradients [grad]), a book of trigonometric tables or a slide rule. They are best demonstrated by illustrative examples followed by practice.

## Example 1

To find a side, given the length of one side and one angle (Fig.1.5)

In this case, we know the length of the hypotenuse and the angle **adjacent** to the side whose length we are trying to find, *b*.

**cos $\theta = b/c$**
**$\Rightarrow$ cos $42° = b/10$**
**$\Rightarrow b = 10 \times$ cos $42° = 10 \times 0.743 = 7.43$ cm**

Note: we could also have used the law of angles to calculate the third angle and then use the formula for sin θ to calculate *b*.

Now that we have two lengths, you can use Pythagoras' theorem to calculate the third {6.69 cm}.

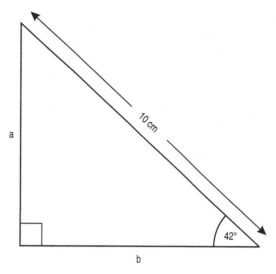

**Figure 1.5** • Example 1.

## Example 2

To find an angle given two sides (Fig. 1.6)
   To find θ:

**sin $\theta$ = opposite/hypotenuse**
**$\Rightarrow$ sin $\theta = 2/9 = 0.222$**

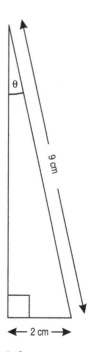

**Figure 1.6** • Example 2.

We can then use the function called **arcsine** to calculate the value of θ (on calculators, this can appear as [inv] [sin], [arc sin] or [$\sin^{-1}$])

$$\Rightarrow \theta = \arcsin 0.222 = 12.8°$$

Note: There are similarly named inverse functions for cosine (arccosine) and tangent (arctangent).

## Conclusion

If most of this material was previously unfamiliar to you, your brain may now be reeling; however, like any new or half-remembered skill, all it takes to become proficient is a little practice so, before proceeding, attempt the quiz below. If you get full marks (the answers are at the end of the chapter), give yourself a pat on the back and move on; if you don't, work out what you have done wrong and restudy the material above until you feel completely confident.

Once you have mastered this section, then you are ready to proceed and should be equipped to deal with (almost) all of the mathematics that you will encounter in this book; however, it is also a section to be revisited if you find yourself at any stage floundering.

## SELF-ASSESSMENT QUIZ

1  If Alf has $a$ bananas and Basil has $b$ bananas, how many more bananas than Basil does Alf have?
2  If $r$ people in a restaurant split the cheque of $\$c$ equally, how much does each person pay?
3  If $p$ physiotherapists each treat $q$ patients and $c$ chiropractors each treat $d$ patients, how many patients get treated?
4  $13x + 4y - 6z + 7y + y - 4x + 2z =$
   a  Simplify this equation.
   b  Express the result in terms of $x =$
5  $3h \times 6i \times h \times 2i =$
   a  Simplify this equation.
   b  Express the result in terms of $i =$
6  Expand $(4x - 7y)^2$
7  $2s(3t - 2u)(3t + 2s)$
   a  Expand this equation
   b  Express the result in terms of $u =$
8  In the diagram below:
   a  What is $x$?
   b  What is $\theta$?

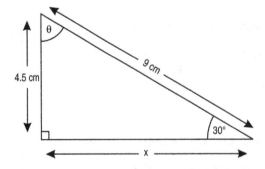

9  In the diagram below:
   a  What is $\theta$?
   b  What is $x$?
   c  What is $\gamma$?

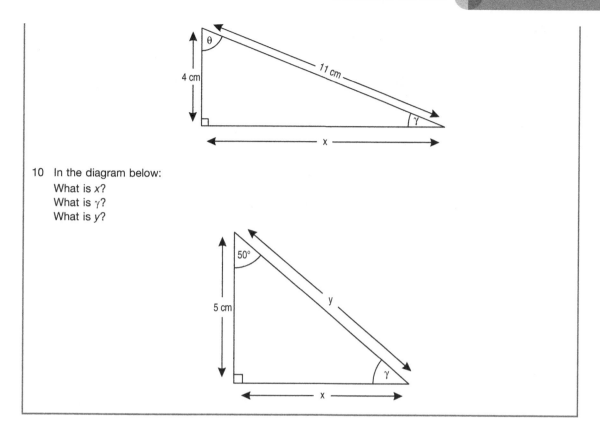

10  In the diagram below:
What is *x*?
What is γ?
What is *y*?

## Vectors and scalars (continued)

### Resolving vectors

Whereas scalar quantities can be multiplied, divided, added and subtracted with impunity to give a scalar answer, when vectors are involved, a different approach is required. Although vectors need not act at 90° to each other, many of those that we encounter are (for reasons that need not concern you yet) going to be doing so.

In typeset print, such as you have in this book, vectors are denoted by bold typeface, so a vector might be written **a** or, if the vector describes translation from point *A* to point *B*, then it would be written **AB**. In handwriting, there are a number of ways to indicate a vector; however, as you only need to know one, probably the simplest to use is the underscore. Thus, **a** is recorded as a̲ and **AB** as A̲B̲ (One can also use an overscore, with or without an arrow or hook at the end.)

So, if an object travels from point *C* to point *D*, in a straight line (Fig.1.7), it is moving from coordinates (1, 2) to (5, 5). We can call this vector **CD** and it can be represented as:

$$\mathbf{CD} = \begin{bmatrix} 4 \\ 3 \end{bmatrix}$$

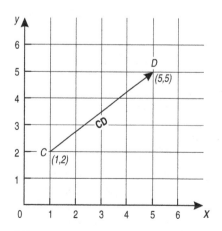

**Figure 1.7** • Translation from *C* to *D* using vector CD.

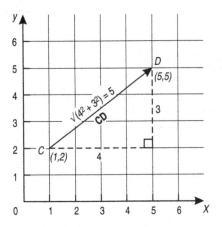

**Figure 1.8** • Solving vector CD using Pythagoras' theorem.

That is, movement of +4 units in the $x$ direction and +3 units in the $y$ direction. We can use Pythagoras' theorem to calculate that the vector must have magnitude 5 units (Fig.1.8).

## Addition of vectors

If

$$\mathbf{a} = \begin{bmatrix} 4 \\ 0 \end{bmatrix} \quad \text{and} \quad \mathbf{b} = \begin{bmatrix} 3 \\ 4 \end{bmatrix}$$

Then $\mathbf{a} + \mathbf{b} =$

$$\begin{bmatrix} 4 \\ 0 \end{bmatrix} + \begin{bmatrix} 3 \\ 4 \end{bmatrix} = \begin{bmatrix} 7 \\ 4 \end{bmatrix}$$

which is represented graphically in Figure 1.9.

From this, we can see that the same rules apply to vector addition (and subtraction) as to normal numbers. In order to resolve the vectors graphically, we construct a triangle of vectors. First we draw **a**, then, starting at the end-point of **a**, we draw **b**. Finally, we draw a line from the start-point of **a** to the end-point of **b**. The dimensions of this line, known as the **resultant** and indicated with a double arrow, give us the answer to the sum **a** + **b**.

## Coordinates and planes

There is a whole new language that needs to be learned when it comes to describing the human body, both in its relationship to the outside world as well as its relationship to other bits of itself. Unfortunately for the student, there is not one but

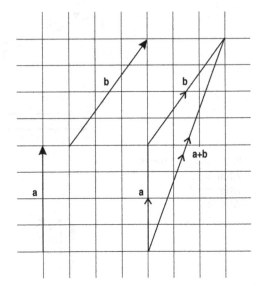

**Figure 1.9** • Graphical addition of vectors. In order to add the vectors **a** and **b**, draw them sequentially, then connect the start and end point with a straight line (called the resultant). The new vector **a**+**b** is indicated with a double arrow.

*two* systems for doing this: the anatomical and the biomechanical and your chosen profession means that you will need to learn both!

The anatomical system is really just a simple matter of memory; in practical terms, the inevitable regular usage in classroom and clinic means that rote learning is not necessary. You can, however, speed the process by deliberately using them as often as possible in your notes – much as you would practise a foreign language; indeed the 4000–6000 new words you are going to acquire during your studies almost constitute a new language – 'Medispeak' – in themselves (by comparison, the average English speaker is said to use between 800 and 1500 words in a typical day).

In contrast, the biomechanical system requires very little memorization, though it is more conceptually challenging.

## The anatomical system

The first thing to understand in both systems is the bodily position to which the terms refer. The **anatomical position** is the starting point for all anatomical references: it doesn't matter if the body to which you are referring is doing a handstand, lying face down or curled up into a ball – the head is still *superior* (or cephalad) to the feet, and the feet *inferior* (or caudal) to the head; the navel *anterior* (or ventral) to the spine, and the spine *posterior* (or dorsal) to the navel. The same is true of medial, lateral, left, right and all the other terms detailed in Table 1.6.

As you can see from Figure 1.10, in the anatomical position, the person is positioned standing upright with the palms facing forwards (supinated). Thereafter, the only real confusion comes from overlap of terms. In older books, and still quite regularly in the USA, the terms ventral and dorsal are

**Table 1.6** Glossary of anatomical descriptive terms

| Term | Meaning |
| --- | --- |
| Abduction | Movement of a joint away from the centre line |
| Adduction | Movement of a joint towards the centre line |
| Anterior | At the front |
| Caudal | Towards the feet |
| Cephalad | Towards the head |
| Coronal plane | The plane running through the body from left to right |
| Cranial | Of, pertaining to, or in the direction of the head |
| Deep | Further from the outer surface |
| Distal | Further from the origin |
| Dorsal | Of, or towards the back |
| Dorsiflexion | Movement of the ankle and foot upwards |
| Eversion | Movement of the foot so that the sole faces outward |
| Horizontal plane | See transverse plane |
| Inferior | Lower |
| Inversion | Movement of the foot so that the sole faces inward |
| Left | Of or to the left |
| Lateral | Away from the centre |
| Lateral rotation | Rotational movement of a joint away from the centre (e.g. in the case of the shoulder, so that the palm faces outward) |
| Medial | Towards the centre |

| Term | Meaning |
| --- | --- |
| Medial rotation | Rotational movement of a joint towards the centre (e.g. in the case of the shoulder, so that the palm faces inward) |
| Median plane | See sagittal plane |
| Palmar | Of, pertaining to or in the direction of, the palm |
| Plantar | Of, pertaining to, or in the direction of, the plantar surface (sole) of the foot |
| Plantarflexion | Movement of the ankle and foot downwards |
| Posterior | Towards the rear |
| Pronation | Movement of the arm so that the palm faces downwards |
| Proximal | Nearer to the origin |
| Right | Of or to the right |
| Rostral | Towards the nose (or, originally, beak) |
| Sagittal plane | A plane through the body from front to back (technically, down the mid-line; planes not in the mid-line are referred to as para-sagittal) |
| Superficial | Nearer to the surface |
| Superior | Higher |
| Supination | Movement of the arm so that the palm faces upwards |
| Transverse plane | A plane running though the body parallel to the ground |
| Ventral | Of, or toward the front of the body |

used. As these terms have dual meanings (dorsal, for example, can mean 'of the back' – as in a fish's dorsal fin – as well as 'toward the back'); internationally, they have been replaced by the less ambiguous *anterior* and *posterior* respectively. The same applies to cephalad (or cranial) and caudal, which have been superseded by *superior* and *inferior*.

When it comes to planes, however, the attempts to replace the traditional transverse, coronal and sagittal planes with horizontal, frontal and median have met with seeming indifference, at least amongst clinicians. We shall, therefore, bow to popular demand and use the former terms.

Movement of joints is also not quite as straightforward as it might be. The terms **flexion** and

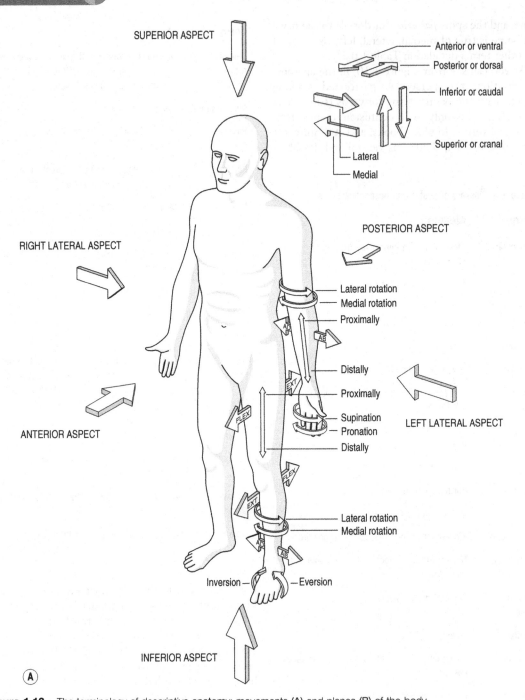

SUPERIOR ASPECT

Anterior or ventral

Posterior or dorsal

Inferior or caudal

Superior or cranal

Lateral

Medial

POSTERIOR ASPECT

RIGHT LATERAL ASPECT

Lateral rotation
Medial rotation
Proximally

Distally

Proximally

Supination
Pronation

Distally

LEFT LATERAL ASPECT

ANTERIOR ASPECT

Lateral rotation
Medial rotation

Inversion — Eversion

INFERIOR ASPECT

(A)

**Figure 1.10** • The terminology of descriptive anatomy: movements (A) and planes (B) of the body.

extension are seemingly unambiguous: flexion of a joint involves approximating (bringing closer together) the surfaces above and below (proximal and distal to) the joint; extension, taking them further apart. However, this isn't always clear – for example in the shoulder, where flexion is considered as movement anteriorly. This can lead the unwary into the trap that *all* flexion is anterior movement and, by corollary, all extension posterior; however, owing to a quirk of embryological development,

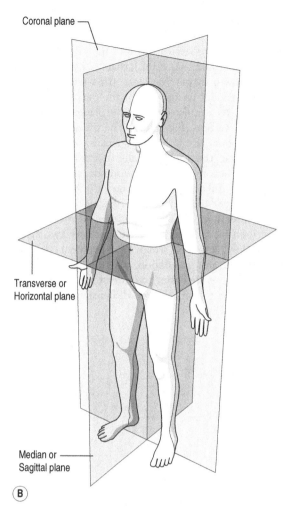

Coronal plane

Transverse or
Horizontal plane

Median or
Sagittal plane

**B**

**Figure 1.10—cont'd**

flexion of the knee (whilst following the rule of approximation) takes place posteriorly. When it comes to the ankle, in order to avoid even more confusion the terms flexion and extension are abandoned: upward movement is termed **dorsiflexion** (the superior surface of the foot is called the *dorsum*) and downward movement is termed **plantarflexion** (the sole is the *plantar* surface).

The terms **abduction** and **adduction** would be completely straightforward if it were not so easy to confuse two words with only one letter different. If we again consider the shoulder, abduction is the movement away from the centreline we make when we lift our arms up sideways; adduction is the movement back down again.

The final pair of movements have also evolved dual terms. Staying with the shoulder and starting with the

anatomical position, turning the palm so that it rests against the thigh is either *internal* or **medial** rotation. Turning it the other way so that the palm faces outwards is *external* or **lateral** rotation. We shall adopt the terms in bold, although as you will now see, there is another way to describe all these movements and planes which was designed to remove all possible confusion, . . . at least, that was the intention!

## The orthogonal system

By describing the body in terms of three orthogonal axes, we can remove all synonyms and ambiguity from the system. Although (in my experience) clinicians much prefer the anatomical system, research papers and biomechanics textbooks not infrequently use the orthogonal system so, as is often the case, it is incumbent upon the manual physician to be bilingual.

Once again, the system begins with the anatomical position. The axes used in a three-dimensional graph ($x$, $y$ and $z$) are then superimposed upon the body. The best way to visualise this (Fig.1.11) is to imagine your own body being impaled by three spears at right angles to each other. The intersection of the three spears (the $x$ axis, the $y$ axis and the $z$ axis) is called the **origin**.

In theory, the system should be wonderful. By referring to the scales on the three axes, it is possible to describe the exact position of any point within or relating to the body. The planes of the body can also be defined: the X-plane is bordered by the $y$ and $z$ axes; the Y-plane, by the $x$ and $z$ axes and the Z-plane by the $x$ and $y$ axes. It is also possible to precisely describe any movement of any part of the body, be it rotation, translation or a combination of the two.

So why is it that this wonderful system, free from the vagaries of linguistics, has not been universally embraced? Because, of course, there is no universal agreement as to which axis should run in which direction or which direction from the origin should be positive and which negative. Conventions seem to vary, not only from country to country, but even from author to author.

This doesn't stop the system being widely used in biomechanics textbooks and, so long as the book is internally consistent, this doesn't stop you from understanding the author – providing they define their orthogonal system at the outset. It does, however, stop you being able to automatically translate a reference to the Z-plane as being the, say, coronal plane or rotation about the $x$ axis as being flexion

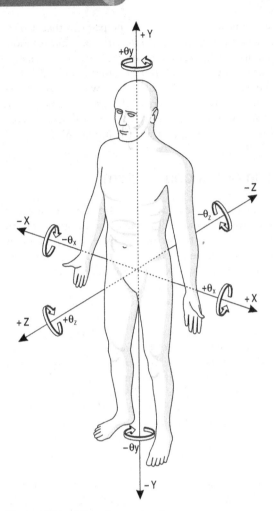

**Figure 1.11 •** The orthogonal system.

its $x$, $y$ and $z$ coordinates $(x, y, z)$: for example, if the origin is at the body's mid-point, level with the second sacral tubercle, the left first ray (big toe) would be at $(0.02, -0.9, 0.2)$, that is 2 cm to the left, 90 cm down, 20 cm forwards (this will obviously vary, dependent on the size of the person and their position). We can also describe the planes of the body using this system (Fig. 1.12). The transverse plane, which is bounded by the $x$ and $z$ axes, now becomes the $Y$-plane; the coronal plane, bounded by the $x$ and $y$ axes becomes the $Z$-plane and the sagittal plane, defined by the $y$ and $z$ axes, is now the $X$-plane.

Movement too can be described in terms of the three directions. However, before we move on to describe this, to a biophysicist there are two types of motion: **rotation**, which is movement about a fixed point, and **translation**, which is movement in a plane. These are easier to understand if we switch for a moment from a three-dimensional to a two-dimensional system.

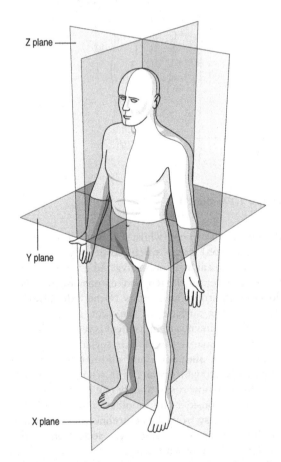

**Figure 1.12 •** Representation of planes in the orthogonal system.

or extension. This is the reason the terms have never become *lingua franca* amongst clinicians.

Therefore, in order to explain the system, we must define our axes. If you subsequently encounter different axial definitions, all the principles you are about to learn remain the same: you will just need to mentally transpose your $x$, $y$, and $z$. So, if you care to imagine yourself as the unfortunate being impaled, in the system we shall be using, the spear running from left to right is the $x$-axis; positive $x$ is to your left, negative to your right. The spear travelling from superior to inferior is the $y$-axis; positive $y$ is upwards, negative $y$ is downwards. Finally, the $z$-axis is represented by the spear transfixing you from front to back (anteroposteriorly); positive $z$ is sticking out forwards, negative $z$ to the rear.

By adding a scale to the axes (say, in metres), we can now map any point in the body in terms of

## Translation

Imagine a ruler, lying on a piece of paper. As well as a numbered scale, the ruler has three letters: *A*, *B* and *C* (Fig. 1.13). If you slide the ruler across the page without altering its alignment, then it has undergone a translation. If the paper is squared and has the *x*-axis running along the bottom and the *y*-axis along the side, you can define the translation in terms of the positive or negative distances travelled by each point:

$$\begin{bmatrix} x \\ y \end{bmatrix}$$

So, in terms of Figure 1.14, the ruler has translated:

$$\begin{bmatrix} +3 \\ -3 \end{bmatrix}$$

in the Z-plane.

## Rotation

This transformation occurs when an object is moved around a single point, known as the centre of rotation. All points within the object move through the same angle, $\theta$. The centre of rotation may lie within the object (Fig. 1.15A) or at a distance from it (Fig 1.15B).

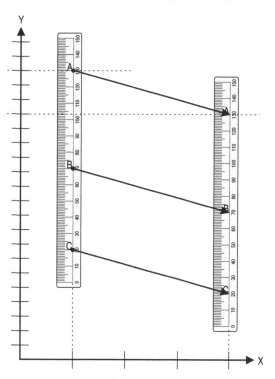

**Figure 1.14** • By adding axes and scales, it is possible to quantify a translation. Here, as movement is bounded by the *x* and *y* axes, it is taking place in the Z-plane. All points in the ruler have moved by +3 units along the *x* axis and −3 units along the *y* axis.

## Multifunctional transformations

Most movements consist of a combination of translation and rotation. For example, Figure 1.16 shows a transformation that would be impossible by either translation or rotation alone. However if we combine the previous two examples and translate the ruler by:

$$\begin{bmatrix} +3 \\ -3 \end{bmatrix}$$

and then rotate through 30°, we arrive at the position shown.

## Three-dimensional movement

Exactly the same rules apply when there are three axes instead of two; by introducing the *z*-axis, we can now describe exactly the same movements using three-dimensional objects (Fig. 1.17). The only difference is that, instead of rotating around a single point, the object moves around a line (axis) and that,

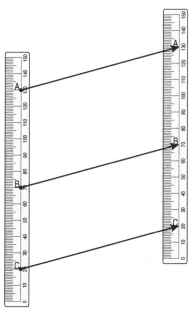

**Figure 1.13** • Translation of an object. Note how all points on the ruler move the same distance along parallel lines.

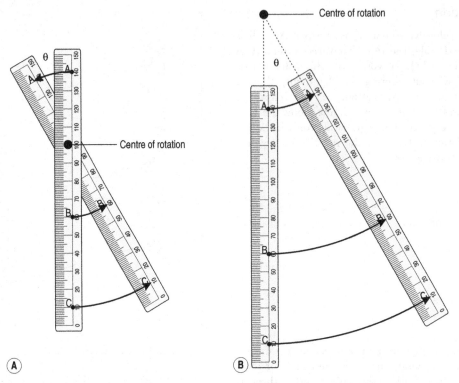

**Figure 1.15** • Rotation of an object. Here, the points move through the same angle, θ, but will move different distances, depending on how far they are from the centre of rotation. This can be located within the object being moved (**A**), in which case the object will spin like the hands of a clock or, at a distance from the object (**B**), causing it to swing.

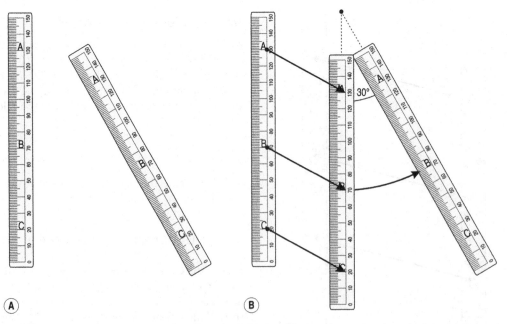

**Figure 1.16** • In order to undergo the transformation pictured below (**A**), the ruler must undergo both translation *and* rotation (**B**).

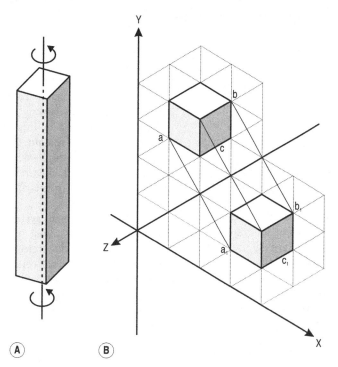

**Figure 1.17** • Exactly the same rules can be extended to three-dimensional objects. They can be rotated, although now this takes place about an axis (the axis of rotation, with all points moving the same angle about the axis, **A**) or translated, again all points move through the same distance in the same direction, **B**).

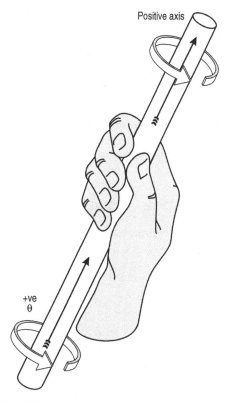

**Figure 1.18** • The right-hand rule for determining the direction of positive rotation about an axis. By gripping a positive axis with the thumb pointing away from you, the fingernails act as arrows to indicate the direction of positive rotation.

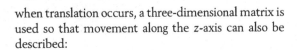

when translation occurs, a three-dimensional matrix is used so that movement along the $z$-axis can also be described:

$$\begin{bmatrix} x \\ y \\ z \end{bmatrix}$$

So this gives a system for describing, highly specifically, translation of the body or any part thereof.

However, most joint movement in the human body consists of rotational movement – that is flexion and extension; abduction and adduction; medial rotation and lateral rotation are all described in terms of positive or negative rotation about a given axis. Positive rotation is *clockwise* movement around a positive axis; negative rotation is *anticlockwise* movement around a positive axis.

To easily remember which is positive, you need to know the **right hand rule**. If you imagine giving a thumbs-up sign using your right hand, and then use the hand to grip any one of the three *positive* axes with the thumb pointing away from the origin, then the fingers indicate the direction of positive rotation about that axis (Fig. 1.18).

So, flexion and extension become positive and negative rotation about the $x$-axis. In most joints, extension is positive $x$-axis rotation $(+\theta_x)$ and flexion, negative $x$-axis rotation $(-\theta_x)$; however, because the knee works 'backwards' these movements are reversed in this joint – the orthogonal system though remains consistent, clockwise movement about the $x$-axis (knee flexion) is still positive, and anticlockwise (knee extension) is negative. In the foot, plantarflexion is $-\theta_x$ and dorsiflexion $+\theta_x$.

In the orthogonal system we have described above, movement about the $y$-axis replaces the terms internal and external rotation; however, in the right arm, internal rotation represents positive $y$-axis rotation $(+\theta_y)$, whilst, in the left, external rotation is $(+\theta_y)$ and vice versa for $(-\theta_y)$. The same variation applies for $z$-axis rotation: abduction is $+\theta_z$ on the left and $-\theta_z$ on the right; adduction $-\theta_z$ on the left and $+\theta_z$ on the right.

This may seem complex but, when you consider the system in its own rights, rather than trying to hold both systems in your mind at the same time, it has a crystal clear purity to it and a concise, universally comprehensible nomenclature.

## Learning Outcomes

- Introduce the methods by which scientists record numbers and units
- Outline the evolution of weights and measures and explain those systems that the clinician is likely to encounter
- Ensure that the student has an adequate knowledge of algebra and trigonometry
- Differentiate between vector and scalar quantities and explain how these may be mathematically manipulated
- Compare and contrast the anatomical and orthogonal systems for describing body movement and position.

## CHECK YOUR EXISTING KNOWLEDGE: ANSWERS

Mark your answers using the guide below to give yourself a score:

**Section 1**

1 $x = (3z - y + 8)$ [2]
2 $2x^2 - xy - y^2$ [2]
3 12 cm [3]
4 22.6° [3]
5 67.4° [3]

**Section 2**

6 1 670 000 000 000 [1]
7 0.000 000 001 76 [1]
8 716 000 metres [1]

9  671 000 000 000 J [1]
10  0.003 004 m (3.004 mm or 3004 μm)   [1]
11  $10^6 = 1\ 000\ 000$   [1]
12  3  [1]
13  $^1/_9 = 0.11$   [2]
14  Kelvin  [2]
15  Ohm  [2]
16  A quantity that has magnitude but no directional dependence (e.g. mass)  [3]
17  a  It will move North East  [2]
    b  5.65 N  [3]
18  Median or sagittal  [3]
19  They are spinning to their right.  [3]

(If you didn't get this answer, it does not necessarily mean that you are wrong, there is variation amongst orthogonal conventions. It does, however, mean that you should read the section on Coordinates and planes to familiarize yourself with the conventions that will be used in this book.)

## How to interpret the results:

36–40:  You have a firm grasp of the basic tools needed to understand the language in this book. As long as you understand any mistakes you may have made, you can move on to the next chapter.

25–35:  Although you have some understanding of the basics, you should revise the areas in which you scored poorly before moving on.

0–34:  You will need to study this chapter in some detail in order to acquire the grounding needed for future chapters.

## A  SELF-ASSESSMENT QUIZ ANSWERS

### Algebra and trigonometry revision section

1  $a - b$
2  $c/r$
3  $pq + cd$
4  a) $9x + 12y - 4z$;   b) $x = (4z - 12y)/9$
5  a) $36h^2i^2 = (6\,hi)^2$   b) $i = \sqrt{(1/36\,h^2)} = 1/6\,h$
6  $16x^2 - 56xy + 49y^2$
7  a) $18st^2 + 12ts^2 - 12uts - 8us^2$
    b) $u = (18st^2 + 12ts^2 - 12uts)/8s^2$. This can be further simplified to $u = 3t\,(3t + 2s - 2u)/4s$
8  a)  7.8 cm b) 60°
9  a)  10.25 cm   b) 21.3°   c) 68.7°
    a)  5.96 cm   b) 40°   c) 7.78 cm

## Bibliography

Allen, R., Schwarz, C. (Eds.), 1998. The Chambers dictionary. Chambers Harrap, Edinburgh.

Alonso, M., Finn, E.J., 1968. In: Fundamental university physics, vol. III. Addison-Wesley, Reading, Mass.

Beiser, A., 1973. The atomic nucleus. In: Concepts of modern physics.

McGraw-Hill Kogakusha, Tokyo, pp. 361–388.

Beiser, A., 1973. Atomic structure. In: Concepts of modern physics. McGraw-Hill Kogakusha, Tokyo, pp. 101–138.

Daintith, J., 1983. Dictionary of physics. Charles Letts, London.

Evans, I.H. (Ed.), 1990. In: Brewer's dictionary of phrase and fable, fourteenth ed. Cassell, London.

Featherstone, N., 2005. In: Reed's Oki nautical almanac, 2006 edition. Adlard Coles Nautical, London.

Garrood, J.R., 1979. Nuclear and quantum physics. In: Physics.

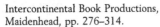
Intercontinental Book Productions, Maidenhead, pp. 276–314.

Green, J.H., Silver, P.H.S., 1981. Exploring the limbs. In: An introduction to human anatomy. Oxford University Press, Oxford, pp. 27–51.

Holderness, J., 1987. Geometry. In: GCSE maths: higher level. Causeway Press, Ormskirk, pp. 35–53.

Holderness, J., 1987. Trigonometry in right-angled triangles. In: GCSE maths: higher level. Causeway Press, Ormskirk, UK, pp. 333–344.

Klein, P., Sommerfeld, P., 2004. Grundlagen und konzepte. In: Biomechanik der Menschlichen Gelenke. Elsevier, Munich, pp. 1–138.

Moore, K.L., 1985. The basis of medical language. In: Clinically oriented anatomy, second ed. Williams & Wilkins, Baltimore, pp. 33–37.

Nicolson, I., 1970. Astronomy. Hamlyn, London.

http://physics.nist.gov/cuu/Units/prefixes.html. Online. 28 September 2006.

http://physics.nist.gov/cuu/Units/units.html. Online. 28 September 2006.

Richardson, R.S., 1960. A survey of the stars. In: The fascinating world of astronomy. McGraw-Hill, Colombus, pp. 195–210.

Schafer, R.C., 1983. The human machine. In: Clinical biomechanics: musculoskeletal actions and reactions. Williams and Wilkins, Baltimore, pp. 3–39.

Schafer, R.C., 1983. Mechanical concepts and terms. In: Clinical biomechanics: musculoskeletal actions and reactions. Williams and Wilkins, Baltimore, pp. 40–56.

Standring, S. (Ed.), 2005. Anatomical nomenclature. In: Gray's anatomy: the anatomical basis of clinical practice. Elsevier, Edinburgh, pp. 3–4.

# Chapter **Two**

2

# Natural philosophy

## CHAPTER CONTENTS

Check your existing knowledge . . . . . . 27

Introduction . . . . . . . . . . . . . . . . 28

Velocity, angular velocity and
acceleration . . . . . . . . . . . . . . . . . 30

Mass and momentum . . . . . . . . . . 31

Force . . . . . . . . . . . . . . . . . . . . 32

Newton's laws and equations of motion . . 33

Workshop . . . . . . . . . . . . . . . . . 36

Gravity . . . . . . . . . . . . . . . . . . . 36

Energy and work . . . . . . . . . . . . . 37

  Heat and temperature . . . . . . . . . . 38

  Pressure and partial pressures . . . . . 40

  The gas laws . . . . . . . . . . . . . . 44

Learning outcomes . . . . . . . . . . . . 46

Check your existing knowledge:
answers . . . . . . . . . . . . . . . . . . 46

Workshop: answers . . . . . . . . . . . 47

Bibliography . . . . . . . . . . . . . . . . 47

## CHECK YOUR EXISTING KNOWLEDGE

1 Separate the following units into vectors and scalars:
   - a Velocity
   - b Speed
   - c Acceleration
   - d Mass
   - e Angular velocity
   - f Momentum
   - g Force
   - h Energy
   - i Work
   - j Temperature

2 Which quantity can be calculated by averaging the gradient of a graph of velocity against time?

3 State Newton's three laws

4 A car starts from rest and accelerates at $3 \text{ ms}^{-2}$ for 8 seconds.
   - a What is its final velocity?
   - b How far has it travelled?

5 A motorcycle travels at $15 \text{ ms}^{-1}$ for 500 m, and then it accelerates constantly for 5 seconds until it is travelling at $30 \text{ ms}^{-1}$.
   - a How long does it take to travel the first 500 m?
   - b What is its rate of acceleration?
   - c How far does it travel whilst accelerating?
   - d Assuming no further acceleration, how long does it take to travel the next 500 m?

6 If two objects have a mutual gravitational attraction of 60 N at a separation of $10^4$ km, what will their attraction be at:
   - a $2 \times 10^4$ km
   - b $10^3$ km

7  If an object of mass 10 kg, is raised to a height of 30 m against a gravitation field of 10 Nkg$^{-1}$
   a  How much work is being done?
   b  If it is being lowered at 0.5 ms$^{-1}$, what is its kinetic energy?

8  Give the SI unit(s) for:
   a  Temperature       f  Weight
   b  Heat              g  Work
   c  Force            h  Pressure
   d  Distance       i  Acceleration
   e  Mass           j  Area

9  20 m$^3$ of gas is at a pressure of 1atm and 20°C. If the temperature remains constant and the volume is increased to 50 m$^3$, what will the pressure be now?

10  If the volume is then decreased to 10 m$^3$, but the pressure is kept constant, what will the new temperature of the gas be?

# Introduction

If algebra and trigonometry owe their origins to the Greeks, then 17$^{th}$ century Europe was the birthplace of modern science … and, quite frankly (in Europe), nothing much came in between – the 'dark ages' were named for their dearth of intellectual enlightenment rather than levels of ambient light. Historians generally regard this period as extending from the fall of the Roman Empire in the 5$^{th}$ century AD to the onset of the mediaeval period in the late 9$^{th}$ century. By contrast, anthropologists have extended it until the European Renaissance (literally 'new birth') in the 12$^{th}$ century; some, indeed, mark it as late as the 15$^{th}$ century – a thousand years of academic regression and stagnation.

Intellectually, the period can be regarded as starting with the destruction of the Royal Library of Alexandria, which, since the 3$^{rd}$ century BC, had held an immense store of knowledge; contemporary accounts suggest hundreds of thousands of scrolls. Ironically, the date of destruction – indeed, whether the library was truly destroyed, broken up into smaller collections or dissipated by lack of patronage and more pressing political concerns – is unknown; one of the more salient features of the Dark Ages was the lack of documentary evidence in a period where perhaps only one person in a thousand was literate.

Outside of Europe, the flame of human development was kept flickering by the Chinese, Indians and Arabs who became sophisticated in astronomy (at that time indistinguishable from astrology) and mathematics (remember that oh-so-useful zero). Indeed, some historians regard the spark that ignited the renaissance as the opening up of the Near and Far East by travellers such as Marco Polo, bringing not just technological innovations including gunpowder, spectacles and pasta but scientific knowledge to augment that from the classical literature extant from the previous millennium.

The principal tributary to which the river of modern science can be traced is probably Roger Bacon (?1214–?1292), a Somerset-born Franciscan friar, philosopher, alchemist and medic; the 'Father of Science', 'Dr Miribalis' (Fig. 2.1). In his most famous work, *Opus Maius*, he outlined his unsurpassed knowledge of gunpowder, optics, mathematics, moral philosophy, theology, grammar … and experimental science, of which he was probably the inventor and certainly an ardent practitioner.

It is Bacon who is credited with having invented the 'Scientific Method' – hypothesis tested by experimentation and observation. This may now

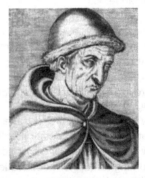

**Figure 2.1** • 'Dr Miribalis', Roger Bacon, a Franciscan monk who lived and died in the 13th century, is regarded by many as the father of modern science for his introduction of the scientific method of hypothesis tested by experimental observation in contrast to the theological argumentation of the day.

seem basic in the extreme but, before Bacon, science was a matter of metaphysical debate and religious dogma; he sowed the seeds from which sprang the randomized controlled trials in today's biomedical journals.

Bacon, though, would not have thought of himself as a scientist but as a philosopher – a lover, and seeker, of knowledge. . .as would those who followed him, culminating with Isaac Newton. They were *natural philosophers*, interested in the secrets of the world around them ('scientists' were not invented until the 18th century) and it was these men who laid down the ground rules for the physics that we still use today.

However, for such men to flourish, two things were needed: freedom of expression and cross-fertilization of ideas (combined, perhaps, with a slight sense of competition). Bacon had little of either and, like other individual geniuses in the centuries that followed him, most notably Leonardo da Vinci (1452–1519) and Galileo Galilei (1564–1642), his work was often curtailed or even destroyed. The all-powerful authority of the Church regarded science as a direct challenge to the fundamentals of the bible and was ruthless in suppressing anything that contradicted that view.

Galileo suffered particularly badly in this respect, suffering imprisonment by the Inquisition, house arrest and finally (under pain of a rather horrible death) being made to recant his 'heretical' support for the Copernican heliocentric system. The Church had determined that it simply wasn't possible for sunspots to rotate about the Sun or Jupiter's moons around Jupiter: the Pope had decreed that the Earth was the centre of the Universe around which *everything* rotated. The Pope was appointed by God, and therefore infallible; the Inquisition took care of anything that might interfere with that, including Galileo.

The opportunity for the requisite level of intellectual freedom and learned discourse came with the Restoration of the British monarchy in 1660, following a protracted Civil War, regicide and Cromwell's puritanical 'Commonwealth', which proscribed everything from Christmas to dancing.

Within months of Charles II regaining the English throne, the finest minds of the day were meeting on a regular basis; two years later, a Society for 'The promoting of Physico-mathematicall Experimentall Learning' was formed and, in 1663, Charles II granted it a royal charter. The Royal Society still exists today and there are few higher accolades in the field of science than the honorific 'FRS'

(Fellow of the Royal Society) after one's name. The membership of the time reads like a 'Who's Who' of physics – Robert Hooke and Christopher Wren (who are probably better remembered as the men behind the rebuilding of London after the Great Fire of 1666, in particular St Paul's cathedral), Robert Boyle and, of course, Isaac Newton. It was these men and their peers who provided much of the groundwork that still forms the basis of physics today and which forms the content of this chapter.

## CLINICAL FOCUS

Many of the terms that you will meet in this chapter are misleadingly familiar. 'Energy', 'Weight', 'Heat' and 'Power' are all words that you hear and use on a weekly, if not daily, basis. However, be warned, in physics they have a specific and highly precise meaning that may well be different from that employed in everyday use and, when you use them in this context, you *must* be aware of this.

This will also be true of areas other than physics and it is important as a clinician that you can differentiate between lay usage of terms and professional usage. Examples of such medical words include 'rheumatism', 'arthritis' and 'sciatica'.

If a patient comes in complaining of 'rheumatism', they almost certainly mean that they have a deep aching somewhere; if you are speaking to a consultant rheumatologist (or, indeed, most healthcare professionals) it means that they have one of a number of rather rare, often inter-related connective tissue disorders such as polymyalgia rheumatica (PMR) or systemic lupus erythematosus (SLE).

'Arthritis', to most people, suggests 'joint pain' or 'wear and tear'; to a manual physician, it means an inflammatory arthropathy such as rheumatoid arthritis, ankylosing spondylitis or Reiter's syndrome (the term 'degenerative joint disease' now tends to be used in preference to the completely separate disease process of osteoarthritis, which frequently coexists with 'true' arthritis).

Similarly, 'sciatica' specifically means pain arising from the damage to the sciatic nerve (there are many other things that can give pain in the back of the leg). Patients will often use the term to mean *any* pain in the leg; general practitioners, usually failing to consider alternative aetiologies, use the term loosely to describe pain in the buttock, posterior thigh and/or leg. Manual physicians – particularly those involved with manipulation – need to use the term with great diagnostic specificity and, more importantly, realize that it describes a symptom and not a condition. There exists a multitude of conditions that can cause sciatica and it is important to treat the cause rather than the symptom.

# Velocity, angular velocity and acceleration

In everyday speech, 'velocity' and 'speed' are interchangeable; in physics, they are (usually) not. Both are measured in units of distance (displacement) per unit time (metres per second; miles per hour etc.); however, **velocity** is a **vector** quantity (having magnitude *and* direction) whilst **speed** is **scalar** (having magnitude alone).

**Acceleration** is change in velocity (deceleration is expressed as negative acceleration; both are measured in metres per second per second $= ms^{-2}$). This can, therefore, be caused by a change in the magnitude of the velocity *or* a change in its direction (or both). Put in terms of driving a car, using the brake or accelerator causes a change in both speed *and* velocity; however, using the steering wheel causes a change in velocity *even if the speed remains constant.*

In terms of graphical representation (Fig. 2.2), if time ($t$) is plotted on the $x$-axis and displacement ($s$) on the $y$-axis, then the slope of the graph represents the velocity: the change in displacement, $\Delta s$, divided by the change in time $\Delta t$. Whereas this is straightforward if the graph is a straight line (i.e. constant velocity). If it is not, then the *mean* velocity needs to be obtained using a method of calculation known as calculus. If you are unfamiliar with this, read the Fact File below before proceeding; if calculus is old hat, then you will easily appreciate that velocity can be written as:

$$v = \frac{ds}{dt}$$

Similarly, if we plot the results of this graph with velocity ($v$) on the $y$-axis and time ($t$) on the $x$-axis, we get a gradient representing acceleration ($a$). If this is a straight line, then acceleration (the rate of

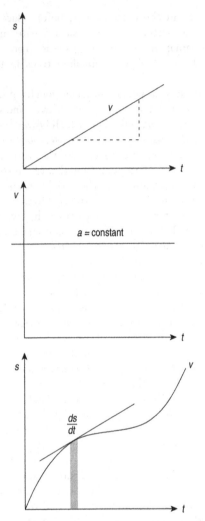

**Figure 2.2** • A graph of displacement against time. The slope (tangent) of the graph represents the velocity. When the value of this tangent is plotted against time, then tangent of the resultant graph represents acceleration. In this case, as the change of velocity (i.e., the acceleration) was constant, the graph is a straight line. The final example demonstrates the case where the velocity is variable. In order to calculate the velocity from the displacement against time graph, we must repeatedly take the tangent and then work out the average. This is done using differential calculus.

change of velocity) is constant; if not, then calculus can calculate the average gradient:

$$a = \frac{dv}{dt} = d^2s/dt^2$$

This, for example, is why the Earth is *accelerating* around the sun, although its speed is constant (bar the loss due to friction of a millisecond per century), its velocity is constantly changing as it describes an ellipse around the sun. This can be inconvenient on occasions; however, if we measure displacement in terms of the number of degrees ($\theta$) traversed per unit time we can measure the **angular velocity** ($\omega$):

$$\omega = {}^{d\theta}\!/_{dt}$$

Because the rotation is about a specific axis, which can be changed, angular velocity is also a vector quantity.

## Fact File

### CALCULUS

The basic premise behind calculus is that, if you look at a small enough piece of a curve, it appears to be a straight line. This is the same reason that, for centuries, people assumed the Earth is flat; the curve is changing so slowly that, when we look around us, the bit we can see appears to be a level plane.

This means that, if our graph of, say, displacement against time (= velocity) isn't a convenient straight line and we can't therefore measure the slope, we can break it down into very small sections. The slope of each section is a straight line and can be measured in the normal way. By adding up the individual gradients and averaging them, we get a result for, in this case, velocity.

We can use the same principle to calculate the area under each very small part of the line; knowing this tells us, in this example, the total distance travelled.

The first instance is called *differential calculus* and, rather than write ${}^{\Delta s}\!/_{\Delta t}$, which would refer to the gradient of the whole of a straight line, we write ${}^{ds}\!/_{dt}$ showing that we have worked out the gradient using calculus.

If we want to calculate the area under a line, we use *integral calculus*.

$$s = \int v.dt$$

This is the shorthand way of saying that the distance travelled is the area enclosed by the line on a graph of velocity against time.

In order to understand this text, you do not need to be able to perform calculus but you will need to know how it is possible to deal with curved lines on graphs (note also that *any* line on a graph is called a 'curve' – even if it is straight!)

# Mass and momentum

In the same way that physicists differentiate speed and velocity, 'mass' and 'weight' are also separate entities. **Mass** ($m$) is a measure of the quantity of matter in an object and, within the SI system, is measured in kilograms. It does not matter where the mass is – outer space, the centre of the Earth, the surface of the sun – the mass remains constant. By contrast, **weight** ($W$) is the force by which a mass is attracted to a gravitationally massive object (such as the Earth):

$$W = mg$$

where $g$ is the acceleration of free fall, which can vary depending on location (Table 2.1). Although we measure our weight in kilograms, it should in fact be measured in newtons; we can get away with it because we are in a (reasonably) constant gravitational field. If we were in free-fall or outer space, our weight would be 0 N, although our mass would be unchanged.

This brings us to another property, **momentum** ($I$), which is dependent on mass rather than weight. If we were to run into a brick wall, it would hurt: how much it hurt would depend on how heavy we are and how fast we are running, so it is no surprise to learn the momentum is the product of these two factors:

$$I = mv \text{ units kg.ms}^{-1} = \text{Ns } (1\text{N} = 1 \text{ kgms}^{-2})$$

However, even if we were weightless – say, in outer space – it would hurt just as much when we hit the wall; our mass is still the same.

**Table 2.1** Gravitational forces on selected astronomical bodies

| Body | Free fall acceleration |
| --- | --- |
| Earth | $9.8 \text{ ms}^{-2}$ |
| Moon | $1.6 \text{ ms}^{-2}$ |
| Jupiter | $25.3 \text{ ms}^{-2}$ |
| Pluto | $0.6 \text{ ms}^{-2}$ |
| Sun | $270.7 \text{ ms}^{-2}$ |
| Neutron star | $1.4 \times 10^{12} \text{ ms}^{-2}$ |

## CLINICAL FOCUS

Weight, is something that is – or should be – of keen interest to any primary contact medical professional. Obesity carries with it an increased risk for a plethora of conditions: diabetes mellitus, with its neurovascular complications; atherosclerosis, the commonest cause of heart disease; hypertension with the increased risk of cerebrovascular incidents; and, probably, asthma, depression and hormonal problems.

To the clinician, weight is a relative measurement and is obviously related to, amongst other things, height. Rather than absolute weight, Body Mass Index (BMI) is used; this is calculated by dividing weight (in kilograms) by the square of the patient's height (in metres).

$$BMI = \frac{W\ (kg)}{h^2\ (m^2)}$$

The results are then interpreted using the scale for adults (see Table 2.2; different scales are used for children and teenagers).

Common sense is needed when applying these scales – a highly muscular athlete or body-builder can easily have a BMI well above normal levels without being obese; the relationship between waistline and chest size is a good secondary marker. Awareness of risk factors (being female, black, middle aged, of lower socioeconomic status and having a familial history) is also helpful as early intervention in a progressively overweight patient offers a better prognosis.

For the manual physician, there are also the biomechanical consequences to consider. Increased weight means increased loading on weight-bearing structures. Back pain is more common in the obese and osteoarthritis is generally twice as common, though this figure is even higher in hips and higher still in knees and ankles.

**Table 2.2** Body mass index

| BMI | Status |
| --- | --- |
| Below 18.5 | Underweight |
| 18.5–24.9 | Normal |
| 25.0–29.9 | Overweight |
| 30.0 and over | Obese |

Entrapment syndromes, such as carpal tunnel syndrome, are also more common in the morbidly overweight owing to decreased subcutaneous space (which is taken up by adipose deposition), and the overweight have a higher incidence of accidents and – because of their increased momentum – tend to suffer greater injury in falls.

The level of the problem has spiralled in the last two decades. In the USA, 20% of adults are obese and 12% of children. This is particularly worrying because, whereas adults become obese by storing fat in subcutaneous cells, which swell accordingly, if a child is subject to an excessive calorific load, their bodies will respond by creating more storage cells. This makes it far more difficult to lose weight – even if the cells are only storing normal levels of fat, their profusion will mean an elevated BMI.

European countries (particularly the UK) and Japan are following in America's – increasingly deep – footsteps. The current generation of schoolchildren is the first in 250 years whose expected lifespan is less than that of their parents; obesity is the principal reason for this.

# Force

Once again, this is a term, the specificity of which, in physics, is in sharp contrast to the generality of meaning in the vernacular. To the scientist, **force** *(F)* is something that changes an object's velocity, remembering that velocity is a vector quantity with both magnitude and direction. As we saw when discussing weight, force is measured in newtons (N) and can be calculated using the formula:

**F = mass × acceleration**

or, more concisely:

**F = ma**

 **DICTIONARY DEFINITION**

FORCE

Although normally defined as 'that which changes a body's *velocity*', you may see alternative definitions of force: 'that which changes a body's *momentum*' or 'that which accelerates a body'. As acceleration is defined as change of velocity and momentum is directly proportional to velocity, these statements are in fact all consistent and all true.

# Newton's laws and equations of motion

Reading this far, you will already have gathered that Sir Isaac Newton (Fig. 2.3) was an important man in the history of physics; arguably, he is the most important. Born in 1642, the year that Galileo died, Newton was something of a prodigy. Although he seems to have been a solitary, reclusive child, preferring introspection to classes (which probably bored him), he flourished whilst at Cambridge University; by the age of just 27, he was Lucasian Professor of Mathematics (the same chair is now held by Stephen Hawking). In 1665, when bubonic plague hit London and Cambridge, he withdrew to the family home in Lincolnshire and devoted himself to developing the ideas that would make him famous.

Typically for Newton, he did not choose to publish them until 1687, and then only because he was afraid someone else might claim credit for them. *Philosophiae Naturalis Principia Mathematica* (The Mathematical Principles of Natural History), commonly referred to as the *Principia*, is probably the most important scientific book of all time, although Darwin's *On the Origin of Species* might give it a close run.

Although he achieved excellence in many other fields: optics (he discovered diffraction), fluid mechanics, history, theology and alchemy and was an able administrator (for 28 years he was master of the Royal Mint) and politician (twice a member of parliament), it is for the work on mechanics and gravitation that he owes his principal fame.

His three laws of motion govern and quantify most of the everyday movement that we observe. Let us consider them in order.

## Fact File

### ISAAC NEWTON 1

Newton, despite being president of the Royal Society from 1703 until his death in 1727, did not appear to be a great believer in scientific collaboration. He was intolerant of criticism, harboured lifelong grudges and was vindictive towards rivals – he tried, and nearly succeeded, in ruining the German mathematician, Liebnitz, who had (whilst Newton kept his own work secret) independently discovered 'differential calculus' (using a much more user-friendly method that Newton's 'fluxions') which we still employ today.

## CLINICAL FOCUS

Both Isaac Newton and Albert Einstein demonstrated classic signs of Autistic Spectrum Disorder: obsessive interests, difficulty in social relationships and problems in communicating. Although many autistic people are intellectually impaired (occasionally with specific 'savant' capabilities), these two physicists had key symptoms of high functioning Asperger's (HFA), where brainpower is not only unimpaired but often appears to be enhanced, at least in areas requiring logical rationale.

Newton in particular seems like a textbook case: as a child, he was a loner and, when engrossed in work, he hardly spoke. He was lukewarm or bad-tempered with the few friends he had and often forgot to eat (one anecdotal tale tells of his landlady insisting he eat and giving him an egg and a watch with which to time it. When she returned, Newton was staring at the egg and boiling the watch).

If no one turned up to his lectures, he gave them anyway, talking to an empty room. He even had a nervous breakdown at 50, brought on by depression and paranoia.

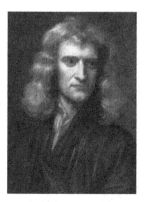

**Figure 2.3** • Newton as he appeared at the time of publication of *Principia* in 1687.

# Newton's first law of motion

*Every body continues in its state of rest or in uniform motion in a straight line unless acted on by an external force.*

You may recognize this as being the definition of force, stated the other way around. Put in simpler terms, things keep on doing what they are already doing (standing still or moving) unless something happens to alter this.

The 'standing still' bit is obvious and completely in accordance with our everyday observations – objects don't spontaneously start moving unless engendered by something or someone (the external force). The 'moving' bit requires a bit more consideration – at first glance it might seem at odds with everyday observation: if we throw a ball into the air, it doesn't carry on travelling in a straight line, it describes a curve (called a parabola) and returns to Earth – we even have the saying 'what goes up must come down'. Similarly, we all know that a freewheeling bicycle will not keep travelling forever; unless we pedal, it will slow and eventually stop.

Newton's flash of genius was to realize that rather than being examples of deviation from this law, such objects are behaving in the observed manner *because* they are being acted on by external forces: the ball's velocity is reduced and reversed by the force of gravity, pulling it towards the centre of the Earth; the bicycle (although post-dating Newton by 200 years) is nevertheless slowed by friction in the wheel bearings, between road and tyre and against the air molecules that must be pushed aside in order to progress. In a world where it is impossible to escape these effects, Newton managed to appreciate these forces for what they were and envisage what would happen if they were removed – indeed, if we threw our tennis ball in the vacuum of outer space, away from gravitational influences, it would keep going indefinitely. The nearest we can come to appreciating this is by reducing friction to a minimum and looking at the behaviour of objects moving on ice. Intuitively, we know that an ice-skater will slow far less than a bicyclist over a similar distance (the sport of curling relies on this) and, over a short distance, an object sliding across a smooth sheet of ice may not appear to slow at all. This tendency for an object to keep on doing what it is already doing (conservation of momentum) is termed **inertia**.

## Fact File

### ISAAC NEWTON 2

The story of Newton sitting in his mother's orchard and asking himself why an apple had fallen downwards rather than upwards is probably apocryphal; however, his intuitive leap regarding his first law may have been due to the fact that his was living during a period, which began in Bacon's time, known as the 'Little Ice Age'. During the time of his confinement to the country, England experienced long, bitterly cold winters – indeed, during this period England recorded its lowest ever recorded atmospheric pressure (931 millibars) and, reputedly, its coldest ever temperature.

The River Thames was frozen sufficiently to bear the weight of not just skaters but of a coach and horses and, in the Fenlands of Lincolnshire, (which, lying below sea level, flooded every winter), there would have been skating aplenty. Had Newton not had access to those now climatically rare natural ice-rinks, perhaps he would never have received the spark that ignited his unique insights into motion.

# Newton's second law of motion

*The rate of change of a body's momentum is proportional to the applied force and takes place in the direction in which the force acts.*

Once again, this law follows what we already know intuitively and can be inferred from what we already know about physics. Let us take once again the analogy of the bicycle (whose mass remains constant and, therefore, whose change in momentum is solely dependent on its change in velocity), being acted upon by an external force (the wind). We know from experience that the change in the bicycle's velocity will depend on the strength of the wind and its direction (a head wind will slow us down; a tail wind speed us up).

We could also have deduced this from our existing knowledge. We know that momentum is proportional to velocity ($I = mv$) and, therefore, that *change* in momentum, $\Delta I$, is proportional to *change* in velocity. We also know that change in velocity is acceleration and that acceleration is proportional to force ($F = ma$).

# Newton's third law of motion

*For every action, there is an equal and opposite reaction.*

This is the shortest, most oft quoted and superficially simple of the three laws. The recoil of a gun in firing is familiar and easy to understand: the bullet (light but very fast) zooms forwards whilst the much heavier gun kicks back a lot more slowly. The momentum of the two objects is equal in magnitude but opposite in direction. Much less intuitive but far more common is the consequence of living on a gravitationally massive spheroid. We are used to seeing a book resting on a table, our feet upon the floor and are aware that both are subject to the force of gravity; however, if it were not for the fact that the table and floor (or, more properly, the molecular bonds therein) were pushing back with an equal and opposite reaction, we – and the book – would plummet towards the centre of the planet to be incinerated in the magma lying a few kilometres below our feet.

## The equations of motion

Newton's laws lay down some fundamental truths about the way the world around us moves and reacts but these are laws of qualification; they tell us how but not how much. From the laws and, with Newton's knowledge of calculus, it is possible to logically derive equations that allow us to accurately calculate an object's velocity, acceleration, distance travelled or time taken. Although these equations of motion have been superseded by Einstein's equations of relativistic motion, unless you are accelerating towards or travelling at the speed of light, the relativistic component of the equations become so small as to be immeasurable and, in the everyday setting of Planet Earth, the equations revert to those of Newton.

If we draw a graph of velocity against time for a car that is already moving and is continuing to accelerate we would end up with the diagram shown in Figure 2.4. At the beginning $(t = 0)$, the car is moving with its initial velocity, $u$ (if it had been stationary, $u$ would have been equal to zero and the line would have started at the origin instead of halfway up the $y$-axis). Now we know that the slope of the graph gives the acceleration $(\Delta v/\Delta t)$ and the area under the graph gives the distance $(\int v.dt)$. As this is a straight-line graph, the calculations are quite straightforward. (Understanding the derivations is not essential, the equations are easy enough to memorize but, if you do understand how they are arrived at, it is always possible to recreate them from first principles if memory fails.)

The velocity at any point is obviously the initial velocity $(u)$ plus the change in velocity

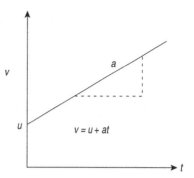

**Figure 2.4** • Velocity. A graph of the changing velocity of a car ($v$) during time ($t$). At the start of the measurements, the car is already travelling with an initial velocity ($u$).

(acceleration, $a$) multiplied by the amount of time for which that acceleration has been occurring $(t)$. Put mathematically:

$$v = u + at$$

To calculate the distance, we need to know the area under the graph. If you are comfortable with calculus, this can be done by integrating:

$$\int v.dt = (u + at).dt = ut + \tfrac{1}{2}at^2$$

If you prefer visual methods we can easily calculate the area under the graph (Fig. 2.5).

The formula for the area of a rectangle is length × breadth $= ut$.

The formula for the area of a triangle is:

$$\frac{\text{height} \times \text{width}}{2} = \frac{t \times at}{2} = \frac{\tfrac{1}{2}at^2}{2}$$

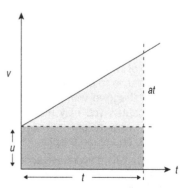

**Figure 2.5** • Distance. A graphical solution to the question of how far the car has travelled ($s$), which is equal to the area under the graph.

The area under the graph is the sum of these two shapes:

$$s = ut + \tfrac{1}{2}at^2$$

The third equation of motion can be obtained by a little juggling. From the first equation, we know:

$$v = u + at$$

Rewriting this in terms of $t$ gives:

$$t = \frac{v - u}{a}$$

If we drop this value of $t$ into the second equation of motion:

$$\begin{aligned} s &= \frac{u \times (v-u)}{a} + \frac{a \times (v-u)^2}{a^2} \\ &= \frac{u \times (v-u)}{a} + \frac{(v-u)^2}{2a} \\ &= \frac{2uv - 2u^2 + v^2 - 2vu + u^2}{2a} \end{aligned}$$

Multiplying both sides by $2a$ gives:

$$\begin{aligned} 2as &= 2uv - 2u^2 + v^2 - 2vu + u^2 \\ &= 2uv - 2uv + u^2 - 2u^2 + v^2 \\ &= v^2 - u^2 \end{aligned}$$

Rewriting this in terms of $v^2$ gives:

$$v^2 = u^2 + 2as$$

## Workshop

The equations of motion, whilst easy to use, may require manipulation to put them into the form you require. If you struggled with the questions at the start of the chapter, you may like to practise on the questions below before moving on. Answers are given at the end of the chapter.

1. A man is in a 100 m sprint. He accelerates at 4 ms$^{-2}$ for the first 20 m and runs at a constant velocity thereafter until the last 10 m when he starts to decelerate at 0.1 ms$^{-1}$.

    a. How fast is he travelling after 1.5 s?

    b. How far does he travel in this time?

    c. How fast is he travelling at 20 m?

    d. How long does he take to cover the next 10 m?

    e. How far can he travel in 1 s?

    f. How long does he take to cover the middle section (20–90 m)?

    g. What is his velocity as he crosses the finishing line?

    h. What was his time for the race?

## Gravity

Of the forces that glue together the universe, gravity, despite being the first to be identified and its effects understood (Sir Isaac Newton again), is the most mysterious. As we have seen above, it is gravity that causes mass to have an associated weight and this is directly proportional to the strength of the gravitational field.

It is also this mutual attraction of masses that keeps the planets orbiting the sun and satellites orbiting planets ... although, in reality, the Earth does not orbit the sun, both bodies orbit a common point; however, because the sun is so much more massive than the Earth, that point is within the volume of the sun itself. In a similar way, not only are we attracted to the Earth, but the Earth is also attracted towards us (although the former is stronger by a factor of $10^{23}$!). When the bodies are of a more similar size, as with the Earth and moon, the mutual attraction is more obvious. When the moon and sun's gravitational fields line up (during the new moon), we get a much larger tidal range (spring tides) than we do when they oppose each other (neap tides). Without the moon, we would have no tides at all; the effect is due entirely to the gravitational pull of the moon on the water of the Earth's oceans.

The mutual attraction of two objects is calculated using **Newton's law of gravitation:**

$$F_g = \frac{GM_1M_2}{r^2}$$

where $F_g$ is the gravitational force produced between two objects of mass $M_1$ and $M_2$ whose centres are separated by distance $r$. G is the Universal Gravitational Constant, which is equal to $6.67 \times 10^{-11}$ Nm$^2$kg$^{-2}$

and, as with other such constants, does not need to be memorized! As the masses of any pair of objects are also likely to be constant, the force is proportional to the inverse of the distance of separation squared. This relationship is known as the **inverse square law** and it is an important one – it is not just a rule of gravitation, you will encounter it again in other fields, so it is worth making sure that you have a thorough understanding of it now.

We intuitively know that, the further you are from an object, the weaker the gravitational field. However, the manner in which it drops in intensity is very specific and relates to the **square** of the distance. Thus, if you double the distance, the field will only be one-quarter as intense; triple it and the field drops to one-ninth of its original intensity; quadruple it, the field is only one-sixteenth of the value and so on. The same is true in reverse: twice as close gives four times the strength of field; eight times as close, sixty-four times the strength.

---

### Fact File

#### GRAVITY

Although its effects are easily calculated, both in everyday and relativistic situations, we are not much nearer to understanding what gravity is and how and why masses are mutually attracted than was Newton. The interactions that bind together molecules and atoms are stronger than gravity by a factor of up to $10^{38}$ although they act over very much smaller distances. This explains, amongst other things, why solids behave as they do (we don't fall though them, nor are we irresistibly attracted towards them) even though they are – as we shall see in later chapters – 99.99% empty space. These forces and their mediating particles (photons, gluons etc.) have been studied for decades; nobody has yet succeeded in identifying a 'graviton', which remains a hypothetical particle.

#### MOON

What is a moon? In fact, our moon and Earth only just stop short of being a binary or twin planetary system. The centre of rotation lies (just) within the planetary mass of the Earth, otherwise there would be a good case for regarding them both as planets orbiting around each other. This argument certainly holds for Pluto and its moon Charon, which is half the size, although considerably less dense. Not only do both orbit a centre of mass that is outside Pluto, but two other, smaller satellites, Nix and Hydra, orbit this same point, i.e. they orbit both the twin dwarf planets rather than Pluto itself.

---

# Energy and work

Energy is defined as: *the capacity of a system to do work.*

It can take many forms; you will be familiar with people talking of 'chemical energy', 'thermal energy', 'electrical energy' or 'nuclear energy'. This differentiation largely relates to the form in which the energy is being stored. For example, chemical energy is the energy stored in the molecular and atomic bonds within substances, which can be released in chemical reactions; nuclear energy, the energy stored within the bonds between the fundamental particles in atomic nuclei, is the source of the energy for nuclear power stations (nuclear fission) and for stars (nuclear fusion). In addition, there is 'mechanical energy', which, at this stage, will be our main area of focus; this, however, can also take several different forms.

Energy is usually given the symbol, $E$, though sometimes you may see it, rather confusingly, as $W$. In this text, we shall be using $E$ for energy and $W$ for work.

As you will recall from the previous chapter, in the SI system, energy is measured in joules – although, as you will also recall from the previous chapter, whereas physicists seldom deviate from SI units, clinicians frequently do and, as discussed below, you will need to have a familiarity with several other ways of measuring energy in order to interact with the society in which you live and will be practising (see below).

Work is also measured in joules and is defined as: *the process of energy transfer.*

It is calculated by multiplying the force *(F)* used and the distance moved in the direction of the force, sometimes called the *displacement (s)*. This fits well with our intuitive knowledge: if we are pushing a heavy object, the amount of work we do will depend on the amount of force that we use and how far we push it. This relationship can be written as:

**$W = Fs$**

So energy can be stored and, when it is transferred, this process is called 'work'. Stored energy is referred to as **potential energy** (because it has the potential to do work).

**Gravitational potential energy** is the energy possessed by a body by virtue of its position in a gravitational field. If a mass, *m*, is lifted through a height,

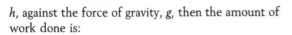

$h$, against the force of gravity, $g$, then the amount of work done is:

**$W = mgh$ joules**

However, energy can never be created or destroyed, a principle known as **conservation of energy**. Therefore the potential energy $(E_p)$ of the mass is also:

**$E_p = mgh$ joules**

The energy is stored and can be used again to do work. This is the manner in which a pendulum clock works. When the clock is wound up, a lead weight is lifted. This weight gradually descends, transferring its energy to the pendulum, which would otherwise slow and stop owing to the effects of friction in its bearings and air resistance. This does not, of course, violate the principle of energy conservation: the gravitational potential energy is converted into mechanical energy (running the pendulum), which, in turn, is converted into thermal energy (heat from friction).

**Kinetic energy** is the energy of movement – obviously, a moving body must have energy, which can do work (although this will slow the body down). The work needed to slow the body to rest can be calculated. We know that $W = Fs$ and also that $F = ma$.

Therefore: $W = (ma)s$
From the equations of motion, you will recall that:

**$v^2 = u^2 + 2as$**

However, as we are slowing the body to rest:

**$v^2 = 0^2 + 2as$ or $as = v^2/2$**

So, if:

**$W = mas$,  $W = m(v^2/2)$**

Or:

**$W = \frac{1}{2}mv^2$**

So, the kinetic energy of a moving object is:

**$E_K = \frac{1}{2}mv^2$ joules**

As stated earlier, there are other forms of mechanical energy, such as elastic energy, which will be dealt with in the following chapter. Other types of energy will be detailed in later sections of the book.

## Heat and temperature

**Temperature** is actually quite a tricky concept to pin down with a definition. It is best defined as: *the 'hotness' of an object (reflected by the intensity of the motion of its constituent particles)* and is a property that determines whether there will be heat flow between two objects (one of the fundamental laws of thermodynamics states that heat will flow from a hotter object to a cooler object until the two are at the same temperature). It is a function of the mean kinetic energy of the particles within a system.

It has symbol $T$ and, in the SI system, is measured in kelvin (K).

**Heat** is defined as: *the internal energy of a system* (i.e. the combined kinetic energy of all the atoms and molecules within the system).

It is given the symbol Q and is measured in joules (J).

Heat, therefore, is not solely dependent on temperature but is the product of temperature, mass and a property called thermal capacity (a substance's ability to store heat).

The difference between heat and temperature is best understood by comparing and contrasting two different systems; let us consider:

• A spark from a fire
• A warm bath of water.

The first of these has a high temperature (perhaps 850 K); indeed, if one were to land on your skin, it would cause a nasty burn as it rapidly transferred its thermal energy (the rate of transfer of thermal energy is proportional to the difference in temperature between the two objects). However, despite its high temperature, a spark does not have much heat. Because it has only a low mass, the amount of energy contained in a spark is fairly insignificant; if you were to put the spark into a cup of cold water, you would probably need a very sensitive thermometer to measure any appreciable change in the temperature of the water. By contrast, a bath has a much lower temperature, perhaps a pleasant 330 K. However, water has a high thermal capacity and mass. Its energy is therefore much greater than a single spark.

There are three temperature scales with which you will need to be familiar: Fahrenheit, Celsius (sometimes still called centigrade) and Kelvin. The problem (for scientists) with the first two scales is that, whilst they are convenient for everyday usage, they are not absolute scales: they don't start at zero; therefore, 70°C is not twice as hot as 35°C. This makes them very inconvenient for use in equations.

Daniel Fahrenheit was a Polish doctor who built and calibrated the first really accurate thermometers, initially using alcohol (in 1709) – the revolutionary (and more practical, though considerably more toxic) mercury thermometer was to follow 5 years later. To avoid regular recourse to negative figures, he eventually set the freezing point of water at 32°F and the average temperature of the human body at 96°F. On the Fahrenheit scale, water boils at 212°C.

Some three decades later, the Swedish astronomer Anders Celsius had the more logical idea of setting 100 degrees between the freezing and boiling points of water (hence the occasional use of 'degrees centigrade') and this scale is now used in most countries of the world in everyday measurements.

## Fact File

### CELSIUS

Although Anders Celsius is credited with the invention of the scale, he originally placed the freezing point of water at 100°C and the boiling point at 0°C, thus creating a scale in which a *decreasing* reading indicated *increasing* temperature. It was a biologist colleague, Carolus Linnaeus, the inventor of the modern taxonomical system of naming living organisms by genus and species, who put the scale into the more logical orientation that we use today.

A century would pass before physicists demanded an absolute scale for temperature, and Sir William Thomson (who became Lord Kelvin for his work on the transatlantic telephone cable) would be the man to provide it. He had observed that, for every 1°C drop in temperature, a gas will contract by $1/273$ of its volume as measured at 0°C. From this, he inferred that there must be a point at which the volume would reach zero, beyond which it would be impossible to go. The actual value of 0 K – 'absolute zero' – is −273.15°C (−459.67°F) at which point, the internal energy of the substance would also be zero. The temperature is a hypothetical one, to reach absolute zero would take an infinite amount of energy; however, scientists have succeeded in creating temperatures just a few ten-millionths of a Kelvin above absolute zero at which strange physical effects can occur: liquids can flow uphill, solids shatter like glass and electricity can flow without any resistance.

Whenever you see the symbol for temperature in an equation, you must use a value in Kelvin – Celsius and Fahrenheit will produce nonsensical results.

To convert Celsius to Kelvin:

$$K = {}^{\circ}C + 273.15$$

To convert Fahrenheit to Celsius:

$$^{\circ}C = \tfrac{5}{9} \times ({}^{\circ}F - 32)$$

Should you need to convert Celsius to Fahrenheit:

$$^{\circ}F = \tfrac{9}{5} \times ({}^{\circ}C + 32)$$

If you are American, there is one other scale that you may encounter, the Rankine scale (°R). This scale does for Fahrenheit what kelvins do for Celsius, i.e. establish a scale that starts at absolute zero:

$$^{\circ}R = {}^{\circ}F + 459.67$$

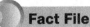

---

**Fact File**

**FAHRENHEIT**

Fahrenheit recognized that mercury – unique in being a metal that is liquid (its freezing point is −39°C (−38°F)) at the range of temperatures experienced climatically – expands at a constant rate in direct proportion to the temperature. By channelling this expansion up a thin, flat capillary tube, he was able to accurately measure temperature change with a device that, unlike the alcohol thermometer, was much less bulky and not significantly affected by changes in atmospheric pressure. He set 1°F as being the expansion of mercury by 0.01% of its volume . . . so, despite all appearances to the contrary, there is a metric element to the Fahrenheit scale!

---

## CLINICAL FOCUS

Body temperature is one of the vital signs monitored by primary contact healthcare professionals in order to gauge their patients' wellbeing. A normal temperature may vary considerably during the course of 24 hours, being at its lowest in the early morning (2 am – 5 am) when it may be down to 35.8°C (96.4°F) and at its highest in late afternoon or early evening (4 pm – 8 pm). These figures though only apply to oral temperatures (rectal readings are usually 0.5° C (0.9° F) higher and axillary temperatures 0.5° C lower) and to adults (infants' rectal temperature is often as high as 38.3°C (101°F) and seldom falls below 37.2°C (99°F) until three years of age).

Measurement of temperature has become a much easier affair since the advent of new types of thermoelectric digital thermometers, which do away with mercury and glass altogether (although it is still worth learning how to use the traditional oral medical thermometer: it has the advantage of never needing new batteries!). Particularly, the tympanic instruments that can be inserted into the ear and give an accurate reading at the click of a button have made the assessment of body temperature far less cumbersome and time consuming and are a particular boon with paediatric patients.

There are two things that it is worth bearing in mind with temperature readings outside of the normal range. Firstly, a person's temperature can be too low as well as too high. **Hypothermia** (a core

temperature of less than 35°C (95°F)) is a not uncommon clinical finding, particularly in the elderly, either in lower socioeconomic groups or with impaired thermoregulation from pathologies such as heart complaints or pneumonia. Secondly, **pyrexia** (an elevated temperature) may tell you that the patient has something wrong with them, but it does not tell you what. The majority of pyrexia is from self-limiting viral infections but a persistently elevated temperature without obvious cause is a cause for concern and further investigation. This is particularly true if manipulative therapy is proposed as a treatment protocol and unexplained pyrexia of more than 100°F for three days or longer is regarded as an indication for radiological investigation prior to adjustment.

The principal causes of pyrexia of unknown origin are:
- Infection.
  - Abscess, TB, bacteria, viruses, parasites etc.
- Neoplasms
  - Especially lymphomas
- Connective tissue diseases
  - Inflammatory arthropathies, SLE, arteritis etc.
- Other
  - Drug reactions, sarcoidosis, inflammatory bowel disease, pulmonary embolism, intracranial pathology.

---

# Pressure and partial pressures

If you have read and understood the section above on temperature, you will hopefully have gained an intuitive feel for the fact that there is a link between temperature and pressure; in fact, many of the definitions given above have the caveat 'at constant pressure' or 'at one atmosphere of pressure' invisibly appended to them.

**Pressure** is defined as: the forces acting at 90° to a unit area of a surface. It is given the unit $p$ and, in the SI system, is measured in pascals (Pa) although, as you will see, there are several systems for measuring pressure in everyday usage.

Although this definition appears a little verbose, it can be summarized as:

$$P = \frac{F}{A}$$

which is consistent with the definition of the pascal that you may recall from Chapter 1 as being 1 newton per metre squared. We use this simple fact on a daily basis without thought. To give maximum pressure, a small point of contact is needed as with drawing pins or sharpened knives; to minimize pressure, as with snowshoes and tractor tyres, a large contact area is employed.

**Atmospheric pressure** is caused by the molecules in the air (i.e. $N_2$, $O_2$, $CO_2$) striking against surfaces (i.e. us!). This is dependent upon:

- The number of molecules hitting at a given moment
- The transfer of momentum when they strike (you will recall that the momentum of a molecule is proportional to both its mass and its velocity).

Because we live with the atmosphere on a daily basis, it is not surprising that 1 atmosphere (1 atm) is sometimes used as a measure of pressure; you will sometimes see experiments or definitions that are 'at standard temperature (0°C) and pressure (1 atm)' or 'STP'. Unfortunately, atmospheric pressure can vary quite considerably both with elevation (which is why atmospheric pressure is always quoted by weathermen at sea level) and with changing weather systems. One atmosphere has, by international agreement, been set to 101 325 Pa – thus removing the vagaries of altitude and altering weather systems.

significantly more painful in low-pressure weather systems (and in colder weather).

Similarly, there is also a link between atmospheric pressure and rheumatoid arthritis (which tends also to be affected by extremes of temperature) and fibromyalgia. Some psychiatric conditions, particularly those involving impulsive behaviour, also worsen when the pressure dips.

Meteorologists and medics both measure pressure in millimetres (or inches) of mercury. The principle on which a mercury barometer works is shown in Figure 2.6. The force of air molecules pushing down on the mercury in the dish in which the open end of the tube is sitting is enough to push up the mercury in the vacuum sealed side of the tube to a height of 760 mm (29.92 inches or 1 atmosphere), plus or minus atmospheric variation. Medics also use millimetres of mercury (mm Hg) to record blood pressure.

There are a number of other units of pressure that you may well encounter when listening to weather forecasts, recording histories from divers or inflating the tyres on your motor car. These are detailed in Table 2.3.

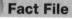

### Fact File

**ATMOSPHERIC PRESSURE**

The highest ever-recorded atmospheric pressure was 814 mm (32.06″) of mercury in Mongolia in 2001, 7% higher than normal; the lowest, 653 mm (25.69″) of mercury, which is 14% lower than normal. This occurred in the Western Pacific during Typhoon Tip in October 2005.

### CLINICAL FOCUS

Atmospheric pressure is an important consideration for the clinician as changes in the barometer reading have implications for our health. You may have heard people claim that they know when bad weather is on the way because their 'gammy leg' or similar ancient injury plays them up. Far from being an old wives' tale, there is considerable evidence that degenerative joint disease (osteoarthritis) is

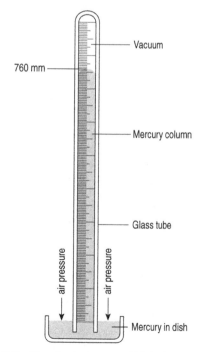

**Figure 2.6** • The classical mercury U-tube barometer.

**Table 2.3** Different units commonly used in the measurement of pressure

| Unit | Comments | Pascal equivalence |
|------|----------|--------------------|
| Pascal (Pa) | The SI unit of pressure = 1 Nm$^{-2}$ | |
| Atmosphere (atm) | Commonly used by divers. Pressure in a fluid = depth × $g$ × density (the pressure at the deepest point on the ocean floor is 830 atm). It is also used to describe the contents of pressurized containers | 1 atm = 101 325 Pa |
| Bar (b) | A unit from the CGS system, more often encountered as the millibar (mb), which is used as a standard on aneroid barometers and by meteorologists (these are the figures you will see on weather charts). The bar is also used for European tyre pressures | 1 b = 10$^5$ Pa |
| Millimetres of mercury (mm Hg) | Used for barometric measurement and in taking blood pressure | 1 mm Hg = 133.3 Pa |
| Inches of mercury (Hg or in Hg) | Used for barometric measurement in the USA (blood pressure is still recorded in mm Hg) | 1 inch Hg = 3386 Pa |
| Kilograms per metre squared (kgm$^{-2}$) | Although at first sight this is the logical SI unit, rather than the derived pascal, it should be remembered that the kg only exerts pressure if in a gravitation field … which accounts for the conversion factor | 1 kg m$^{-2}$ = 9.8 Pa |
| Pounds per square inch (psi) | The imperial unit of pressure, encountered on filling station forecourts – most care tyres are filled to about 30 psi, around twice atmospheric pressure | 1 psi = 6895 Pa |
| Torr | Equal to the mm Hg | 1τ = 133.3 Pa |

## CLINICAL FOCUS

Blood pressure is made up of two components: **systolic** pressure (the surge created when the heart pumps) and **diastolic** pressure (the residual pressure in the arteries when the heart is resting between beats). The apparatus used to measure blood pressure is called a **sphygmomanometer** (pronounced sfig-mo-man-om-meter) comprising an inflatable cuff, which is placed around the patient's arm and pumped up to the point where it constricts the arteries sufficiently to prevent arterial flow (Fig. 2.7). Modern, electronic cuffs (Fig. 2.8) are self-inflating and give a digital readout in seconds; however, the traditional manual method is still an important skill for the clinician to master.

Once the pulse has been occluded, the cuff is then slowly deflated until a pulse is detected using a stethoscope; this is the systolic pressure. As the cuff continues to deflate, the sounds become muffled and then rapidly disappear, this is the point at which turbulent flow ceases, the diastolic pressure. Blood pressure classification is detailed in Table 2.4. It is worth noting that blood pressure is frequently elevated through anxiety and 'white coat syndrome' on the first visit to a clinician and hypertension should only be diagnosed if the readings remain high on two or more consecutive visits.

All primary healthcare workers should be involved in the monitoring of blood pressure; high blood pressure is one of the great silent epidemics of the Western world and predisposes towards heart failure, cerebrovascular incidents, renal failure and atherosclerosis. With malignant hypertension, there is a 50% chance of death within 12 months.

On average, one-quarter of the Caucasian and one-third of the black population will have essential (primary) hypertension, which accounts for 95% of all cases, the incidence increasing with age. Only half of sufferers are aware they have the condition and, of those who are aware, only half manage adequate control; in other words, 75% of hypertensives and one-fifth of the general adult population are damaging their health with an elevated blood pressure. Detection and monitoring at the primary care level is a major public health concern.

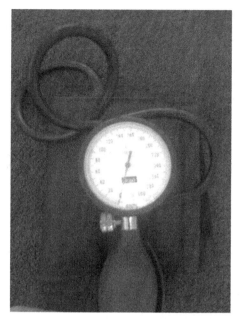

**Figure 2.7** • The traditional sphygmomanometer. Portable versions, such as this, use dials. Desktop systems tend to still employ a mercury column to indicate pressure.

**Table 2.4** Classification of adult blood pressure*

| Category | Systolic (mm Hg) | Diastolic (mm Hg) |
|---|---|---|
| Optimal | $< 120$ | $< 80$ |
| Normal | $< 130$ | $< 85$ |
| High–normal | 130–139 | 85–89 |
| Stage I hypertension (mild) | 140–159 | 90–99 |
| Stage II hypertension (moderate) | 160–179 | 100–109 |
| Stage III hypertension (severe) | 180–209 | 110–119 |
| Malignant | $\geq 210$ | $\geq 120$ |

*Where systolic and diastolic fall into different categories, the higher category is used.

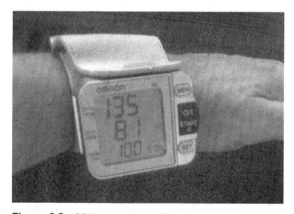

**Figure 2.8** • Modern electronic blood pressure cuffs inflate automatically and give a digital readout in seconds.

Although we have discussed 'air molecules' when considering atmospheric pressure, this is in fact a misnomer; there are no such things as 'molecules of air', rather the molecules that comprise the stuff we breath are, as we have already said, a mixture of gases. Each one of those gases contributes to the overall pressure of the atmosphere; each has a **partial pressure**, the total of which add up to atmospheric pressure:

$$P_{N_2} + P_{O_2} + P_{CO_2} + P_{other} = P_{atmosphere}$$

$$0.78\,atm + 0.21\,atm + 0.03\,atm + 0.07\,atm = 1\,atm$$

So the partial pressure of each gas is related to the concentration of that gas in the mixture and to the total pressure of the mixture. The partial pressure of any constituent gas can be calculated by determining the pressure that that gas would exert if all other gases were removed. This is known as **Dalton's Law**.

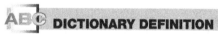 **DICTIONARY DEFINITION**

**DALTON'S LAW**

Dalton's law, which is also sometimes known as Dalton's law of partial pressures was formulated in 1801 and states that the total pressure exerted by a gaseous mixture is equal to the sum of the partial pressures of each individual component in a gas mixture. Mathematically, it can be expressed by the formula:

$$P_{total} = P_1 + P_2 + P_3 + \dots P_n$$

The partial pressure of a gas in a liquid is directly related to the amount of that gas dissolved in the liquid. This, in turn, is determined by the partial pressure of the gas in the atmosphere adjacent to that liquid. The gases will form an equilibrium whereby the partial pressure of the gas in solution becomes equal to its partial pressure in the atmosphere adjacent to the solution. This is known as Henry's Law. If this equilibrium is changed – the proportion of a substance in the gas alters or the pressure of the gas itself is modified – then a new equilibrium will be reached with the new partial pressures of the dissolved gases reflecting this. This situation is reflected in Figure 2.9.

## CLINICAL FOCUS

In the lungs, the air in the alveoli constitutes the environment surrounding pulmonary capillaries through which blood moves. Separating the blood and the air are the extremely thin alveolar and capillary membranes, both of which are highly permeable to carbon dioxide and oxygen.

This means that gases can move in both directions through the respiratory membrane. Oxygen enters blood from the alveolar air because the $Po_2$ of alveolar air is greater than the $Po_2$ of the incoming, deoxygenated blood. Simultaneously, carbon dioxide molecules exit from the blood into the alveolar air – the $Pco_2$ of venous blood is much higher than the $Pco_2$ of alveolar air. This two-way exchange of gases between alveolar air and pulmonary blood converts deoxygenated blood to oxygenated blood.

By the time blood leaves the pulmonary capillaries as arterial blood, equilibration of oxygen and carbon dioxide across the membranes has occurred, or as near to equilibration as can be obtained in the time available. Arterial blood $Po_2$ and $Pco_2$ therefore usually equal or very nearly equal alveolar $Po_2$ and $Pco_2$ (Table 2.5).

## The gas laws

Given their relationship to the velocity of interacting particles, and recalling that temperature is a function of the kinetic energy of a substance, you will hopefully be unsurprised to learn that there is a direct link between temperature and pressure. This link has been quantified in the gas laws, of which there are three:

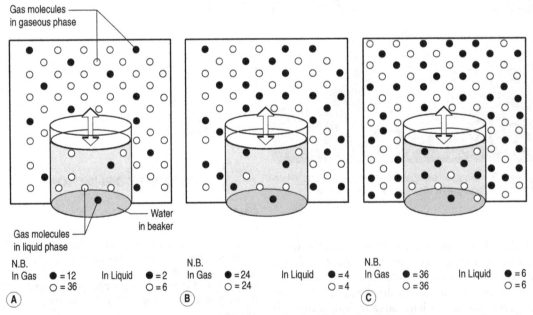

Figure 2.9 • Relative pressures. The partial pressure of gases dissolved in a liquid will form the same proportions as is found in the gases adjacent to the liquid once equilibrium has been reached (A). If the partial pressures in the atmosphere change, the partial pressures in the liquid rapidly reach a new equilibrium as more particles will dissolve into the liquid that evaporate away from it (or vice versa) until a new balance has been obtained (B). If the overall pressure of the atmosphere changes, the gaseous partial pressures will all increase by the same amount and, thus, so will the liquid partial pressures (C).

**Table 2.5** Partial pressures of gases in the pulmonary-cardiovascular system. Despite the constant diffusion across the alveolar/capillary membranes, the partial pressures of the gases in the alveoli remain approximately constant owing to the regular reventilation occurring by breathing. Atmospheric pressure is assumed to be mean, dry, sea level

|  | Atmosphere | Alveolar air | Arterial blood | Venous blood |
|---|---|---|---|---|
| $P_{O_2}$ | 160 mm Hg = 0.21 atm | 100 mm Hg = 0.13 atm | 100 mm Hg = 0.13 atm | 40 mm Hg = 53 matm |
| $P_{CO_2}$ | 0.2 mm Hg = 2.6 matm | 40 mm Hg = 53 matm | 40 mm Hg = 53 matm | 46 mm Hg = 60 matm |
| $P_{H_2O}$ | 0 | 47 mm Hg = 62 matm = | 47 mm Hg = 62 matm = | 47 mm Hg = 62 matm = |

**Boyle's law** states that the volume of a fixed mass of a gas is inversely proportional to pressure (if the temperature remains unchanged).

## DICTIONARY DEFINITION

### BOYLE'S LAW

Robert Boyle (1627–91), whom we have already encountered as one of the founding members of the Royal Society, formulated the first of the gas laws in 1662. It was also discovered independently by Edme Mariotte four years later and is therefore sometimes referred to as the *Boyle-Mariotte law*. It is defined as: *for a fixed amount of gas kept at a fixed temperature, pressure and volume are inversely proportional*. This can be expressed mathematically as:

$$V \propto \frac{1}{p} \quad \text{or} \quad pV = \text{constant} = \Re_1$$

As we have already defined the pressure of a gas (the atmosphere) as being due to the number of collisions of its constituent molecules against an opposing surface, it should not come as any surprise that by doubling the volume (and thus halving the number of molecules per cubic metre), we also halve the pressure.

By contrast, **Charles' law** states that, if the pressure is kept constant, the volume of a gas will be proportional to the temperature (which, you will recall, we are measuring in kelvin). If you imagine a syringe with a frictionless plunger containing a gas, then if the molecules are given more thermal energy, they will move faster. This will mean they hit the plunger with greater momentum and push it backwards (thus increasing the volume), until the pressure has returned to its previous level.

## DICTIONARY DEFINITION

### CHARLES' LAW

Charles' law was actually first published in 1802, but the author Joseph Gay-Lussac cited unpublished work by Jaques Charles (who also invented the hydrogen balloon) dating back to 1787. It states: *for a fixed amount of gas kept at a fixed pressure, temperature and volume are directly proportional.* This can be expressed mathematically as:

$$V \propto T \quad \text{or} \quad \frac{V}{T} = \text{constant} = \Re_2$$

Having laws that cover situations whereby the temperature and pressure are kept constant, the third law deals with keeping the volume constant and is known as the **Gay-Lussac law**. This states that, for a fixed mass of gas at a constant volume, the pressure is directly proportional to the (absolute) temperature. This can be visualized by imagining that the syringe plunger is fixed. As the gas cannot now expand, it hits the walls of the syringe with increasing force (per unit area) and the pressure increases.

## DICTIONARY DEFINITION

### GAY-LUSSAC'S LAW

Sometimes known as the pressure law, in order to differentiate it from another law formulated by the same French chemist, Joseph Gay-Lussac published the third gas law in 1802. It states that: *for a fixed volume of gas, temperature and pressure are directly proportional.*

This can be expressed mathematically as:

$$p \propto T \quad \text{or} \quad \frac{p}{T} = \text{constant} = \Re_3$$

By combining these three equations, we arrive at the **ideal gas equation**, this states that, if we take a gaseous system and make changes to it, then the start (*s*) and end (*e*) states will be related as follows:

or

$$\frac{pV}{T} = \text{constant}$$

$$\frac{p_s V_s}{T_s} = \frac{p_e V_e}{T_e}$$

## Learning Outcomes

If you have understood the contents of this chapter, you should now understand:
- The concepts of velocity and acceleration
- The effects of mass, momentum and force
- Newton's laws and the associated equations of motion
- The relationship between energy, work, heat and temperature
- The behaviour of gases and their response to changes in pressure, volume and temperature.

## CHECK YOUR EXISTING KNOWLEDGE: ANSWERS

Mark your answers using the guide below to give yourself a score:
1  Vectors: a, c, e, f, g; Scalars: b, d, h, i, j [1 each]
2  Acceleration [3]
3  I  Each body continues in its state of rest or in uniform motion in a straight line unless acted on by an external force
   II  The rate of change of a body's momentum is proportional to the applied force and takes place in the direction in which the force acts
   III  For every action, there is an equal and opposite reaction [2 each]
4  a 24 ms$^{-1}$ [3]   b 96 m [3]
5  a 33.3 s [3]   b 3 ms$^{-2}$ [3]   c 112.5 m [4]   d 16.7 s [3]
6  a 15 N [2]   b 600 N [2]
7  a 3000 J [2]   b 1.25 J [2]
8  a kelvin b joule c newton d metre e kilogram f newton g joule h pascal i metres per second squared j square metres [1 each]
9  0.4 atm [2]
10  1465 K (1192°C) [2]

## How to interpret the results:

55–60: You have the necessary grasp of the basic physics that you need to understand the biomechanical principles in this book and should be able to proceed without difficulty.

40–54: There are some important gaps in your knowledge, which need to be filled before proceeding.

0–39: You will need to study this chapter fully before proceeding; the contents represent some of the fundamentals on which your future understanding will be based.

## Workshop: Answers

1a  $v = u + at$.
   Therefore $v = 0 + (4 \times 1.5) = 6\ \text{ms}^{-1}$

1b  $s = ut + \frac{1}{2}at^2$.
   Therefore $s = (0 \times 1.5) + (0.5 \times 4 \times 1.5^2)$
   $= 4.5\ \text{m}$

1c  $v^2 = u^2 + 2as$.
   Therefore $v^2 = 0^2 + (2 \times 4 \times 20) = 160$
   Therefore $v = \sqrt{160} = 12.7\ \text{ms}^{-1}$

1d  If he is travelling at $12.7\ \text{ms}^{-1}$, it will take him $10/12.7 = 0.79\ \text{s}$ (you should not need the equations of motion for this)

1e  Trick question! As his velocity is now constant and you calculated it in 1c, the answer is 12.7 m

1f  Same procedure as 1d. $70/12.7 = 5.51\ \text{s}$

1g  $v^2 = u^2 + 2as$. At 90 m we know his velocity is $12.7\ \text{ms}^{-1}$; this now becomes his initial velocity for the last 10 m

   Therefore $v^2 = 12.7^2 + (2 \times -0.1 \times 10) = 161.3 - 2 = 159.3$
   Therefore $v = \sqrt{159.3} = 12.6\ \text{ms}^{-1}$

1h  This needs to be calculated in three sections. For the first 20 m: $v = u + at$. Therefore $t = (v - u)/a$.
   We know from 1c that, at 20 m, he is travelling at $12.7\ \text{ms}^{-1}$.
   Therefore $t = (12.7 - 0)/4 = 3.18\ \text{s}$.
   For the constant velocity section: (20–90 m) $t = 5.51\ \text{s}$ (1f).
   For the last 10 m: $t = (v - u)/a$.
   From 1c, $u = 12.7\ \text{ms}^{-1}$; from 1g, $v = 12.6\ \text{ms}^{-1}$.
   Therefore $t = (12.6 - 12.7)/0.1 = -0.1/0.1 = 1\ \text{s}$.
The total time taken is $3.18 + 5.51 + 1 = 9.69\ \text{s}$ . . . congratulations, you have just equalled the world record!

## Bibliography

Allen, R., Schwarz, C. (Eds.), 1998. The Chambers dictionary. Chambers Harrap, Edinburgh.

Bates, B., 1995. The general survey. In: A guide to physical examination and history taking, sixth ed. J B Lippincott, Philadelphia, pp. 123–130.

Bates, B., 1995. The cardiovascular system. In: A guide to physical examination and history taking, sixth ed. J B Lippincott, Philadelphia, pp. 259–312.

Beers, M.H., Berkow, R. (Eds.), 1999. In: The Merck manual of diagnosis and therapy, seventeenth ed. Merck, West Point, PA.

Buie, M.W., Grundy, W.M., Young, E.F., Young, L.A., et al., 2008. Orbits and photometry of Pluto molecules of air's slowing rotation. Online.

Available from: novan.com/earth.htm 30 September 2008, 12:15 BST.

Hamilton, R.L., Charon. Available online: http://www.solarviews.com/ eng/charon.htm 3 Nov 2006, 14:51 GMT.

Hart, J.T., 1970. Semicontinuous screening of a whole community for hypertension. Lancet 2 (7666), 223–226.

Hebra, A., 2003. Hot stuff: temperature, pressure and thermodynamics. In: Measure for measure: the story of imperial, metric and other units. Johns Hopkins University Press, Baltimore, pp. 98–118.

Hebra, A., 2003. The missing link: energy. In: Measure for measure: the story of imperial, metric and other units. Johns Hopkins

University Press, Baltimore, pp. 119–140.

Hope, R.A., Longmore, J.M., Hodgetts, T.J., et al., 1993. In: Oxford handbook of clinical medicine, third ed. Oxford University Press, Oxford.

Isaac Newton Institute for Mathematical Sciences. Isaac Newton's Life. Online: www.newton.cam.ac.uk/ newtlife.html 25 Oct 2006, 10:14 BST.

James, P.B., 1993. Dysbarism: the medical problems from high and low atmospheric pressure. J. R. Coll. Physicians Lond. 27 (4), 367–374.

Koenigsberg, R. (Ed.), 1989. In: Churchill's Illustrated medical dictionary. Churchill Livinstone, New York.

Mackowiak, P.A., Wasserman, S.S., Levine, M.M. 1992. A critical appraisal of 98.6°F, the upper limit of the normal body temperature, and other legacies of Carl Reinhold August Wunderlich. JAMA 23-30;268 (12), 1578–1580.

Matthew, H.C.G., Harrison, B. (Eds.), 2000. Bacon, Roger. In: Oxford dictionary of national biography: in association with the British Academy. From the earliest times to the year. Oxford University Press, Oxford. Online: www.oxforddnb. com/articles/1/1008-article.html 24 Feb 2005, 5:31pm BST.

Pallen, C.B., Wynne, J.J., Wemyss Brown, et al. (Eds.), In: The New Catholic Dictionary; Vatican edition (a complete work of reference on every subject in the life, belief, tradition, rites, symbolism, devotions, history, biography, laws, dioceses, Missions, centers, institutions, organizations, statistics of the Church, and her part in promoting science, art, education, social welfare, morals and civilization). Online. Available: www.catholic-forum.com/saints/ ncd00954.htm 24 Oct 2006, 12:02 BST.

Petrie, J.C., 1998. Hypertension: the United Kingdom experience. Am. J. Hypertens. 11 (6 Pt 1), 754–755.

Price, G., A historical outline of modern religious criticism in western civilization. Online. Available: www.rationalrevolution.net/articles/ religious_criticism.htm; 10 Sep 2005 24 Oct 2006, 10:19 BST.

Royal Society. A brief history of the society. Online. Available: www.royalsociety.ac.uk 24 Oct 2006, 16:58 BST.

Schauf, C.L., Moffett, D.F., Moffett, S.B., 1990. Gas exchange and gas transport in the blood. In: Human physiology: foundations and frontiers. Mosby, St Louis, pp. 426–445.

Schory, T.J., Piecznski, N., Nair, S., et al., 2003. Barometric pressure, emergency psychiatric visits, and violent acts. Can. J Psychiatry 48 (9), 624–627.

Scott, S.K., Rabito, F.A., Price, P.D., et al., 2006. Comorbidity among the morbidly obese: a comparative study of 2002 US hospital patient discharges. Surgery for Obesity and Other Related Diseases 2 (2), 105–111.

Shoemaker, A.L., 1996. What's normal? Temperature, gender, and heart rate. Journal of Statistics Education 4, 2.

Singh, S., 1997. I think I'll stop here. In: Fermat's last theorem. Harper Perennial, London, pp. 1–36.

Thibodeau, G.A., Patton, K., 2006. Physiology of the respiratory system. In: Anatomy and physiology, sixth ed. Elsevier, Philadelphia, e-book.

Thorne, J.O., Collocott, T.C. (Eds.), 1984. Chambers biographical dictionary. Chambers, Edinburgh.

Turley, M., Tobias, M., Paul, S., 2006. Non-fatal disease burden associated with excess body mass index and waist circumference in New Zealand adults. Aust. N. Z. J. Public Health 30 (3), 231–237.

Tuthill, A., Slawik, H., O'Rahilly, S., et al., 2006. Psychiatric co-morbidities in patients attending specialist obesity services in the UK. QJM 99 (5), 317–325.

Verges, J., Montell, E., Tomas, E., et al., 2004. Weather conditions can influence rheumatic diseases. Proc West Pharmacol Soc 47, 134–136.

Weathers, L., 2006. Einstein and Newton showed signs of high functioning Asperger's syndrome. Online. Available: www. aspergerssyndrome.net/einstein.htm 1 Nov 2006 15:49 GMT.

Wingstrand, H., Wingstrand, A., Krantz, P., 1990. Intracapsular and atmospheric pressure in the dynamics and stability of the hip. A biomechanical study. Acta. Orthop. Scand. 61 (3), 231–235.

Wong, L., Temperature of a healthy human (body temperature). In: Elert, G. (Ed.), The physics factbook. Online. Available: hypertextbook. com/facts/LenaWong.shtml 4 October 2008 10:35 BST.

# Chapter Three

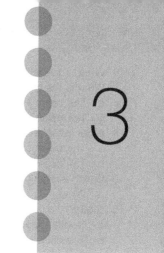

# Applied physics

## CHAPTER CONTENTS

Check your existing knowledge . . . . . . . . 49
Levers, beams and moments . . . . . . . . . 50
   First order lever . . . . . . . . . . . . . . . . . . . 51
   Second order lever . . . . . . . . . . . . . . . 52
   Third order lever . . . . . . . . . . . . . . . . . . 52
   Muscle action . . . . . . . . . . . . . . . . . . . 52
   Moment of inertia . . . . . . . . . . . . . . . . 53
Workshop . . . . . . . . . . . . . . . . . . . . . . 57
Bending moments and torsion . . . . . . . . 58
Second moment of area . . . . . . . . . . . . 60
Polar moment of inertia . . . . . . . . . . . . . 62
Centre of gravity . . . . . . . . . . . . . . . . . . 63
Instantaneous axis of rotation . . . . . . . . 64

Property of materials . . . . . . . . . . . . . . 65
   Elasticity . . . . . . . . . . . . . . . . . . . . . . . . 65
   Plasticity . . . . . . . . . . . . . . . . . . . . . . . . 65
   Viscoelasticity . . . . . . . . . . . . . . . . . . . . 65
   Creep . . . . . . . . . . . . . . . . . . . . . . . . . . 66
Stress and strain . . . . . . . . . . . . . . . . . 66
Moduli of elasticity . . . . . . . . . . . . . . . . 66
Learning outcomes . . . . . . . . . . . . . . . . 68
Check your existing knowledge:
answers . . . . . . . . . . . . . . . . . . . . . . . . 68
Workshop: answers . . . . . . . . . . . . . . . 68
Bibliography . . . . . . . . . . . . . . . . . . . . . 69

## CHECK YOUR EXISTING KNOWLEDGE

1 An object weighs 50 N. Using a lever, it can be moved using a force of 10 N
   a What is the mechanical advantage of the lever?
   b If you want to raise the object by 10 cm, how far will the other end of the lever have to move?
2 Identify the class of lever associated with the following systems
   a A wheelbarrow
   b The biceps muscle moving the elbow
   c A seesaw
3 A balanced seesaw has total length 4 m. A child weighing 150 N climbs on one end
   a What moment do they generate?
   b A second child climbs on the other end. How far from the pivot must they sit if they weigh 250 N and wish to balance the seesaw?
4 The forearm weighs 20 N and its centre of mass acts at 0.15 m from the elbow.
   a What moment does it generate if held horizontal?
   b What moment does it generate if held at 45°?
   c If the arm remains stationary, what moments are generated by the elbow flexors?
5 Construct diagrams to demonstrate:
   a A positive bending moment
   b Negative shear force

6  What is the relationship between shear force and bending moment?
7  What is the relationship between the intrinsic shear forces and:
  a  The beam's own weight
  b  The beam's length
8  What is the relationship between the intrinsic bending moment and:
  a  The beam's own weight
  b  The beam's length
9  Which is stronger, a steel I-beam or a solid steel beam with the same external dimensions.
  a  Why?
10 State:
  a  Hooke's law
  b  The class of material to which it applies

# Levers, beams and moments

The lever is perhaps the simplest of all machines; its existence pre-dates the wheel and is testified to by the existence of the Pyramids and Stonehenge. "Give me a fulcrum and a lever long enough and I will move the earth," boasted Archimedes in the 3rd century BCE. Stone Age technology was less prosaic, but – together with rollers and ramps – enabled the movement and erection of blocks of stone weighing over 10 tonnes at sites such as Stonehenge, Avebury and Carnac.

It is important for us to understand levers, and the mathematics associated with them: the biomechanics of the human body is fundamentally little more than a series of interconnected levers.

Three elements make up a lever system: the **load** (the thing that is being moved), the **fulcrum** (the point around which the lever turns) and the **effort** (the force used to move the lever).

Two factors define a lever. The first of these is the **mechanical advantage** (MA), also known as the **force ratio**. A lever is a magnifying force – the amount by which it magnifies the force is given by the MA:

$$MA = \frac{load}{effort}$$

For example, if an object weighs 30 N but the lever allows a person to move it using just 5 N (Fig. 3.1):

$$MA = \frac{30}{5} = 6$$

Note: the MA does not have any units; it is, in effect, a ratio. Of course, it is not possible to do this without a

trade-off, otherwise we would be getting energy for free and violating pretty much every law of physics. The payback comes with the fact that, although we don't have to push so hard, we do have to push further. The ratio of the distance moved by the effort ($S_E$) to the distance moved by the load ($S_L$) is called the **distance ratio** (DR), also known as the **velocity ratio**:

$$DR = \frac{S_E}{S_L}$$

If a system is 100% efficient, which, of course, is only ever hypothetically possible, then these two factors will balance each other out: moving the load using the lever in Figure 3.1 will require only $^1/_6$ of the effort but the load will only move $^1/_6$ of the distance compared with the effort.

---

**Fact File**

**EFFICIENCY OF A SYSTEM**

The fact that systems are never 100% efficient means that these two factors can be used to calculate the actual efficiency of a system ($\eta$):

$$\eta = {}^{MA}/_{DR}$$

This conversely means that, if we know the efficiency of a system, we can (if we know the weight of the object) calculate the force needed to move it given a set lever or the size of lever/fulcrum position needed to move it given a set force.

---

Levers come in three flavours, depending on the relative position of the elements that make up a lever system:

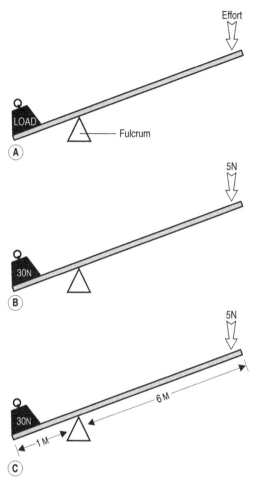

**Figure 3.1** • A lever system comprises the *lever* itself, which is raised on a *fulcrum* around which it turns so that a *force* (effort) can be used to move a *load* (A). If the distance from the fulcrum to the effort in one direction is greater than the distance from the fulcrum to the effort in the other, the effect of the effort is magnified. This effect, called the mechanical advantage, is calculated by dividing the load (30 N) by the effort (5 N). In this example (B), the mechanical advantage is 6; that is, the effort is being multiplied six-fold; however, although this enables us to lift a load six times as heavy, the ratio of the distances from the load to the fulcrum compared with the effort to the fulcrum will also be 1:6 (C). This, in turn, means that for every centimetre we want to raise the load, we must move the other end of the lever by 6 cm – this is the distance ratio.

## First order lever

These are the type of system that most people envisage when the word 'lever' is mentioned – a crowbar moving a heavy rock is an example of a first order lever whereby the fulcrum lies between the effort and the load (Fig. 3.2). Other examples

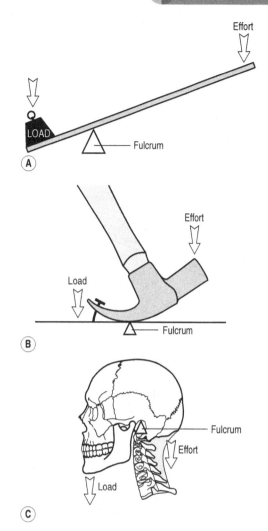

**Figure 3.2** • In a first order lever, the fulcrum lies between the effort and the load (A) as is the case with a claw hammer pulling out a nail (B). Examples of first order levers in the human body are rare, but the action of the anterior or posterior cervical muscle on the head, with the atlanto-occipital joint acting as the fulcrum, comprises such a system (C).

include a children's seesaw, pliers cutting a wire or a claw hammer pulling out a nail.

Although this form of lever is perhaps the most familiar, and is the most efficient for moving heavy loads, it is not, in general, a practical arrangement for the human body. However, the action of the intrinsic muscles of the upper cervical spine in moving the head either backwards or forwards (the atlanto-occipital joints acting as the pivot) does constitute a first order system.

## Second order lever

In this type of system, the load lies between the effort and the fulcrum (Fig. 3.3). The most obvious example of such an arrangement is the wheelbarrow: the pivot is the wheel axle; the load is in the barrow and the effort applied to the handles. Again, this is not usually a practical arrangement for the

musculoskeletal system; however, one example of a second order system is the action of the gastrocnemius and soleus muscles on the foot and ankle. When we stand on tiptoe, the load is transmitted via the ankle joint, the pivot is the metatarsophalangeal joints and the effort is applied via the tendinous insertion of the muscles into the calcaneus (the Achilles' tendon), which lies posterior to the ankle joint.

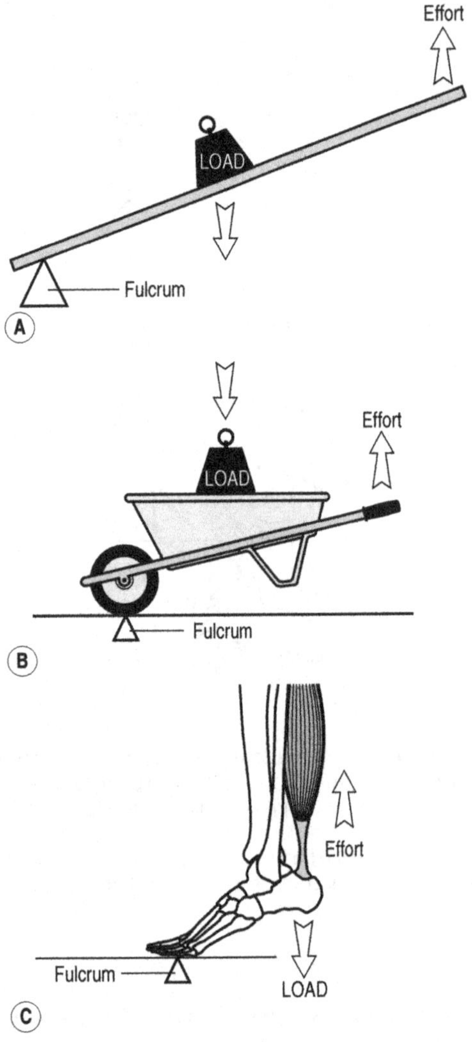

## Third order lever

In a third order lever, we have the one remaining permutation of load, fulcrum and effort: the effort lies between the fulcrum and the load. This is the system in which we are most interested as it used to move almost every joint in the body. If we flex our elbow to lift a pint of beer to our lips, the fulcrum is the elbow, the load is the beer and the effort is provided (primarily) by the insertion of the biceps muscle into the bicipital aperneurosis, approximately 4 cm distal to the elbow joint.

Another example of a third order lever is a pair of tweezers: the fulcrum is the meeting point of the two arms, the load is the object being gripped by the two ends and the effort is provided by your fingers squeezing together the two arms.

## Muscle action

Not all muscles act directly on the bones they move to articulate a given joint. Although most do – called **direct action** – there are muscles that precipitate movement indirectly, called **indirect action**. Examples of direct action are seen all over the body: think of the action of biceps brachialis (Fig. 3.4) as a classic example. Some muscles, however, do not insert directly in to the two bones that they articulate. Perhaps the best – and most easily understood – example of this is the action of the four quadriceps muscles, which, in this circumstance, can be considered as a functional whole.

The quadriceps (Fig. 3.5) arise from the femur and act to extend the knee. The muscle faces a problem, however: if the knee is flexed, it has to somehow 'get round the corner'. It achieves this by inserting into the superior pole of the patella, a large sesamoid bone that acts as a pulley, its reciprocally curved deep surface sliding between the two condyles of the femur. A tendon then runs from the inferior pole of the patella to the tibial tuberosity, so that contraction of the muscle will extend the knee: the quadriceps move the patella; the patella moves the tibia.

**Figure 3.3** • In a second order lever, the load lies between the effort and the fulcrum (A). Everyday examples of this include the classic wheelbarrow (B). Examples of second order levers in the human body are almost non-existent; however, the action of the gastrocnemius and soleus muscles of the calf (which insert into the calcaneus) in raising the foot on to 'tiptoe' (the metatarsophalangeal joints acting as the pivot) and the body's centre of gravity (which lies anterior to the line of action of the calf muscles) acting as the load can be said to comprise such a system (C).

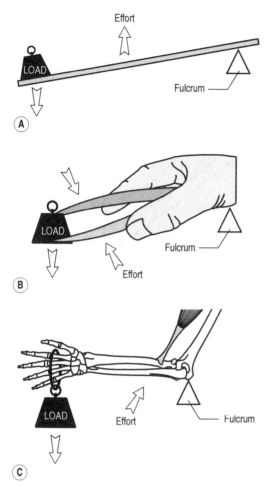

Figure 3.4 • A third order lever is one in which the effort lies between the load and the fulcrum (A). The fingers operating on a pair of tweezers to lift an object is a good example of an everyday third order system (B). Third order levers have the disadvantage of having a mechanical advantage of less than 1, although the distance ratio will correspondingly be greater than one. In the human body, this has the consequence that a small amount of muscle contraction will cause a larger amount of joint movement, albeit at the expense of strength. Third order systems are widely employed in the human body, a classic example being the action of the biceps brachialis muscle (C). The biceps exerts a direct action between the arm and the forearm.

## Moment of inertia

The direction of pull of a muscle – called its **line of action** – is an important consideration when considering the turning force created in a joint by a muscle. This turning effect is known as a **moment of inertia** (*moment* for short) and applied to any object that is able to rotate about an axis such as the forearm, which

rotates about the elbow or, in the first instance, a door, which rotates about its hinge (Fig. 3.6).

In Figure 3.6, we see four ways in which a force could be applied to the door and we know intuitively from our daily experience what will happen if we push the door in each of the instances A–D. Force A will not move the door as it is not generating a turning force, merely pushing the door into its hinges. Force C will move the door with all of the force directed in the right direction but we all know the door will move much more easily if we push further away from the hinge, exactly as is the case with a lever and its fulcrum, as is the instance with Forces B and D.

So, from this we can deduce that there are two factors that govern the size of the turning force or *moment*. The first is the distance from the pivot to the point where the force is being applied; the second is the direction in which the force is being applied, the *line of action*. The formula from which we can calculate a moment ($I$) is obtained by multiplying the force ($F$) by the perpendicular distance ($d$) from the line of action of the force to the axis:

$$I = Fd$$

NOTE: Remember, however, that force is a *vector* quantity and, therefore, only the component of force *perpendicular* to the door need be considered.

This is best understood by reconsidering the four examples on an individual basis. If we consider example C (Fig. 3.7) first, we do not need to resolve the vector of forces because all of the force is being directed at right angles to the door. The distance, $s$, from the line of action of the force ($F = 10$ N) is 20 cm; therefore, the moment is:

$$I = Fd = 10 \times 0.2 = 2 \text{ Nm [note the units]}$$

In example D (Fig. 3.8), the force is again acting perpendicularly to the door but this time the perpendicular distance from the line of action of the force to the axis of rotation is 80 cm.

$$I = Fd = 10 \times 0.8 = 8 \text{ Nm}$$

When we consider example C (Fig. 3.9), we have a more complex situation as the calculation of the perpendicular distance from the line of action of the force to the pivot now requires some consideration and a little bit of trigonometry. If we look at the situation in (A), we can see the distance that we need to calculate, $d$. In order to do this, we need to construct a short series of right-angled triangles

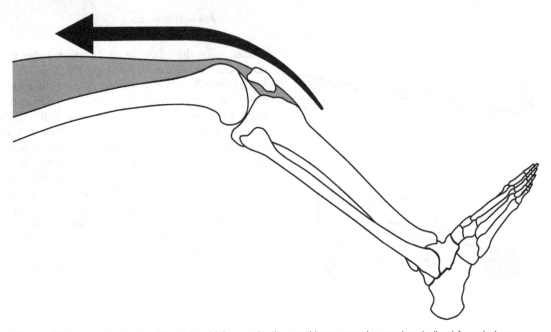

**Figure 3.5** • In contrast to the biceps brachialis muscle, the quadriceps muscles exert an indirect force between the thigh and the shin with the patella acting as an intermediary, enabling the muscle tendon to cope with the biomechanical problems created by operating with the knee in flexion.

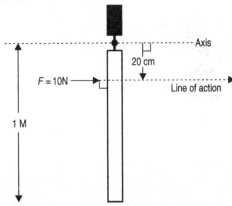

**Figure 3.7** • A force of 10 N being applied at right angles to a 1 m door at a distance of 20 cm from the axis (hinge).

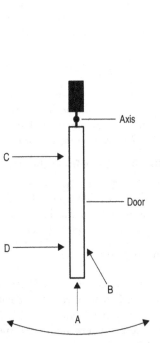

**Figure 3.6** • Four different forces being applied to a door. Each creates a turning force known as a moment, which can be calculated as the product of the applied force and the perpendicular distance from the line of action of the force to the pivot.

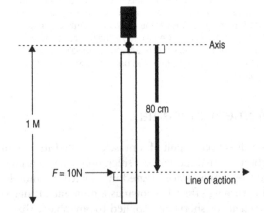

**Figure 3.8** • A force of 10 N being applied at right angles to a 1 m door at a distance of 80 cm from the axis (hinge).

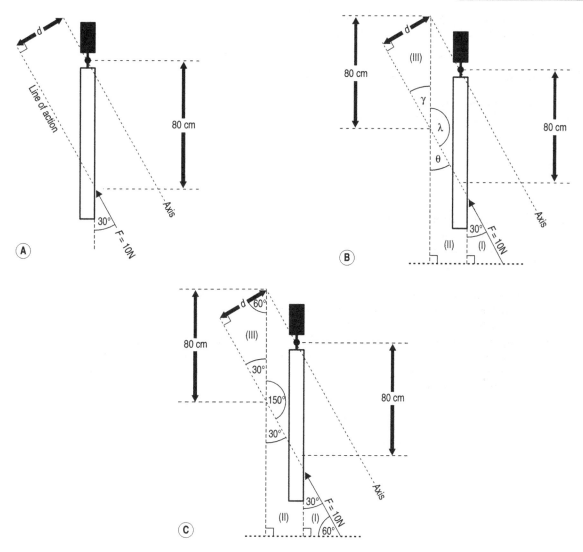

**Figure 3.9** • A force of 10 N being applied at 30° to a 1 m door at a distance of 80 cm from the axis (hinge) **(A)**. In order to calculate the moment of inertia, it is necessary to calculate the perpendicular distance from the line of action of the force to the axis, *d*. To do this, we draw a vertical line from the extension of the axis of rotation and construct a second line perpendicular to it to create three triangles I, II and III **(B)**. As I and II are exactly the same shape, we know that θ = 30° **(C)**. This means that λ = 180° − 30°= 150° and that, likewise, in III γ is also 30° (those of you familiar with all the rules of triangles will have spotted this at once). Therefore *d* = 80 × sin 30° = 40 cm. *I* = *Fd* = 10 × 0.4 = 4 Nm.

so that we can use basic trigonometry to calculate the angles and lengths required.

If we draw a vertical line from the intersection of *d* and the extension of the axis and a perpendicular to this, which intersects *F*, there are now three right-angled triangles, I, II and III.

As triangles I and II are exactly the same shape, their internal angles must be the same and so θ must be 30°. As there are 180° on a straight line, this means λ must be 180°− 30° = 150°. The same principle

shows that γ = 180° − 150° = 30°. This means that we now have the ability to calculate all the dimensions of triangle III: we know it is a right-angled triangle with hypotenuse of 80 cm and internal angles 90°, 30° (and, by rule of internal angles, 60°). Therefore:

**d = sin 30 × 80 cm = 0.5 × 80 cm = 40 cm**

Therefore the moment:

**I = 0.4 × 10 = 4 Nm**

In the final example, A (Fig. 3.6), the line of action *is* perpendicular to the axis; therefore, the distance is zero:

$$l = Fd = 0 \text{ Nm}$$

From the standpoint of the manual physician, doors have only a limited interest: they can be closed to allow privacy and opened to admit a patient. Let us therefore take an example that instead relates to the human body.

## Example 1

In Figure 3.10, the biceps brachialis muscle is holding the arm stationary against two forces, a 20 N weight held in the hand and the weight of the forearm itself, which is regarded as operating through its **centre of gravity**. We wish to know what force the muscle needs to generate in order to maintain this posture.

All the moments acting on a body are summative (that is, they can be added and subtracted); however, it is necessary to realize that those acting in a clockwise direction (in this case the action of the muscle) will counter those acting in an anticlockwise direction. It is convenient to regard those moments acting in a clockwise direction as being positive and those acting in an anticlockwise direction as negative. This is by no means essential, so long as you make one direction positive and the other negative, the maths will come out right. Because this is a purely voluntary notion, it is always a good idea to state your convention at the outset, so, in this case: *clockwise* = +*ve*.

If the arm is stationary, then the sum of the positive moments must be equal to the sum of the negative moments:

$$l_{weight} + l_{forearm} + l_{biceps} = 0$$

which can be written as:

$$\Sigma l = 0 \text{ Nm}$$

Calculating the moments created by the mass and the forearm weight is quite straightforward as the perpendicular distance from the lines of actions of the forces to the axis is simply the distance from the elbow at which the forces act. In the case of the forearm's centre of gravity, this is 12 cm; in the case of the weight held in the hand, 20 cm (remember that these quantities will need to be converted into metres). As the weight is given in newtons rather than kilogrammes, it will not need to be converted; therefore:

$$l_{weight} = F_{weight} \times d_{weight} = -20 \times 0.2 = -4 \text{ Nm}$$
$$l_{forearm} = F_{forearm} \times d_{forearm} = -10 \times 0.12 = -1.2 \text{ Nm}$$

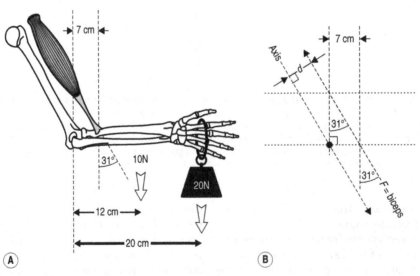

**Figure 3.10** • Example 1: the biceps brachialis muscle is countering a negative (anticlockwise) moment produced by the combined forces of the weight of the forearm – acting through its centre of gravity – and a weight being held in the hand (A). What force is generated by the muscle (B)?

So:

$$\Sigma I_{anticlockwise} = (-6 + 1.2) \, \text{Nm.} = -5.2 \, \text{Nm.}$$

So, the anticlockwise (−ve) moment being generated by the action of the biceps brachialis muscle is −5.2 Nm (assuming, of course, for the sake of simplicity, that this is the only muscle involved in flexion of the elbow). We can construct a second diagram (B) showing the dimensions pertinent to the biceps brachialis muscle. We know that:

$$I_{biceps} = F_{biceps} \times d_{biceps}$$

As it is the force that we are trying to calculate, we can rearrange this as:

$$F_{biceps} = I_{biceps} \div d_{biceps}$$

$$= -5.2 \div (\cos 31° \times 0.07)$$

$$= -5.2 \div 0.06 = -86.7 \, \text{N}$$

## Workshop

If your mind is reeling slightly after that or, indeed if it is not but you didn't actually work the example through, it would be as well to use the following example to test your skills. The answers can be found at the end of the chapter.

Consider the following scenario:

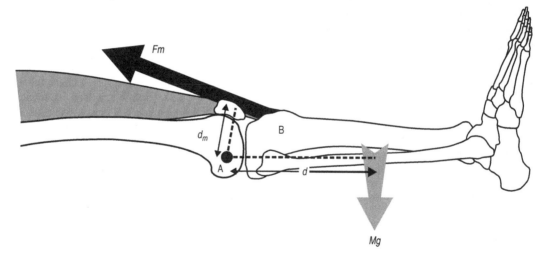

- The centre of rotation is in the femoral condyles (A)
- The weight of the leg (= $Mg$) is 80 N
- The distance, $d$, is 300 mm
- The leg is held horizontal and stationary
- The quadriceps muscles insert 60 mm from the centre of rotation (A) to the tibial tuberosity (B) at an angle ($d_m$A$d$) of 25°
- The line of action of the muscle is 75° anticlockwise from the vertical.

**Question 1:** Determine the moment due to the weight of the leg.

**Question 2:** If the person was wearing a shoe weighing 3 N and the length of the leg (distance from A to the centre of mass of the boot) was 40 cm, what force is required by the quadriceps muscles to resist this new moment of inertia?

Manipulation creates moments of inertia and the size of the moment is not just dependent upon the force of the thrust but also on the position of the hands, the *contact point*. The greater the distance from the axis of rotation, the greater the moment of inertia. This means that manipulative adjustments are not so much dependent on the strength of the physician but rather on their skill.

For the clinically experienced manipulator, the adjustment itself becomes largely intuitive – the hand position; the direction and degree of force; the decision to use assisted or resisted techniques; the employment of gentle, long lever releases or more specific short lever adjustments are all arrived at by experience, the individual patient and personal preference.

However, for the student intern, this lack of past practice on which to draw needs to be compensated for by a thorough grounding in the anatomy and biomechanics of all of the body's articulations and complete understanding of the relationship between applied force and its rotational and translational consequences.

It has been estimated that the average manipulative physician – whether chiropractor, manipulative physiotherapist or osteopath – causes one iatrogenic fracture during their career, usually without significant complications. However, no reliable epidemiological data exist, and estimates of frequency vary between 1:85 000 and 1:400 000 manipulations. Like many uncommon events, they are hard to research and often remain undiagnosed – the patient will merely report feeling 'sore' for several weeks after an adjustment.

The most commonly affected bones are the ribs, where fractures can remain radiologically occult, and for which there is no remedial treatment. These are usually due to undiagnosed bone pathology, affecting the integrity of the underlying bone (most commonly osteoporosis but there have also been cases involving osteomalacia, Paget's disease, tumours and infection).

# Bending moments and torsion

A **beam** – in engineering terms – is a long, slender structural element that can support both transverse and axial loads. For physical therapists, we may admire the beams in a half-timbered mediaeval house but it is bones – the beams that support the

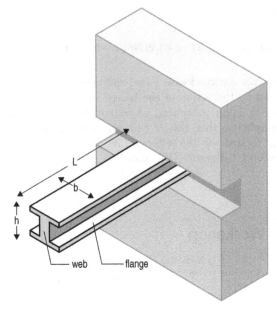

**Figure 3.11** • The standard nomenclature of a cantilevered I-beam.

body – in which we are interested. However, the mechanics of hollow tubes are a lot more complicated than those of the solid rectangular beams used by the architects of yore, so let us begin there.

Beams have a fairly standard nomenclature (Fig. 3.11), although you will occasionally see height, $h$ referred to as depth, $d$. In this example, the beam is **cantilevered**, that is fixed at one end. The force, $F$, generates a turning force in the beam but, as the beam is fixed, it cannot turn; instead, the beam can bend, giving rise to a **bending moment**. A **shearing force** is also generated within the beam. As with moments of inertia, these have conventions as to which direction is positive and which is negative (Fig. 3.12).

Returning to our example, it is possible to generate simple diagrams that show the shear force and bending moment at any point along the length of the beam (Fig. 3.13). As with moments of inertia, multiple forces are summative.

A *shear force diagram* is constructed by moving along the beam from its origin and summing the forces distal to any given position. A bending moment diagram is obtained in much the same way, except that the moment is, as we would expect from our previous experience with moments of inertia, the sum of the product of each force ($F$) and its distance ($x$) from the origin.

We can also consider a non-cantilevered beam (Fig. 3.14). Exactly the same process is employed to

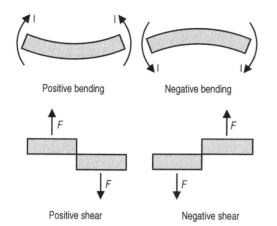

**Figure 3.12** • Sign conventions for bending moments and shear forces in beams.

generate the diagrams, though the sign convention will, of course, be different. In both cases, the shear force or bending moment is calculated by determining the area of the graph at the appropriate point.

There is, however, a problem with these beams: we have assumed that the beams themselves are weightless. Anyone who has tried to lift a solid oak beam of the type we are considering will know that this is far from being the case. We can construct diagrams that show the shearing force (S) and bending moment (M) generated by the weight of the beam itself, both for cantilevered and simply supported beams, by considering the beams as still being weightless, but now with weights at regular intervals all along them (Fig. 3.15).

The mathematical laws by which we can calculate and relate these two quantities are, unsurprisingly, given that they relate to the area enclosed by a line on a graph, governed by calculus.

$$\frac{dM}{dx} = S$$

Therefore:

$$-\int F.dx = \int dS = S \text{ and } \int S.dx = \int dM = M$$

To put this into English (and don't worry, you're not going to be asked to start calculating actual forces, it's the concept that you need to grasp):

• The shear force is equivalent to the rate of change in the bending moment as you move along the beam

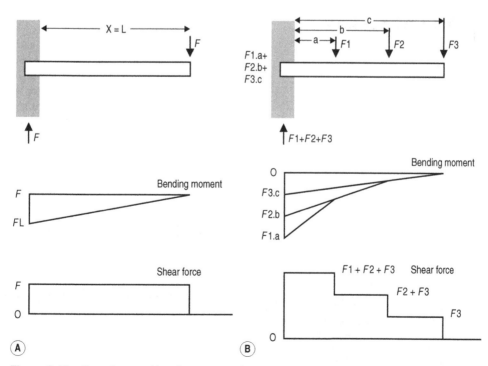

**Figure 3.13** • Shear force and bending moment diagrams for cantilevered beams with simple (A) and complex (B) load combinations.

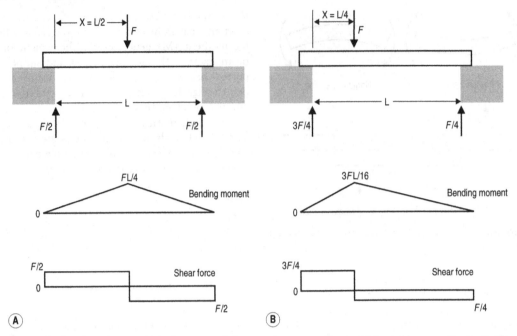

**Figure 3.14** • Shear force and bending moment diagrams for non-cantilevered ('simple') beams with simple **(A)** and complex **(B)** load combinations.

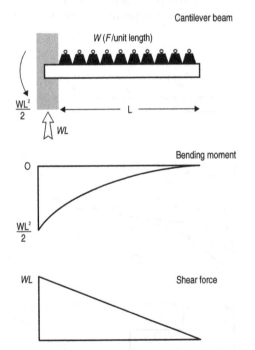

**Figure 3.15** • The self-loading characteristics of a beam can best be understood by considering a 'weightless' beam with succession of closely packed small loads. This means we can use calculus to determine the bending moment and shear force at any point.

• The areas contained in the diagrams of shear force and bending moment are equal and opposite
• In addition to external forces, the intrinsic weight of the beam also generates shear forces and bending moments. In the case of the former, these are directly proportional to the weight and to length of the beam; however, the bending moment is proportional to the *squares* of the weight and length.

This means that, if you double the length of, say, a 15th century, well-seasoned oak beam, you will also double its weight; therefore, the shearing force will increase four-fold. However, the bending moment will increase *sixteen-fold*.

## Second moment of area

This brings us to the next physical property that we need to consider. The second moment of area, $I_x$, is a measure of how well the geometry of a beam resists bending. It is defined as:

$$I_x = \int y^2 dA$$

and has units $m^4$

As before, our understanding of this needs to be intuitive rather than mathematical, the implications of this formula are that the contribution to the rigidity of a structure by any part of it is proportional to the *integral of the square* of the area's distance from the neutral axis (Fig. 3.16).

This leads to a very interesting phenomenon. For those of you who thought that engineers used I-beams (Fig. 3.17) in order to save money by reducing the amount of steel employed in their girders and lintels, think again – an I-beam is actually *stronger* than an equivalent piece of solid steel. This

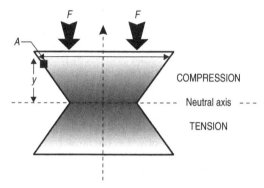

**Figure 3.16** • The second moment of area of a beam is much more dependent of the material furthest from the neutral axis. I = ∫y² dA

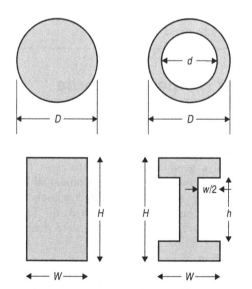

**Figure 3.17** • Solid beams can actually be less rigid than their hollow, lighter, engineered counterparts.

seems such a counterintuitive concept that it is worth investigating a little further. The formula for the moment of area for a solid rectangular cross-section is given by:

$$I_x = WH^3/12$$

If we put in some typical figures for a girder of, say, height 0.4 m and width 0.3 m this gives a value for $I_x$ of 0.0016 m⁴.

Now let us consider the I-beam. Here, we can take away the contribution to the second moment of area given by the 'cut out' sections. We should remember though that these don't contribute much to the rigidity as they are close to the neutral axis of the beam. The two crosspieces of the 'I' by contrast contribute much more significantly. The formula for an I-beam is given by:

$$I_x = (WH^3 - wh^3)/12$$

Again, using typical values for $w$ and $h$ of 0.2 m and 0.35 m respectively, $I_x = 0.00088$ m⁴. So the second moment of area is only 55% *but* if we consider what has happened to the weight of the beam, it has decreased by a factor of 2.4. This significantly diminishes the self-loading from the beam's own weight; therefore, for a beam of fixed length in the case we have just considered, the resistance to shearing increases by 32% and the bending moment decreases by 74%.

The same argument can be used to calculate the second moment of area for a hollow rectangular beam and, most importantly for us in our consideration of bones, of the relative rigidities of a circular cross-section of a solid and a hollow tube. If we put in figures typical of, say, a human femur whereby $D = 0.05$ m and $d = 0.015$ m, then the second moment of area for the solid shaft is:

$$I_x = \pi D^4/64 = 3.1 \times 10^{-7} m^4$$

Whereas for the hollow bone:

$$I_x = \pi (D^4 - d^4)/64 = 3.0 \times 10^{-7} m^4$$

You can see that, in the case of the tube, there is almost no difference between the values of a solid cylinder and its hollow equivalent yet, in the example above, the cylinder has only half the weight.

Of course, human bones are not actually hollow. The outer layer of cortical bone, composed mainly of calcium hydroxyapatite, its surface corrugated by reactions to stress patterns (trabercular lines) and ridged by the pull of the Sharpey fibres that anchor tendons and ligaments, does contain a hollow tube; however, this tube is packed with a lightweight lattice of cancellous bone (Fig. 3.18).

These needle-like spicules, oriented along lines of stress, honeycomb the internal area of bone and support the marrow. They add to the overall strength of the bone but, more importantly, give the brittle cortical bone the flexibility it needs to resist loading and shearing forces without shattering.

As ever, shape specifies function and there are five main types of bone within the body:

**Long bones** are distinguished by the presence of a longitudinal axis (diaphysis), flared ends (metaphysis) and specifically adapted articular ending (epiphysis). It is this shape that defines long bones rather than their actual size – although the longest bones in the body (the femur, tibia, fibula, humerus, ulna and radius) are long bones, so are some of the shortest, the phalanges that form the fingers and toes.

**Short bones** lack this traditional appearance and often have no obvious longitudinal axis, instead possessing a cuboid appearance – indeed, one short bone is actually called the cuboid (the most lateral tarsal bone). Most short bones are found in the tarsi of the feet and carpi of the wrist and are often named for their distinctive shapes – the *navicular* (from the Latin meaning 'little ship', the same root from which we get *navy*) has the shape of a boat hull; the lunate looks like the crescent moon, from which it gets its Latin name (still recalled in the adjectival form, *lunar*); the cuneiforms are wedge-shaped (from the Latin *cuneus*).

**Flat bones** are usually broad and thin and often have a protective rather than a load-bearing function. Many skull bones (particularly those of the calvarium), the scapulae (shoulder blades), sternum (breast bone) and ribs are all examples of flat bones.

**Irregular bones** are often clustered together in groups and, as the name suggests, have unusual shapes and a variety of sizes. The facial bones and the vertebrae that form the spine (Fig. 4.6) are good examples of irregular bones.

**Sesamoid bones** often form spontaneously, embedded in the tendons of muscles that are being subjected to articular stresses or friction. The patella (kneecap) is the largest of these bones – and the only one that is universally present, although they are common in the hallux (big toe) and occasionally found in the thumb or fingers.

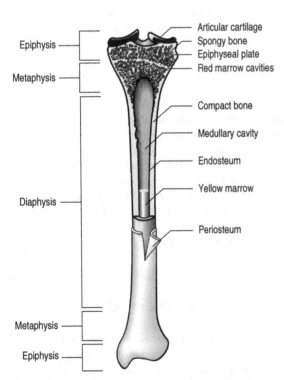

Figure 3.18 • A longitudinal section of the right tibia showing the relationship between compact and cancellous bone.

Epiphysis
Metaphysis
Diaphysis
Metaphysis
Epiphysis

Articular cartilage
Spongy bone
Epiphyseal plate
Red marrow cavities
Compact bone
Medullary cavity
Endosteum
Yellow marrow
Periosteum

# Polar moment of inertia

Having established the rules for the behaviour of structures in bending and shearing, there is one final stressor that we need to consider – torsion. The ability of a geometric structure to resist twisting forces is measure by its **polar moment of inertia**, J, a property, as you might expect, closely related to second moment of area. Indeed, the formulae for the two are very similar; for a solid shaft:

$$J = \pi D^4/32$$

and for a hollow one:

$$J = \pi(D^4 - d^4)/32$$

Therefore exactly the same arguments apply to the increasing importance to the torsional rigidity provided as one moves away from the axis of rotation. As with second moment of area for a cylinder, this increased with the *fourth* power of the distance; therefore a hollow shaft will have almost the same polar moment of inertia as a solid one, but with a fraction of the weight.

## CLINICAL FOCUS

A little bit of mathematics quickly demonstrates exactly why bones are hollow. Let us consider two shafts with the same cross-sectional area, one solid, the other hollow, in this case the femur from the previous example whereby $D_h = 0.05$ m and $d = 0.015$ m. This has the same cross-sectional area as a solid shaft of bone with $D_s = 0.017$ m. The torsional angle, $\theta$, is given by the formula:

$$\theta = TL/JG$$

We have already defined $J$ as the polar moment of inertia; $T$ is the **torque**, the turning force; $L$ is the length (for a femur we shall take this as 0.4 m); and $G$ is the **shear modulus**, a concept we shall be exploring in more detail later in the chapter but which for the moment can be regarded as a measure of a given material to shear strain. For bone, the figure is typically around 5 GPa. If we assume the femur is subjected to a torquing force of 10 Nm:

For the solid shaft:

$$J_s = \pi D_s^4/32 = 8.2 \times 10^{-9} m^4$$
$$\theta_s = TL/J_sG = (10 \times 0.4)/(8.2 \times 10^{-9} \times 5 \times 10^9)$$
$$= 0.00975\,rad = 3.5°$$

For the hollow shaft:

$$J_h = \pi(D_h^4 - d^4)/32 = 6.1 \times 10^{-7} m^4$$
$$\theta_h = TL/J_hG = (10 \times 0.4)/(6.1 \times 10^{-7} \times 5 \times 10^9)$$
$$= 0.00026\,rad = 0.9°$$

For the same weight and expenditure of material, the difference is that between a crippling spiral fracture and normal function – something worth remembering the next time you pivot on your foot to kick a football!

## DICTIONARY DEFINITION

**TORQUE**
Torque is a twisting force, also called the *moment of force* as it produces a moment of inertia. If the body to which it is applied is fixed, it will twist rather than turn the body.

# Centre of gravity

In our previous example of a moment of inertia acting on a limb, we considered the whole mass of the extremity to be acting through a single point – from a mathematical standpoint, this concentration of mass makes calculations far simpler. This imaginary point is known as the **centre of gravity**, although physicists generally refer to it as **centre of mass** as they also wish to consider bodies acting outside gravitational fields or large cosmic bodies that exert gravitational forces upon each other. When it comes to patients, the terms are interchangeable.

In simple, homogeneous, symmetrical structures, the location of an object's centre of gravity may coincide with the geometrical centre of the body. An asymmetrical object composed of a variety of materials with different densities, such as a human being, may well have a centre of gravity located at some distance from its geometrical centre. In some extreme cases, such as irregularly shaped objects or hollow bodies, the centre of gravity may occur at a point that is actually external to the physical material, for example between the legs of a chair or in the hollow centre of a football.

Although calculating an object's centre of gravity involves summation of the moments acting on the body using integral calculus, there is (fortunately) an easier, practical method. When an object is suspended from a single point, its centre of gravity lies directly beneath that point. Therefore, by suspending the object from three separate points and marking the vertical from those points using a plumb line, cross-triangulation will give us the centre of gravity (Fig. 3.19).

As this procedure can involve ethical difficulties with humans, it is useful to note at this point that, in the average person, the centre of gravity lies approximately 4–5 cm anterior to the second sacral tubercle.

Published tables and handbooks list the centres of gravity for most common geometrical shapes. For a triangular metal plate such as that depicted in

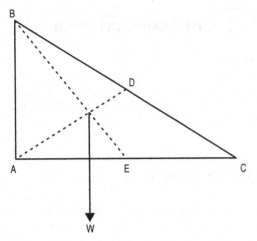

**Figure 3.19** • Whenever an object is suspended from a single point, its centre of gravity lies directly beneath that point. Therefore, the centre of gravity, G, of an object such as a triangle can be located by suspending the plate by a cord attached at point A, and then by a cord attached at point B. When suspended from A, the line AD is vertical; when suspended from B, the line BE is vertical. The centre of gravity is at the intersection of AD and BE. Although G can also be calculated mathematically, for complex, irregular objects, the suspension method is frequently more practical.

Figure 3.19, the calculation would involve a summation of the moments of the weights of all the particles that make up the metal plate about point A. By equating this sum to the plate's weight W, multiplied by the unknown distance from the centre of gravity G to AC, the position of G relative to AC can be determined. The summation of the moments can be obtained easily and precisely by integral calculus.

The point G can be located by suspending the plate by a cord attached at point A, and then by a cord attached at point C. When suspended from A, the line AD is vertical; when suspended from C, the line CE is vertical. The centre of gravity is at the intersection of AD and CE. When an object is suspended from a single point, its centre of gravity lies directly beneath that point.

## Instantaneous axis of rotation

When a rigid object rotates in a plane, at every instant of time there is a point, either within that body or at a distance from it, which does not move. An axis perpendicular to the plane through this point is called the **instantaneous axis of rotation (IAR)**. It is a concept that is more easily understood visually than descriptively (Fig. 3.20A).

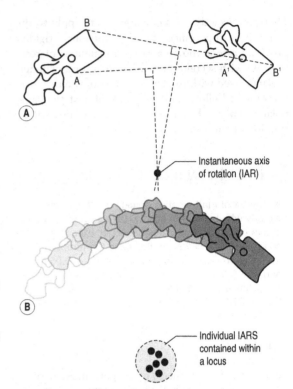

**Figure 3.20** • When an object such as a human vertebra moves between two points, it rotates about an instantaneous axis of rotation (IAR) **(A)**. In reality, this movement comprises an infinite number of smaller movements, each with their own IAR **(B)**. If enough of these are plotted, it is possible to establish a locus that contains all of the IARs for each possible movement in that plane.

The reason that it is termed *instantaneous* axis of rotation is that, at every instant, the axis of rotation can be different. If Figure 3.20A represents the end points of a vertebra's range of motion in flexion and extension, then there exists an infinite number of points representing every possible rotation therein. If sufficient of these points are mapped, which can be done using a technique known as videofluoroscopy, a locus of points can be formed (Fig. 3.20B) and these represent the IARs of normal ranges of motion. These loci alter with degenerative changes and other pathology and are useful in understanding both normal and abnormal motion, particularly in the spine where the three-joint complex between each functional spinal unit creates motion much more complex than in single articulation – a concept that is explored in more detail in the following chapters.

# Property of materials

There are four properties of materials in which we are interested, demonstrated in varying degrees by different types of material found within the human body.

## Elasticity

**Elasticity** is the tendency of a material to return to its original shape once a deforming stress has been removed. Crystalline structures, such as the calcium hydroxyapatite from which cortical bone is made, have only a small degree of elasticity from **slip planes**, areas where atoms can slip over each other and from **edge dislocations**, natural faults within the crystal structure that can 'give' when stretched, sheared or compressed. By contrast, polymeric structures, such as the collagen from which our soft tissues (skin, tendon, cartilage, muscle, blood vessels, fascia etc.) are formed consist of long-chain molecules. These molecules often have a degree of curl or bend to them; application of stress will straighten out the molecules causing them to lengthen – in the case of elastic by up to thirteen times its original length. When the stress is removed, the molecule will return to its 'natural' shape ... and, therefore, its original length.

Truly elastic materials obey **Hooke's law**, named after the inaugural member of the Royal Society whom we encountered in Chapter 2. This states that, for an elastic material, the extension, $x$, is proportional to the force applied, $F$:

$$F \alpha x$$
$$\therefore \quad F = kx$$

where k, the constant of proportionality is called the **spring** or **force constant**.

So, for an elastic material, if we plot force against extension, we will get a straight line whose gradient is k. In reality, most materials only exhibit this idealised behaviour during the first stages of elastic deformation (Fig. 3.21). The point at which this occurs is called the **limit of proportionality** (because, beyond it, extension is no longer proportional to the force applied); however, the material still demonstrates elastic behaviour in that it will return to its original length when the force is removed.

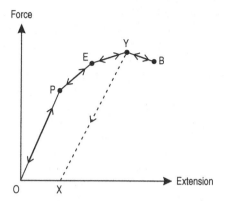

**Figure 3.21** ● Graph of force against extension. During the ideal elastic phase, the extension is proportional to the force applied. When the limit of proportionality (P) is reached, this ideal behaviour is no longer demonstrated although the material's deformation remains reversible up to the elastic limit (E). After this, the material becomes plastic; further deformation has a degree of irreversibility about it such that, when the force is removed, there has been a degree of permanent deformation of length OX. When the yield point (Y) is reached, the material will continue to extend without the application of additional force until it fails at its breaking point (B).

## Plasticity

**Plasticity** is the tendency for a material to suffer permanent deformation – that is, *not* to return to its original dimensions once a deforming stress has been removed. Plastic behaviour begins once a material has reached its **elastic limit**. In an ideal plastic material, the additional deformation is *all* permanent; however, few materials are ideal and there will often be some degree of return until the material reaches its **yield point**. After this, it will continue to lengthen spontaneously until it fails at its **breaking point**. You will most likely have seen this behaviour in bubble gum, where a big blob at the end of a thin strand will stretch away under its own weight causing an increasingly thin connecting strand that will eventually snap, frequently causing the gum to land on an unsavoury surface that renders it subsequently unchewable.

## Viscoelasticity

Another property that we need to consider, which is particularly prevalent in living, organic materials, is the tendency of constantly loaded materials to deform elastically over time. This is known as viscoelasticity. With the development of modern materials, we are all much more familiar with such substances, which are now commonly used in orthopaedic mattresses and pillows. It you have ever lain on such a mattress, you will know that it gives a rather odd sensation: at first, the mattress seems rather uncomfortably hard but, after a few seconds, you feel yourself sinking into it as it deforms to your body's shape ... that is, the heavier you are, the greater the deformation. When you get up, it takes a while for the dent left by your body to vanish but again, after a few seconds, it does until the mattress is again a smooth surface. This property is demonstrated by many of the body's soft tissues.

## Creep

The final property in which we are interested is also time-dependent, though this time is over hours, days or years rather than seconds and minutes. **Creep** is the slow deformation of a solid over a period of time as the result of a continuous applied stress.

# Stress and strain

So far in this section, we have been using the terms 'force' and 'stress' as apparent synonyms; however, they are only equivalents in certain circumstances. Stress – another one of those words that have a very specific meaning to physicists, different to its lay meaning – is actually defined as the force per unit area applied to a body. As such, its units are newtons per metre squared, which, as you may recall from Chapter 1, is the definition of a Pascal (Pa). So, in fact, the terms 'force' and 'stress' are only synonyms when applied to either the same body or a body with identical dimensions.

Stress may be described in a number of different ways. **Tensile stress** is a deforming stress that tends to stretch an object; **compressive stress**, that which tends to shorten it. **Bulk stress** refers to overall force per unit area (pressure) from the environment surrounding an object and **shear stress** is that which produces an angular deformation, the tangential force per unit area.

In addition to the stress applied to an object, we also need to know the amount of deformation that has occurred. This is known as the **strain** and is the fractional change in dimension produced by a stress. In the simplest case, where the stress is uni-dimensional (as is the case in both **tensile strain**

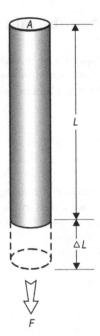

**Figure 3.22** ● The effects of tensile stress. A force, $F$, per unit area, $A$, has produced a deformation causing a change in length, $L$, by $\Delta L$ (i.e., to a new length of $L + \Delta L$).

and **compressive strain**) this is the simple ratio of the change in length divided by the original length (Fig. 3.22). There are equivalent ratios for **bulk strain** (change in volume/original volume) and **shear strain** (the angular displacement produced).

# Moduli of elasticity

The spring constant of Hooke's Law is of limited value as it is unique for any given specimen and is dependent on the dimensions of the object as well at the material from which it is made. Of more use is a standardized measure of the 'stiffness' of a material and such a measure was defined by Thomas Young in the early 19th century. It is after him that the best know and most commonly used modulus of elasticity, **Young's modulus**, is named.

Young's modulus ($E$) is defined as:

$$E = \frac{\text{tensile stress}}{\text{tensile strain}}$$

or

$$E = (^F/_A)/(^{\Delta L}/_L)$$

Because strain is a ratio and, as such, is dimensionless, the units of Young's modulus are the same as for those

**Table 3.1** Values of Young's modulus for a variety of materials

The values are approximate as this value can vary considerably depending on the purity and quality of the material. In the case of human materials, there are other factors to consider: $E_{collagen}$ will decrease by 10% with age; osteoporotic bone can decrease to the point where it can no longer withstand the stress of the body's weight; pH has an effect as does load duration – bone and collagen are both viscoelastic materials

| Material | Young's modulus (GPa) |
| --- | --- |
| Steel | 200 |
| Brass | 100 |
| Aluminium | 70 |
| Glass | 65 |
| Concrete | 30 |
| Cast Iron | 27 |
| Bone | 25 |
| Nylon | 20 |
| Wood (oak)* | 12 |
| Spider silk | 11 |
| Wood (cedar)* | 6 |
| Collagen | 4 |
| Polystyrene | 3 |
| Rubber | 0.001 |

*along the direction of the grain

of stress, pascals. Typical values for Young's modulus for a range of materials are given in Table 3.1.

As with stress and strain, there are other moduli of elasticity. Compression is treated in the same way as tension – the **bulk modulus** is calculated by dividing bulk stress by bulk strain (fractional change in volume).

The ability of a material to resist a turning force is given by the **shear modulus**, $G$ or $\mu$, (also known as the modulus of rigidity). This is defined in terms of the amount of rotation produced by a given stress:

$$G = (F/A)/\tan \theta$$

There is one further feature of which you need to be aware. When most substances elongate, they also become thinner (similarly, when they compress, they become thicker). The degree to which this happens is called **Poisson's ratio.** As a ratio, the quantity has no units and is quantified as the ratio of the transverse strain to the longitudinal strain – the proportional change in width ($w$) divided by the proportional change in length ($l$):

$$\sigma_p = (\Delta w/w)/(\Delta l/l).$$

 CLINICAL FOCUS

As the tendons of fusiform muscles will visibly decrease in diameter as the force of the muscular contraction increases, this means that we not only have to consider the strength of the muscular contraction but the reduction in Young's modulus as the force of the contraction increases and the tendinous diameter decreases.

We must also consider that tendons and cartilage are viscoelastic materials and, as such, respond variably over time; therefore, their response to loading and unloading and repetitive loading is non-linear. For example if we consider tension of the articular cartilage of the knee, we find that rapid, body-weight tension increases its effective Poisson's ration (EPR) from typical values of 0.16 to 0.5. By comparison, typical values for steel are 0.28 and the average for aluminium compounds is 0.33.

However, this figure continues to increase after the loading has been removed, reaching 0.7 some 20 seconds later. It then decreases relatively slowly; after ten minutes, the value is still 0.3 and it does not approach its starting value again for almost half an hour (under compression this return is achieved in 8–10 minutes).

This means that, with repetitive loading and/or tension, the starting EPR will be higher each time and, consequently, the effective strain will also be greater and the effective Young's modulus less.

The combination of these factors explains why tendinous and cartilaginous injuries are most common at the start of exercise and when the musculoskeletal structures are fatigued and emphasizes the importance of warm-up and warm-down regimes in athletic training.

## Learning Outcomes

- Introduce the concepts of levers, beams and moments and their application to the human body
- Outline the part that bending moments, torsion and shear have to play in musculoskeletal biomechanics
- Ensure that the student has an adequate knowledge of second and polar moments of area as they apply to skeletal architecture
- Differentiate between various properties of materials and synthesize these with anatomical structures within the body
- Develop the concepts of centre of gravity and instantaneous axis of rotation.

## CHECK YOUR EXISTING KNOWLEDGE: ANSWERS

1  a   5 [2]           b   50 cm [2]
2  a   2nd class [3]   b   3rd class [3]   c   1$^{st}$ class [3]
3  a   600 Nm [5]      b   2.4 m [5]
4  a   3 Nm [5]        b   2.12 Nm [5]   c   equal and opposite to b [2]
5  See Figure 3.13 [5 each]
6  The shear force is equivalent to the rate of change of the bending moment (or you have expressed this mathematically): $\int F.dx = \int dS = S$ and $\int S.dx = \int dM = M$ [5]
7  a   Directly proportional [2]   b   Directly proportional [2]
8  a   Moment proportional to square of weight [2]
   b   Moment proportional to square of length [2]
9  a   The I-beam [1] b It has less preloading and only a slightly smaller moment of area [5]
10  a   Force and extension are proportional [2]
    b   Elastic materials [2]

### How to interpret the results:

60–65:  You have a firm grasp of the basic tools that you need to understand the language in this book. As long as you understand any mistakes you may have made, you can move on to the next chapter

40–60:  Although you have some understanding of the basics, you should revise the areas in which you scored poorly before moving on

0–40:   You will need to study this chapter in some detail in order to acquire the grounding needed for future chapters

## Workshop: Answers

Rather that simply state the answers, it might be helpful to indicate how they were obtained, just in case you didn't get them right . . . or were uncertain how to get them at all.

- The first thing that we are required to do is to state our sign convention: clockwise = positive

### Question 1

- We know that the sum of moments, $\Sigma l = 0$, therefore $l_{muscle} + l_{mass} = 0$ or $l_{mass} = -l_{muscle}$
- We also know that $l = Fd$ where $F$ = force and $d$ = perpendicular distance from the line of action of the force to axis. In this case, we have already been given $d$, which, as the leg is being held horizontally and gravity is acting vertically, is 300 mm = 0.3 m
- Therefore, $l = Fd = 80 \times 0.3 = 24$ Nm

## Question 2

- Once again, we begin with the knowledge that the sum of moments must equal zero:

$\Sigma l = 0$, therefore $l_{muscle} + l_{mass} + l_{shoe} = 0$, or
$(l_{mass} + l_{shoe}) = - l_{muscle}$

- We can calculate $l_{shoe}$ in exactly the same way as we just calculated $l_{mass}$

$l_{shoe} = Fd = 3 \times 0.4 = 1.2 \, Nm$

- Therefore, the total clockwise moment $= 24 + 1.2 \, Nm = 25.2 \, Nm$ and the total anticlockwise moment $= - 25.2 \, Nm$.

- $l_{muscle} = F_m d_m$, so $F_m d_m = - 25.2$

- To calculate $d_m$:

$\cos\theta$ = opposite/hypotenuse
$\cos 40° = d_m/600$
Therefore $d_m = 60\cos 40° = 46 \, mm$

- $F_m d_m = - 25.2$

Therefore $F_m = - 25.2/d_m = - 25.2/0.046 = -548 \, N$

# Bibliography

Daintith, J., Deeson, E. (Eds.), 1983. Dictionary of physics. Charles Letts, London.

Eformulae.com. Engineering formulae: strength of materials. Online. Available: www.eformulae.com/engineering/strength_materials.php 11 September 2007 12:10 BST.

Efunda. Moment of inertia. Online. Available: www.efunda.com/math/areas/MomentOfInertia.cfm 10 September 2007, 11:55 BST.

Ernst, E., 2001. Prospective investigations into the safety of spinal manipulation. J. Pain Symptom Manage. 21 (3), 238–242.

French, M., 2007. Polar moment of inertia. Online. Available: www2.tech.purdue.edu 8 September 2007 19:05 BST.

Hayes, N.M., Bezilla, T.A., 2006. Incidence of iatrogenesis associated with osteopathic manipulative treatment of pediatric patients. J. Am. Osteopath. Assoc. 106, 605–608.

Hurd, D.C., 2004. Measuring basic wood properties. In: Using physics and engineering concepts for building guitar family instruments: an introductory guide to their practical application. Bold Strummer, Westport, CT.

Johnson, K., 1986. Machines. In: GCSE physics for you, revised ed. Hutchinson, London (Chapter 18), pp. 138–147.

Kiviranta, P., Rieppo, J., Korhonen, R.K., et al., 2006. Collagen network primarily controls Poisson's ratio of bovine articular cartilage in compression. J Orthop. Res. 24, 690–699.

Knowles, E. (Ed.), 2004. In: The Oxford dictionary of quotations, sixth ed. Oxford University Press, Oxford.

Köhler, T., Vollrath, F., 1995. Thread biomechanics in the two orb-weaving spiders *Araneus diadematus* (Araneae, Araneidae) and *Uloboris walckenaerius* (Araneae, Uloboridae). J. Exp. Zool. 271, 1–17.

Li, L.P., Herzog, W., Korhonen, R.K., et al., 2005. The role of viscoelasticity of collagen fibres in articular cartilage: axial tension versus compression. Med. Eng. Phys. 27, 51–57.

Lynch, H.A., Johannessen, W., Wu, J.P., et al., 2003. Effect of fiber orientation and strain rate on the nonlinear uniaxial tensile material properties of tendon. J. Biomech. Eng. 125, 726–731.

Middleton, D.B., 1993. Comparison of digital videofluoroscopy and 3-space isotrack in the measurement of sagittal plane flexion of the lumbar spine. Anglo-European College of Chiropractic, part requirement for BSc Chiropractic, Bournemouth.

Nave, R., Young's modulus. Department of Physics and Astronomy, Georgia State University. Online. Available: www.hyperphysics.phy-astr.gsu.edu/hbase/permot3.html 17 September 2007 10:35 BST.

Pins, G.D., Huang, E.K., Christiansen, D.L., et al., 1997. Effects of static axial strain on the tensile properties and failure mechanisms of self-assembled collagen fibers. Journal of Applied Polymer Science 63, 1429–1440.

Roylance, D., 2000. Statics of bending: shear and bending moment diagrams. Massachusetts Institute of Technology, November 15, 2000. Online. Available: web.mit.edu/course/3/3.11/www/modules/statics.pdf 10 September 2007, 11:45 BST.

Roymech. Shear force and bending diagrams. Online. Available: www.roymech.co.uk/Useful_Tables/Beams/Shear_Bencing.html 10 September 2007, 11:50 BST.

Schwartz-Dabney, C.L., Dechow, P.C., 2002. Edentulation alters material properties of cortical bone in the human mandible. J. Dent. Res. 81 (9), 613–617.

Silver, F.H., Christiansen, D.L., Snowhill, P.B., et al., 2001. Transition from viscous to elastic-based dependency of mechanical properties of self-assembled type I collagen fibers. Journal of Applied Polymer Science 79, 134–142.

Silver, F.H., Seehra, G.P., Freeman, J.W., et al., 2002. Viscoelastic properties of young and old human dermis: a proposed molecular mechanism for elastic energy storage in collagen and elastin. Journal of Applied Polymer Science 86, 1978–1985.

Standring, S. (Ed.), 2005. Functional anatomy of the musculoskeletal system. In: Gray's anatomy: the anatomical basis of clinical practice. Elsevier, Edinburgh, pp. 83–135.

Standring, S.(Ed.), Connective and supporting tissues. In: Gray's anatomy: the anatomical basis of clinical practice. Online. Available: www.graysanatomyonline.com 20 October 2008, 12:05 BST.

Stroud, K.A., 1982. Integration applications, part 3. In: Engineering mathematics: programmes and problems, second ed. Programme 20. MacMillan, London, pp. 581–614.

Stroud, K.A., 1982. Polar co-ordinate systems. In: Engineering mathematics: programmes and problems, second ed. Programme 22. Macmillan, London, pp. 637–662.

Thorne, J.O., Collocott, T.C. (Eds.), 1984. Chambers Biographical Dictionary. Chambers, Edinburgh.

Thibodeau, G., Patton, K., The organization of the body. In: Anatomy and physiology, sixth ed. Elsevier e-book. (Chapter 1). Online. Available: www.elsevier.com

Thibodeau, G., Patton, K., Tissues. In: Anatomy and physiology, sixth ed. Elsevier e-book. (Chapter 5). Online. Available: www.elsevier.com

Thibodeau, G., Patton, K., Skeletal tissues. In: Anatomy and physiology, sixth ed. Elsevier e-book. (Chapter 7). Online. Available: www.elsevier.com University of Cambridge.

University of Cambridge. Second moment of area. Online. Available: www.doitpoms.ac.uk/tiplib/BD1/secondmoment.php 8 September 2007, 10:50 BST.

# Chapter Four

4

# The anatomy of physics

## CHAPTER CONTENTS

Check your existing knowledge . . . . . . 71
The classification of joints . . . . . . . . 72
Fibrous joints . . . . . . . . . . . . . . . 74
  Sutures . . . . . . . . . . . . . . . . . . 74
  Syndesmosis . . . . . . . . . . . . . . . 75
Cartilaginous joints . . . . . . . . . . . . . 76
  Primary cartilaginous joints . . . . . . . 76
  Secondary cartilaginous joints . . . . . 76
Synovial joints . . . . . . . . . . . . . . . 77
  Hinge joint (ginglymus) . . . . . . . . . 79
  Plane joint (gliding joint) . . . . . . . . 80
  Pivot joint (trochoid) . . . . . . . . . . 80
  Ball and socket joint
  (spheroidal joint) . . . . . . . . . . . . 81

Saddle joint (sellaris) . . . . . . . . . . 81
Condyloid joint (ellipsoid) . . . . . . . . 81
Bicondylar joint . . . . . . . . . . . . . 83
Structural classification . . . . . . . . . 83
Ligaments . . . . . . . . . . . . . . . . . 83
The classification of muscle . . . . . . . 84
  Skeletal muscle . . . . . . . . . . . . . 84
  Tendons . . . . . . . . . . . . . . . . . 86
Learning outcomes . . . . . . . . . . . . 97
Check your existing knowledge:
answers . . . . . . . . . . . . . . . . . . 97
Bibliography . . . . . . . . . . . . . . . . 98

## CHECK YOUR EXISTING KNOWLEDGE

1. What is an amphiarthrosis?
2. Dentate, serrate and limbus are all examples of what type of joint?
3. What type of joints are the following (use functional as well as anatomical descriptors in your answers)?
   a. knee (femorotibial)
   b. shoulder (glenohumeral)
   c. interphalangeal
   d. intervertebral disc
4. Give an example of a saddle (sellaris) joint?
5. How would you manage a Grade III ligamentous sprain?
6. Which two molecules combine to give muscle its contractile strength and which other molecule is required for this to happen?
7. Why are the following muscles so named?
   a. sternocleidomastoid
   b. flexor digitorum profundus
   c. rhomboid

8 Describe the arrangement of the muscle fibres in the following types of muscle:

a Unipennate

b Strap

c Fusiform

Now check your answers against those given at the end of the chapter.

# The classification of joints

Various attempts have been made at classifying joints in order to bring a degree of generalization from which we can gain understanding. Unfortunately, the different systems – often using Latin terminology – can intimidate the novice with a bewildering array of complex, unrelated, polysyllabic labels.

 ## CLINICAL FOCUS

Many anatomical terms – which naturally tend to spill over into biomechanics – are of Latin or Greek origin, subjects that are seldom taught in schools today but were the universal language of the natural philosophers who first categorized and classified the human body.

Becoming a clinician requires you to learn a whole new terminology of several thousand words; however, if you can understand the etymology – where the roots of the word come from – you will find it far easier.

For example, the Greek word for 'joint' is *arthron*. Once you know this, then understanding words derived from this root becomes much easier:

- **Arthrosis** is a joint (the plural is arthroses)
- **Arthritis** is inflammation of a joint, just like appendic*itis* is inflammation of the appendix
- **Arthropathy** is disease of a joint, just like *path*ology means the study of disease
- **Arthralgia** is joint pain, just like neur*algia* is nerve pain

For this reason, this book will regularly give the roots of a new word to help you build your clinical vocabulary. It also helps to invest in decent medical and English dictionaries; that way you can understand terms rather than having to learn them by rote.

The first thing to realize is that there are, in effect, two ways in which you can organize joints: by their structure or by their function. Which way you chose largely depends on whether you are an anatomist (structuralist) or an orthopaedist (functionalist). As a student of manual medicine, you are, at various times, required to be either or both and therefore familiarity with both systems is required. Figure 4.1 summarizes these two different approaches.

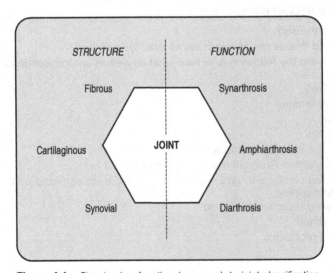

**Figure 4.1** • Structural vs functional approach to joint classification.

In reality, there is considerable overlap between the two systems. In a **fibrous joint**, two adjacent bones are held tightly together by strong connective tissue. Obviously, such an arrangement does not allow for any significant movement so, functionally, this type of joint is termed a **synarthrosis,** from the Greek *syn* (together) and *arthron* (a joint). Therefore, as a rule, fibrous joints are synarthroses.

## CLINICAL FOCUS

Cranial osteopaths, craniosacral therapists and chiropractors using cranial treatment methods would all take issue with the standard classification of sutural joints as 'unmoveable' synarthroses. However, such a debate is really about semantics; the amount of flexion in the cranial sutures, once fully formed, is minimal and, in later life, becomes still further reduced.

The significance of this movement – what might best (to avoid misunderstanding and controversy) be termed 'synarthrotic cranial micro-motion' – remains a matter of speculation and, often heated, debate.

Other joints have **cartilaginous** elements to them, an arrangement that usually allows a degree of flexibility within the joint without free movement. A joint that allows limited movement in this way is called an **amphiarthrosis**, again from the Greek (*amphi*, on both sides; *arthron*, a joint). In general, cartilanginous joints are amphiarthroses.

Finally, joints that have a **synovial** capsule (Fig. 4.2) have all the elements required for free movement, restricted only by the joint anatomy and the soft tissue holding elements. A joint that is freely moveable is referred to as a **diarthrosis** (Greek: *dia*, through; *arthron*, joint), although the amount of movement can vary considerably: take, for example, joints of the upper and lower limbs. In a quadrupedal animal, there is relatively little difference between the joints of the fore and hind limbs. In humans, although the template is the same, the joints of the lower extremity are much less flexible but able to bear the weight of the body; the joints of the upper limb allow a remarkable degree of dexterity, but at the expense of stability – try walking on your hands or writing with your toes!

This is the trade-off that must always be made: high mobility equals low stability; high stability

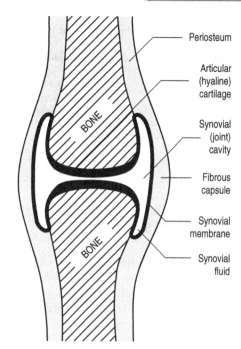

**Figure 4.2** • Components of a synovial joint.

equals low mobility. It is at the extremes that these classifications start to become blurred: at what point do you differentiate 'some movement' from 'free movement'? How little movement is 'no movement'? In practice, an intervertebral disc (a cartilaginous joint) has more movement than the proximal joint between the tibia and fibula (a synovial joint); craniopaths would disagree that cranial sutures are immobile. As ever, when you try to classify something, there will be exceptions that do not fit the generalizations; as ever, it is always best to know the rules and then understand the exceptions.

## CLINICAL FOCUS

Although you might assume that the number of joints in the adult human body is fixed (at 360), this is not the case. The manual physician needs to be aware that up to one patient in 20 will have been born with extra or fewer joints than normal. This is particularly true in and around the vertebral column and spinal manipulative therapists need to be cognisant with the biomechanical implications and consequences of this.

See Table 4.1 for common causes of extra or fewer joints.

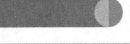
**Table 4.1** Common causes of extra and fewer joints

| Extra joints | Fewer joints |
|---|---|
| • Sacral lumbarization | • Lumbar sacralization |
| • Spinal accessory joints | • Costotransverse fusion |
| • Supernumerary ribs | • Congenital block |
| • Polydactyly |   vertebrae |
| • Luschka's rib | • Syndactyly |
| • Psuedoarthroses | • Srb's anomaly |
| • Sesamoid bones | • Agenesis |

# Fibrous joints

The most consistent feature of fibrous joints is the absence of a joint space; any cavity between the two articulating bones tends to be filled with fibrous connective tissue. There are three types of fibrous joint found in the human body:

## Sutures

Found between the bones of the skull, sutures show significant change throughout a lifetime. In infants, the bones of the skull do not make contact with each other and the dura mater, the outer lining of the brain, is directly palpable in the gaps between the bones. These gaps are called **fontanelles**. The most prominent of these is the anterior fontanelle (Fig. 4.3), bounded by the frontal and parietal bones. This fontanelle (the 'soft spot') has gone by the age of 24 months and, by the age of 6–7 years,

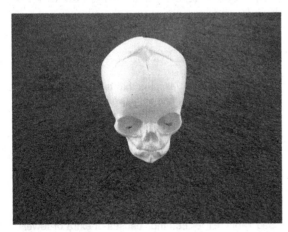

**Figure 4.3** ● A model of an infant skull demonstrating the anterior fontanelle.

the cranial sutures are, for the most part, united. From the third decade onwards, the fibrous interosseous tissue starts to ossify, forming an osseous union of the adjacent bones known as a **synostosis** (Greek: *syn*, together; *osteon*, bone).

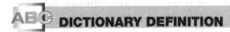
## DICTIONARY DEFINITION

**FONTANELLE**

The word *fontanelle* comes from the French meaning *little fountain*. The most probable aetiology for the word is from cases where the intracranial pressure was raised from, say, hydrocephalus. The fontanelles would therefore bulge and, if they burst, either accidentally or as part of treatment, blood and cerebrospinal fluid would spurt out in a fountain. There is more than one type of suture; unfortunately, there is no official agreement as to their classification. However, the system detailed below offers the best understanding as to the types of sutural joint that have been identified.

### True sutures

With 'true' sutures, margins of opposing bone are connected by a series of interlocking processes and indentations that fit together like a jigsaw puzzle.

• **Dentate sutures**
  ○ Deep interdigitations, similar to meshing cogs. Examples include the sagittal suture.
• **Serrate sutures**
  ○ Fine, tooth-like, serrated interdigitations, similar to interlocking combs. Examples include the metopic suture.
• **Limbus sutures**
  ○ These complex sutures are best understood by breaking down the articulation between two bones into thirds. In the first third, bone A will overly bone B; in the last third, bone B will overly bone A, and in the middle third, the two bones interlock. Examples include the lamboid and coronal sutures.

### False sutures

Not all opposing cranial bones lock together; some merely lie adjacent to each other with the sum of the articulation being the interosseous fibrous attachment. Such joints are therefore generally less rigid than true sutures. There are two types of false suture:

- **Squamous sutures**
  - The bevelled edges of the articulating bones overly each other. Examples include the temporoparietal suture.
- **Plane sutures**
  - The flat edges of the bone do not overlap but instead buttress each other. Examples include the joint between the two maxillae.

## Schindylesis

This Greek word means 'cleft' or 'fissure' which accurately describes the union of a ridged bony prominence with a similarly shaped cleft. A good example of this is the way in which the triangular rostrum of the sphenoid locks into the alae of the vomer.

 CLINICAL FOCUS

Clinical conditions can arise when sutures close prematurely. If the coronal suture closes early, it will not allow further anteroposterior skull development and there will be compensatory lateral growth; this is termed **brachycephaly**. If the sagittal suture closes early, the converse is true and an elongated head is called **dolichocephaly**. Early closure of the metopic suture between the two frontal bones leads to a cone-shaped forehead, **trigonocephaly**.

Unilateral closure of a paired suture causes cranial asymmetry known as **plagiocephaly**. Depending on how early closure occurs and how many sutures are involved, a child can be left with a reduced cranium, **microcephaly**, with mental retardation and other cranial disorders (epilepsy, nerve palsies etc.) from compression of neurological structures.

The most common failure of closure is the midline of the palate (palatines and/or maxillae) causing a cleft palate. In **cleidocranial dysplasia**, there is general midline failure, usually including failure of sutural closure, clavicular agenesis, spinal changes and pubic symphysis defects as well as digital hypoplasia and shortness of stature.

## Peg and socket

The correct anatomical term for a peg and socket joint is a **gomphosis** (Greek: *gomphos*, a bolt). The only place in the human body where such joints are found is the insertion of the roots of the teeth

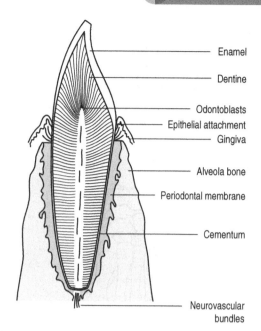

**Figure 4.4** • A peg and socket joint (gomphosis).

into the sockets (alveoli) of the jaw (mandible and maxilla). The details of this arrangement are shown below (Fig. 4.4).

## Syndesmosis

In this type of fibrous joint, two bones are united by a sheet of fibrous tissue. The term syndesmosis again has Greek origins: *syn* means together; *desmos*, a bond. It is at this point that the relationship between fibrous joints and synarthroses begins to break down. Some syndesmoses are aimed at giving rigidity: for example, the interosseous membrane between the tibia and fibula forms, in the ankle, part of the mortice into which the tenon of the talus fits (Fig. 4.5). If this were not solidly immobile, then it would be impossible to stand – the talus would simply separate the two bones above it and slide upwards towards the knee!

By contrast, the equivalent membrane between the ulna and radius allows the two bones to supinate and pronate – over 180° of movement! The degree of movement is dependent on a number of factors: the distance between the bones, the angle of insertion of the membrane and the flexibility of the membrane itself. Despite the mobility of the radio-ulnar syndesmosis, it is still strong enough to act as an anchor point for the tendinous insertions of several forearm muscles.

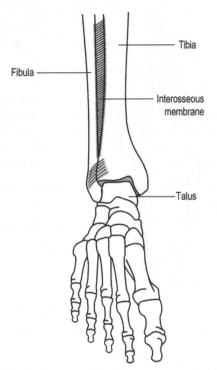

**Figure 4.5** • Schematic diagram of the ankle joint: the interosseous membrane renders the distal talofibular joint a syndesmosis.

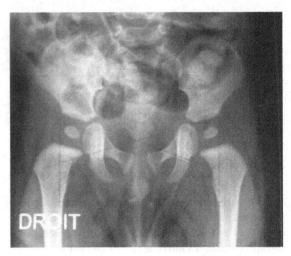

**Figure 4.6** • In this x-ray of a child, the growth plates are clearly evident Unlike bone, cartilage is radiolucent; therefore, the femoral heads and bones of the pelvis appear to be floating in space, the interconnecting cartilage growth plates are radiologically invisible. Image reproduced courtesy of Michelle Wessely, IFEC, France.

## Cartilaginous joints

As suggested by the name, these joints are united by cartilage rather than by fibrous matter. As with fibrous joints, you will discover that there are several ways in which these joints can be classified; however, once you can understand the terminology, which system you decide to use then becomes a matter of informed choice.

### Primary cartilaginous joints

These joints, mainly found in the immature skeleton, are also known as **synchondroses** (Greek: *syn*, together; *khondros*, cartilage). In order for a long bone to grow, the shaft of the bone (diaphysis from Greek: *dia* meaning through; *phyesthai*, to grow, therefore 'to grow through') and the end of the bone (epiphysis: as above but *epi* meaning upon, therefore 'to grow upon') are united by the epiphyseal growth plate, which allows an actively growing zone in which a cartilaginous template ossifies to allow bone expansion (Fig. 4.6). When full growth is achieved, the growth plate also ossifies, forming a synostosis and uniting the bone.

### Secondary cartilaginous joints

By contrast, secondary cartilaginous joints are amphiarthrotic, allowing a biomechanically significant amount of movement. In these joints, which are more commonly called **sympheses** (Greek *syn*, together; *phyesthai*, to grow), we also see, for the first time, the appearance of hyaline cartilage, lining the articular surfaces of bone. This cartilage can either be continuous, as it is in the joint between the sternum and manubrium, or it can be interrupted by articular discs, as is the case in the anterior intervertebral joints of the spine (Fig. 4.7) and the pubic symphysis (Fig. 4.8).

Sympheses are all found in the midline and are, for the most part, confined to the axial skeleton. Although more concerned with the transmission of forces than with movement, they are still prone to the types of injury that are frequently seen by manual physicians.

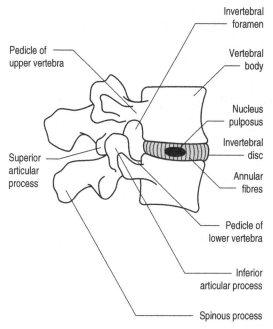

Figure 4.7 • A functional spinal unit showing the intervertebral disc and facet (zygoapophyseal) joints. The disc is an example of a secondary cartilaginous joint and is amphiarthrotic, being primarily concerned in distributing the forces associated with weight bearing; the facet joints are plane (gliding joints) and their combined diarthrotic motion allows considerable movement within the spinal column.

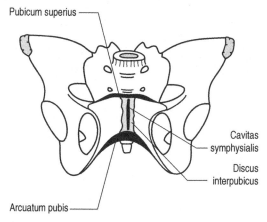

Figure 4.8 • The pelvis showing key features of the pubic symphysis.

## CLINICAL FOCUS

The commonest injury to a secondary cartilaginous joint – and one that is often treated by chiropractors, physiotherapists and osteopaths – is a 'slipped disc'.

In reality, the disc, which can be regarded as a nucleus of glycoproteins contained within concentric rings of fibrocartilage (called 'annular fibres' because of their resemblance to annular tree rings), slips nowhere. Rather, damage to the annular fibres (Grade I) can allow the nucleus to track outwards forming a bulge (Grade II) or herniating into the spinal column causing damage either to a single nerve root (Grade III, Fig. 4.9) or to the spinal cord and/or multiple nerve roots (Grade IV).

Because the spinal cord stops growing before the axial skeleton is mature, it finishes at the level of L2/L3 and the lower nerve roots hang down like a horse's tail, in Latin *cauda equina*, before exiting the spine at the appropriate level. Compression of these can cut off the nerve supply to the legs, bladder and lower bowel, causing paralysis and incontinence, and requiring urgent decompressive surgery.

# Synovial joints

The commonest joints in the body – and the ones, generally, of most interest to the manual physician – are the freely moveable (diarthrotic) synovial joints. The components that make up a synovial joint are detailed in Figure 4.2. As with cartilaginous joints, the bone of the articular surfaces is lined with a smooth coating of hyaline cartilage (except in the temporomandibular joint, the sternoclavicular and the acromioclavicular joint where the articular surfaces are covered with dense fibrous tissue instead). Here, however, the similarity stops.

## Fact File

### SYNOVIUM

The term *synovium* was introduced by the 16th century physician, Paracelsus (born Theophrastus Bombastus von Hoenheim), whose abilities in other fields have since been eclipsed by his reputation as an alchemist. Although some sources regard the coinage of the word as arbitrary, it is possible that it comes from a hybridization of the Greek word *syn,* with and the Latin, *ovum* meaning egg. Synovial fluid is clear but has a higher viscosity than water and it has been suggested that Paracelsus thought that it resembled egg white (albumen).

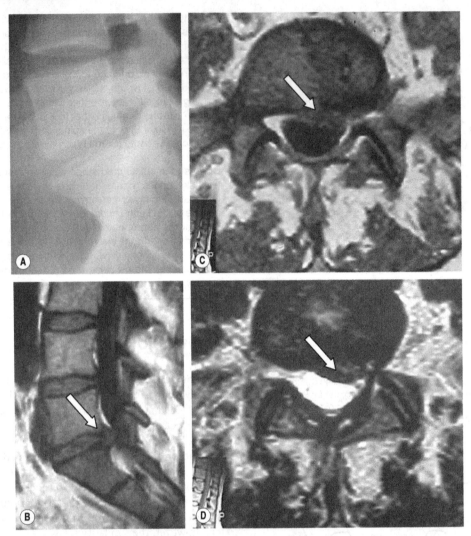

**Figure 4.9** • Because discs are not visualized on plain film x-ray (A), magnetic resonance (MR) imaging is the modality of choice to assess damage to discs. (B) A sagittal T1-weighted MR image shows a disc extrusion on the left at L5 (arrow). (C) A T1-weighted axial image and (D), a T2-weighted sagittal image, demonstrate that the large paracentral extrusion is occluding the left lateral recess and compressing the anterior aspect of the thecal sac (arrows). The disc has also lost some of its height. Image reproduced courtesy of Michelle Wessely, IFEC, France © *Clinical Chiropractic*, 2006.

The key feature of a synovial articulation is the joint space (in reality, more a potential than an actual space, particularly when weight bearing). Unlike the two classes of joints that we have previously examined, there is no connecting tissue between the two (or more) bones involved in a synovial joint. Instead, the joint is contained with a ligamentous capsule, the interior surface of which has cells that secrete synovial fluid, which acts to lubricate the joint's surfaces and allows them to glide smoothly across each other. As a consequence, most synovial joints have considerably more movement than their fibrous and cartilaginous counterparts and are thus classified as **diarthrodial**. Their movement is restricted by the anatomical parameters of the joint, the supporting ligaments and the biomechanical limitations of the articulating muscles.

The major classification system for synovial joints is based on the anatomical relationship between the two articulating surfaces. This is useful for the clinician because, as we shall see later, there are rules of movement associated with these different types of joint that have clinical implications. Unfortunately, you will see a variety of terms used to describe each type of joint. In this text, the descriptive English terms will be used (as they are much easier to remember and actually tell you something about the joint – much as 'peg and socket' is a more useful term than 'gomphosis'), although the variants that you may discover in other sources are also given. The classification of synovial joints, with examples of each type, is detailed below and summarized in Table 4.2.

## Hinge joint (ginglymus)

The simplest and, most probably, the easiest type of synovial joint to understand, the hinge joint or ginglymus (Greek: *ginglymos*, a hinge) is also the second most common in the body – all you have to do is to use a finger to beckon and you will understand why: the interphalangeal joints of the fingers and toes are all simple hinge joints.

In a hinge joint, the articulating bones act, as the name suggests, in the same manner as the hinge of a

**Table 4.2** Classification of synovial joints

| Hinge | (Ginglymus) | Interphalangeal joints<br>Elbow (compound) |
|---|---|---|
| Plane | (Gliding) | Zygoapophyseal joints<br>Acromioclavicular (complex) |
| Pivot | (Trochoid) | Proximal radio-ulnar joint<br>Atlanto-odontoid joint |
| Ball & socket | (Spheroidal) | Hip<br>Shoulder (humeroscapular joint) |
| Saddle | (Sellaris) | $1^{st}$ metacarpophalangeal joint<br>Sternoclavicular joint |
| Condyloid | (Ellipsoid) | Radiocarpal (compound)<br>$2^{nd} – 5^{th}$ metacarpophalangeal joints |
| Bicondylar | (Condylar) | Knee (complex, compound)<br>Temporomandibular (complex, compound) |

door, allowing the joint to move from extension (straight) to a flexed position that is usually limited by approximation of the soft tissues on the flexor surfaces (Fig. 4.10). Sideways motion is precluded

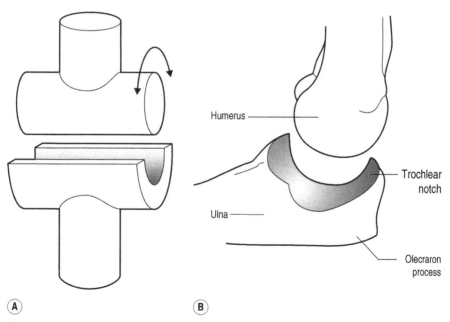

**Figure 4.10** • A hinge joint (ginglymus). A schematic representation (A) and anatomical example, the elbow (humero-ulnar joint) (B).

by strong collateral ligaments, which are usually continuous with the joint capsule.

In reality, the motion of these joints is slightly more complex than a simple mechanical hinge as we shall see later.

## Plane joint (gliding joint)

A plane joint is no more than a simple apposition of two flat surfaces whereby the articular surfaces slide over each other in order to facilitate a, normally small, amount of movement. This movement is often limited by strong ligaments – as is the case in the intracarpal and intratarsal joints, which are, effectively, amphiarthroses – and, even was it not, the surfaces are unable to slide far in opposing directions without becoming disassociated.

Although it is easiest at this stage to regard the surfaces of plane joints to be flat, in reality most have slight curvatures that affect and modify the dynamics of the joints. Plane joints are the most common synovial joints found in the human body: the majority of intervertebral joints are plane joints (Fig. 4.7), as are those found between the bones of the ankle (tarsi) and wrist (carpi).

### CLINICAL FOCUS

The biomechanical disadvantage of a gliding joint is that only its supporting ligaments provide its strength; there is frequently no anatomical limitation to its movement. As a result, partial or full dislocation of such a joint is almost invariably unstable and will require surgical intervention (Fig. 4.11).

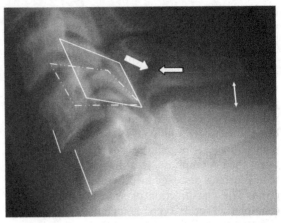

**Figure 4.11** • There is partial disassociation of one of the articular facets of C6–C7 (rectangles) with a resultant increase in the interspinous distance owing to the forward tilt of the 'perched' vertebra (arrow line). The forward position of C6 in relation to C7 is also clearly seen (lines). Also visible is a fracture line involving the spinous process and lamina of C6 (arrows). Image reproduced courtesy of Michelle Wessely, IFEC, France © *Clinical Chiropractic*, 2006.

For spinal manipulators, it is particularly important to identify such injuries as adjustment to 'perched facet' syndrome or to a dislocated spine could have catastrophic consequences.

## Pivot joint (trochoid)

By comparison, the pivot joint is highly specialized, complex and uncommon. As can be seen from the schematic (Fig. 4.12), a cylindrical projection of bone

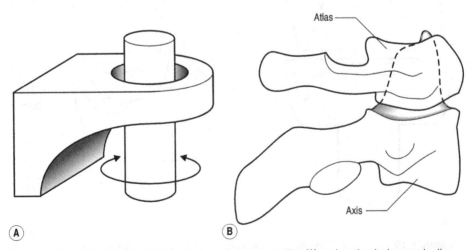

**(A)**       **(B)**

**Figure 4.12** • A pivot (trochoid) joint. A schematic representation **(A)** and anatomical example, the atlanto-odontoid joint **(B)**.

is held against a concave opposing surface by means of a robust ligament. This arrangement allows for maximum rotation with a minimum of translation.

Examples of pivot joints include the proximal radio-ulnar joint and the joint between the atlas and the dens (odontoid process) of the axis.

# Ball and socket joint (spheroidal joint)

These highly mobile joints – the body's equivalent to the universal joint – consist of an (almost) round 'ball' that sits in a hollow socket (Figure 4.13). The two most obvious examples are the shoulder and hip.

# Saddle joint (sellaris)

The way in which a saddle joint articulates is far easier to understand when visualized (Fig. 4.14) than when described; however, technically the joint consists of two concavo-convex surfaces with the direction of maximum concavity occurring at right angles to the direction of maximum convexity. The concavity of the larger surface is opposed to the convexity of the smaller surface and the concavity of the smaller to the convexity of the larger.

In order to hold this image in your mind, imagine two horse riding saddles. If you were to turn the second saddle upside-down and turn it through 90° and then place it on top of the first saddle, then you would have a good approximation both of the appearance of the joint and the way in which it functions, although this is dealt with in greater detail later in this chapter.

Saddle joints are relatively uncommon; the classic example usually given is the joint between the first metacarpal and the trapezium, although the calcaneocuboid and ankle are also sellar joints.

# Condyloid joint (ellipsoid)

The easiest way to appreciate a condyloid joint is to think of a shallow ball and socket joint where the two surfaces are oval rather than round (Fig. 4.15). Because of the oval (or ellipsoidal) shape of the joint, the rotational aspect of the joint's movement is very much more restricted that it is in a ball and socket joint; this is discussed in great detail later on. The wrist joint between the ulna and radius distally and lunate and scaphoid proximally is an example of a condyloid joint.

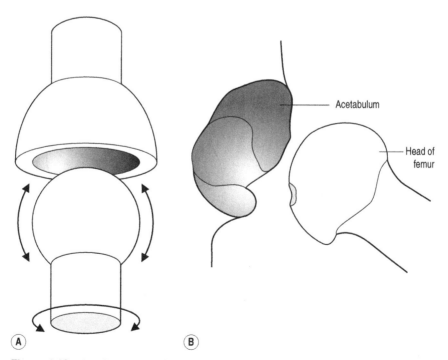

Figure 4.13 • A ball and socket (spheroidal) joint. A schematic representation (A) and anatomical example, the iliofemoral joint (B).

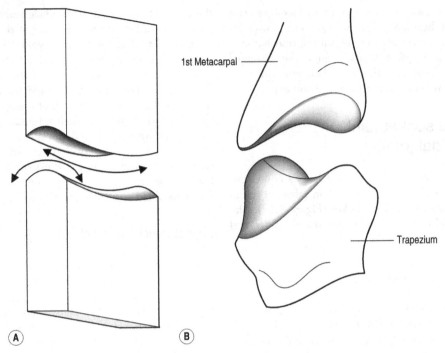

**Figure 4.14** • A saddle joint (sellaris). A schematic representation (**A**) and anatomical example, the first carpometacarpal joint (**B**).

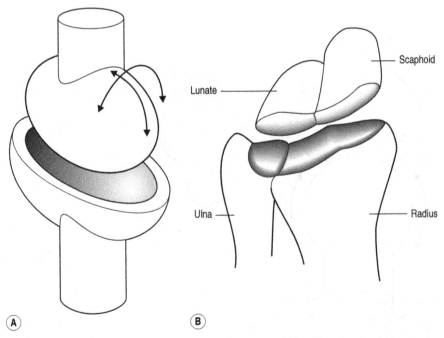

**Figure 4.15** • A condylar joint (ellipsoid). A schematic representation (**A**) and anatomical example, the radiocarpal joint (**B**).

## Bicondylar joint

Many anatomical and even biomechanical texts do not include this classification of synovial joint, preferring to lump the knee and the jaw (temporomandibular joint) in with hinge joints. However, because these joints have convex condyles (knuckles) articulating with flat or slightly concave surfaces, they are anatomically quite distinct from hinge joints and – to a manual therapist – their biomechanical function is also quite different; therefore, it is essential that the distinction be made between the two. Bicondylar joints are further complicated by the presence of fibrocartilaginous structures (menisci) within the joint capsule.

## Structural classification

In addition to the classification system above, there is a secondary system for classifying synovial joints. The two systems are used in conjunction rather than being opposing systems. As we have seen from the examples above, most synovial joints are the simple approximation of two bones with the features typical to such an articulation: fibrous capsule; ligamentous support; synovial membrane and fluid; articular cartilage. These joints, without any complicating features, are called **simple** joints.

If the joint contains additional features, such as an articular disc or a meniscus, then it is said to be **complex**. The acromioclavicular joint, which often contains a rudimentary disc, is an example of a complex synovial joint.

If the articulation involves more than two bones (or one of the bones has more than one articular process), it is termed a **compound joint**. The ankle joint (Fig. 4.5) and the wrist (Fig. 4.15) are examples of compound joints.

It should be noted that joints can be both compound *and* complex. The knee is an example of such a joint. Although only two bones are involved, the femur has two separate condyles making it compound and the menisci qualify it as a complex joint.

## Ligaments

Ligaments are often represented as the internal struts that give biomechanical rigidity to otherwise floppy joints; however, this is both an over-representation of the intrinsic strength of most ligaments and an over-simplification of the way in which joints gain their stability.

Although we have seen that this can be the case in some joints where there is unidirectional instability, such as plane joints, these joints are generally small, as are the muscles that move them (if any; several tarsi and carpi only move as part of a larger functional unit). Although ligaments yield little to tension, they are pliant and do not resist normal joint movement; they are designed to help check abnormal or excessive movements. However, the way in which they do this is only partly through their intrinsic strength; indeed, if the stability of larger, more powerful joints was dependent only upon the strength of their ligaments, they would have to be so bulky and cumbersome that the joints would become unwieldy and so restricted in movement as to be useless.

Instead, joints gain their stability in part from their shape and angulation and, in the case of complex joints, from the additional structures within, such as the menisci ('cartilages') of the knee and, in part, from an additional feature of ligaments, without which many of them would snap every time your body was subjected to physical stress.

Obviously, this does not happen and the reason is because the ligament has within it nerve endings that are sensitive to stretch. As the ligament tightens, these mechanoreceptors increase their firing activity sending fast signals to the brain. In part (and together with the information from Golgi tendon organs, see below), this endows the body with a highly useful sense: proprioception, or the ability to know where our body is in space. Without this sense, not only would you not be able to put your finger on your nose with your eyes shut, but you would also find walking impossible without staring intently at your feet and, even then, you would tend to lurch as if you were drunk.

In addition we have a complex array of neuromuscular reflexes, which provide our joints with much of their stability. If, say, you start to turn over on your ankle, the information from the ligaments on the outside of the ankle cause the ankle's evertors to reflexively contract and help pull the ankle straight again, thus preventing a sprain.

The classification of ligaments is easy: they are either **intrinsic**, a thickening or condensation of the synovial joint capsule; **extrinsic**, separate from the joint capsule; or, occasionally, a mixture of the two. The nomenclature of ligaments is now, mercifully, a much more simple matter than once it was and a good reason for ensuring your anatomy and biomechanics texts are relatively modern. Until quite recently, ligaments frequently had eponymous names – such as the *'Y'-shaped ligament of Bigalow* or the *ligament of Struthers* – which often varied from one part of the world to another and told you nothing about the ligament except the name of the anatomist who discovered it or the surgeon who first found out how to sew it back together again. Now, all ligaments are named for their attachments with modifiers (anterior, superior, medial etc.) where confusion might otherwise arise.

 CLINICAL FOCUS

Injury to a ligament (a sprain) is graded according to severity:

- A Grade I sprain consists of damage to the microfibres of the ligament with no obvious visible deficiency
- A Grade II sprain involves a tear of partial thickness; the ligament still has some residual integrity – the severity of the condition, and its recovery, is dependent on the proportion of damaged to undamaged fibres
- A Grade III sprain involves a complete rupture of the ligament, which will require surgical reattachment (if possible or appropriate)

Such injuries usually benefit from rehabilitation once biomechanical integrity has been re-established. This will involve treatment not merely to the ligament but retraining of the nerves and their stabilizing reflexes and well as the joint and its associated muscles

# The classification of muscle

Muscles consist of fibres, which are actually individual cells called **myocytes** (Greek: *myos*, muscle; *kytos*, hollow). These are grouped together into the **fasciculi** (Latin: *fascis*, bundle) that, in turn, make up muscle sections that are compartmentalized by containing fascia. The individual cells contain myofibrils (approximately 1μm in diameter) that can be thought of as very thin ribbons. These ribbons are, in turn, made up of myofilaments, interlocking strands of actin and myosin that are the powerhouse of muscles (Fig. 4.16).

It is important to remember that the number of cells we have is fixed early in life. When we 'bulk up' at the gym we are not increasing the number of myocytes; rather, we are increasing the number of myofilaments, enlarging the muscle fibres and thus allowing more powerful contractile forces of $100\,\mathrm{Wkg^{-1}}$ or more to be generated.

In **smooth muscle**, which is typically found in visceral structures such as the gut wall, where its slow, peristaltic contractions move food along the alimentary tract, the actin and myosin are not organized in any particular manner. In other parts of the body, however, they form regular, repeating units that, under the microscope, form stripes or bands called striations. This type of muscle is thus called **striated muscle**.

There are two types of striated muscle. **Cardiac muscle** is found only in and around the heart and is peculiar in generating its own intrinsic contractile impulses and for its resistance to fatigue – a heart will beat, on average, once per second for the whole of your life without pausing for rest. However, the heart, and its muscular structure, is only of interest to the manual therapist when its function impinges on treatment and is the province of physiology and pathology textbooks. **Skeletal muscle** by contrast, is a matter of the keenest interest for those involved in manual medicine.

It should be noted that some sources call smooth muscle 'involuntary' (its actions are controlled by the autonomic nervous system and are not ordinarily under conscious control) and skeletal muscle 'voluntary'. These terms are misleading, although much skeletal motion is under our conscious control, there is plenty (breathing, blinking etc.) that is not.

# Skeletal muscle

Most of the muscle in the body is skeletal muscle; in fact, the average human body comprises 43% of the stuff! The function of muscles is intimately related to that of joints, so much so that, from a clinical standpoint, it is almost pointless to separate them. A dysfunctional joint will develop dysfunctional muscles; dysfunctional muscles will cause a dysfunctional joint – and both require optimal neurological control, adequate vascular supply and unimpeded lymphatic drainage to work properly. Understanding this is what (in part) is meant by taking an holistic approach (we shall discuss one of the other parts under kinematic chains in the next chapter).

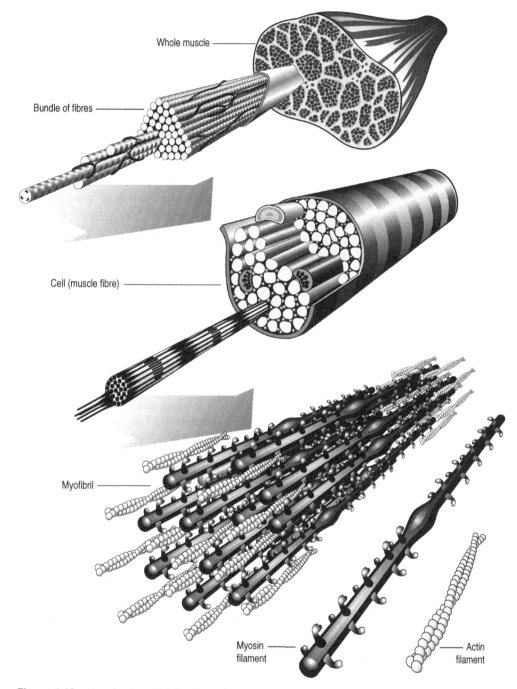

**Figure 4.16** • The structure of skeletal muscle.

Having already looked at the way in which joints are organized, it will come as little surprise to learn that similar classifications exist for muscle: we have already seen that there are different types of muscle, in much the same way that there are different types of joint – there are also further sub-classifications of skeletal muscles and these can be by the way they attach themselves, by the way in which they receive their vascular supply or by their shape, which is intrinsically linked to their function.

# Tendons

Most skeletal muscles move joints. The forces that they develop are transferred to bones, occasionally by means of aponeuroses or fascia, but primarily via tendons. These take the form of straps or cords, usually of round or oval cross section. Made of type I collagen – which has sufficient elasticity to allow the tendon to stretch by up to 6% of its length without damage – tendons are continuous with the muscle fasciculi at one end whilst, at the other, they send down deep anchoring **Sharpey fibres** into the periosteum and cortex of the bone. If the tendon is particularly long, or has to bypass other structures, it travels through synovial sheaths, as is the case with many of the muscles of the hands and feet, which are located in the forearm and leg (if you use your fingers to pretend to play the piano, you can see these synovial sheaths moving under the skin of the back of the hand).

## CLINICAL FOCUS

Although synovial sheaths protect tendons from damage and help lubricate them to ease their sometimes lengthy and tortuous passage, they are not without problems. Trauma, repetitive strain or other pathological factors can often lead to inflammation within the tendon and a vicious circle develops: the inflammation causes swelling, the swelling causes the tendon to rub against the sheath, the rubbing causes inflammation ... and so on.

This condition is known as **stenosing tenosynovitis** (a bit of a mouthful, but stenosis means narrowing; tenosynovitis is a compound word: (Greek) *tenon*, tendon; synovitis, inflammation of a synovial membrane). The commonest site for this condition, which can often be very resistant to treatment, is in the tendons of abductor policis longus and extensor policis brevis – the tendons share a common sheath. The condition is known eponymically as **de Quervain's disease**.

Where the tendinous attachment is broad-based like a sheet, it is termed an **aponeurosis**. These types of tendon often don't attach to bone but instead anchor into interosseous membranes or broad, fibrous bands known as **raphés**.

# Nerve supply

Tendons appear white because their vascular supply is sparse; however, they are rich in sensory nerve endings, primarily Golgi tendon organs, which transmit proprioceptive information to the brain to augment that from **muscle spindles**. The efferent nerves to muscles run to the neuromuscular junction, where the α-motor neuron reaches the muscle fibre. Several short fibres are given off, ending in elliptical areas called the **motor end plate**. In muscles where fine control is required, such as the muscles of the hands and fingers, only a few myocytes are served by a single axon; in large, powerful muscles, several hundred fibres will be served, a more economical arrangement but one that leads to coarser control. The motor neurone, and the fibres it controls, is called a **motor unit.** When an action potential is propagated along the axon, it causes the muscle to contract.

# Physiology

Muscle contraction is, at the molecular level, an extraordinary and fascinating phenomenon involving double-hinged molecular cross-bridges between the myofilaments of actin and myosin (Fig. 4.17). When muscle is relaxed, the cross-bridges are detached; during contraction, they attach and the necks of the cocked heads pivot on their hinges providing

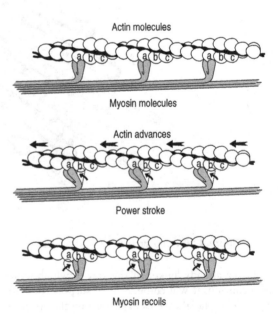

**Figure 4.17** • The action of myosin and actin molecules, producing contractile forces in muscles.

the power stroke that moves the two myofilaments in relation to each other and shortens the muscle. The energy for these actions comes from splitting adenosine triphosphate (ATP). Shortage of ATP means that the myosin is unable to detach from the actin, causing cramp – it is also the mechanism that causes rigor mortis in death.

 CLINICAL FOCUS

With regard to muscle, the term 'relaxed' is a relative one; even at rest, a muscle has some degree of contractile force – this is what 'muscle tone' is, the amount of contraction in a muscle when it is not being used. Only if the nerve to a muscle is severed – or damaged in a disease such as poliomyelitis – will the muscle become truly flaccid (and completely paralysed). Without any neurological input to maintain tone, the muscle will quickly start to waste away.

A certain amount of ATP is stored in muscle cells and, once this is exhausted, the mitochondria of the muscle cells can oxidise creatine phosphate, fatty acids and glucose to produce more ATP. Because oxygen is required for these metabolic processes, they are termed **aerobic** (Greek: *aer*, air; *bios*, life). During prolonged, vigorous exercise, the blood cannot supply oxygen fast enough and the cells have to rely on **anaerobic** metabolism of glucose and glycogen to rapidly supply ATP. Although rapid, the process is much less efficient, producing much less ATP per molecule and making the unwanted waste product, lactic acid. It is this chemical that makes muscles feel 'stiff' after unaccustomed exercise.

## Vascular supply

The way in which a muscle receives its blood supply has important implications for both its function – as we have just seen above – and, in cases of injury, its rate of healing. This is particularly true in older patients who may have a compromised vascular system; this can lead to areas that are relatively avascular that can be resistant to healing. The arterial supply to muscle can be classified into five basic mechanisms given, with examples, in Table 4.3.

The venous drainage has approximately the same territories as the arterial supply. It is known that an important factor in venous drainage is the pressure exerted on the walls of the vein by contraction of the muscle surrounding it; another reason why mobilization and appropriate usage of a muscle is a factor in healing.

## Types of skeletal muscle

Not all skeletal muscle is the same; not surprising really when you consider the difference in demands between, say, the postural muscles of the back (sustained activity, coarse motion) and those of the hand (fine control, intermittent activity). These differing types have been – as, by now, you will not be surprised to learn – classified in several different ways.

First of all, there is a neurophysiological differentiation. When a nerve activates a motor end plate, it elicits a 'twitch', peak force being reached in 25–100 milliseconds, depending on the type of muscle involved. If the nerve can deliver a second impulse within this time, an additional twitch can be produced, adding to the first and building the contractile force to a higher level. This mechanical summation can, up to a point, continue; therefore, the higher the frequency of nerve impulses, the more force is produced. Muscles that rely on 'rate recruitment' to generate their contractile force are known as **fast twitch** (or phasic) muscles.

There is, however, a second strategy for increasing the amount of contractile force within a muscle and that is to recruit more muscle fibres – obviously, a response that involves all of the fibres within a muscle rather than just a few will be more powerful. Muscles that employ this technique are called **slow twitch** (or tonic) muscles.

A second, anatomical classification is used so commonly that we don't even tend to think of it in physiological terms: have you ever stopped to wonder why red meat is red and white meat, white? The answer lies in the presence of **myoglobin**, a substance similar to haemoglobin that can store oxygen in muscle cells (and is red in colour). Muscle that is required to sustain moderate workloads for a sustained length of time utilizes this oxygen storage capacity, together with well-developed mitochondria and dense vascularization, to produce a steady, adequate, efficiently generated supply of ATP to its myofibrils.

At the other extreme are myocytes that meet their energy requirements through anaerobic glycolysis, which enables large amounts of energy to be liberated quickly but is less efficient. These cells are capable of short bursts of intensive activity but rely on periods of relative quiet in between to allow

**Table 4.3** Classification of muscles according to their blood supply

**Type I** Single vascular pedicle supplies whole of muscle belly

**Example**
Tensior fascia lata

**Vascular supply**
Ascending lateral circumflex femoral artery

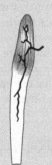

**Type II** Major vascular pedicle supported by minor pedicles that can also support the muscle

**Example**
Gracilis

**Vascular supply**
Medial circumflex femoral artery

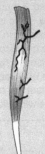

**Type III** Two separate dominant pedicles with separate supplies

**Example**
Gluteus maximus

**Vascular supply**
Superior and inferior gluteal artery

**Type IV** Multiple small pedicles that cannot, in isolation, support the muscle

**Example**
Sartorius

**Vascular supply**
Muscular branch of the femoral artery

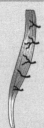

**Type V** Dominant vascular pedicle with multiple secondary pedicles

**Example**
Latissimus dorsi

**Vascular supply**
Thorocodorsal artery + thoracolumbar Perforators

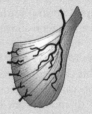

Illustrations reproduced from *Gray's Anatomy* (online edition), 2004, edited by Susan Standring, with permission from Elsevier.

**Table 4.4** Features of skeletal muscle variants

|  | Type I | Type IIA | Type IIB |
|---|---|---|---|
| Colour | Red | Red | White |
| Function | Sustained, postural forces | Powerful, fast movements | Powerful, fast movements |
| Twitch speed | Slow | Fast | Faster |
| ATP production | Aerobic | Aerobic | Anaerobic |
| Capillaries | High density | High density | Low density |
| Fatigue resistance | High | High | Low |
| Power output | Low | Intermediate | High |
| Fibre diameter | Small | Intermediate | Large |

glycogen reserves to be replenished and intracellular pH to be restored.

Red muscle can be slow or fast twitch but, obviously, it would be little use in having slow twitch white muscle. This has led to the development of the current labelling system for skeletal muscle:

- Type I. Red/slow twitch
- Type IIA. Red/fast twitch
- Type IIB. White/fast twitch.

Their differing properties are summarized in Table 4.4.

Although some textbooks will refer to certain muscles as being of these various types, it is important to remember that, in humans, *all* muscles contain *all three* types of fibre, although not in equal ratios. It should also be borne in mind that this ratio can – and does – change in response to the type and regularity of the demands placed upon it: different ratios will be found in those training for the marathon compared to sprinters compared to 'couch potatoes'. Remember, the overall number of myocytes will remain the same but it is possible for a Type I to change into a Type IIA or IIB; if the body demands required it, the innervation and internal cell physiology can adapt accordingly. The mechanism for this change is gene expression.

## Naming of skeletal muscle

You have, by now, encountered the names of several muscles, most with rather unwieldy names from dead languages and none with any of the promised explanations as to aetiology. The reason for this is that muscle naming is far simpler than it might

actually seem and it is better to understand the system before learning several hundred separate etymological origins.

 CLINICAL FOCUS

As with joints, the number of muscles in the human body is not fixed, there are several muscles that appear to be optional design features. Most muscles are consistently present, although occasional individuals may suffer from congenital absence. There are also a number of muscles that have only ever been found in a very few cadaveric dissections; again these individuals were rare exceptions rather than the rule.

Between these two extremes lie a surprising number of muscles that you may or may not have, depending largely on your genetic inheritance. For example, there is a comparatively large muscle that runs from your thoracolumbar junction to the region of your hip by the name of psoas minor ... or at least, there is in about 60% of us; the remainder simply don't have one, its absence doesn't seem to have any adverse effect; in fact, nobody seems entirely certain as to what the purpose of the muscle is (or was).

By contrast, palmaris longus appears to once have been a muscle that was of use in brachiating (swinging from branch to branch); however, one in eight of us have rightly decided that, as a species, this is a habit we are unlikely to be adopting much in the evolutionary future and have dispensed with it altogether. A further 9% have anomalous variants with odd attachments: extra or missing muscle

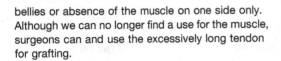

bellies or absence of the muscle on one side only. Although we can no longer find a use for the muscle, surgeons can and use the excessively long tendon for grafting.

Other variable muscles include those for abducting the first and fifth toes and rolling the tongue.

---

Most muscles are named in one of three ways: for their shape, their action or their attachments. Muscles have a minimum of two attachments (many have more) and cross a single joint (or, occasionally, two). As they contract, they move the joint. Usually, one end of the muscle remains stationary whilst the other moves towards it. The stationary end (as a rule, the proximal end) is called the **origin**; the moving end, the **insertion**. In some muscles – such as latissimus dorsi – the muscle can function in either direction and so the origin and insertion are reversible.

You are probably already aware of several muscles named for their shape, even if you weren't aware that this was the case. The deltoid muscle is named for its triangular shape (from the same Greek root as describes a river delta or delta-wing jet); the rhomboid muscle after a rhombus, a geometric shape that is approximately diamond-shaped. There are several others: 'quadratus' means square (as in quadrangle); 'rectus' means straight; 'teres', round.

Shape-related names can also refer to the anatomical features of a muscle. For example, 'biceps' means that the muscle has two heads (similarly, 'triceps' means three heads and 'quadriceps' four); 'digastric' tells you that the muscle has two (*di-*) bellies (*gastric*, the same adjective we use to describe the stomach or belly).

Then there are muscles whose name merely describes their attachments. These can be a particular mouthful until you understand their composite nature. Sternocleidomastoid, a muscle in the neck, attaches to the *mastoid* process of the skull at its proximal end and to the *sternum* and *clavicle* at the other (now you know to what the *cleido* in cleidocranial dysplasia – see above – refers). A slightly easier example is coracobrachialis, a muscle that runs from the **coracoid process** (a projection of bone from the scapular, just below the midline of the clavicle) to the *brachii* (the anatomical name for the arm, which is why swinging from handhold

to handhold by your arms – with or without palmaris longus to help you – is called brachiating).

Finally – well, almost finally – there are the most usefully named muscles. Naming a muscle for its shape tells you little or nothing about what it may do; naming for attachments allows you to infer what it might do by visualizing what happens when the muscle contracts between the two attachments, but only if you know your anatomy in detail. However, a large number of muscles are named for their action, which is particularly useful to manual medics as it saves having to memorize the information. So, for example, it is fairly obvious that, if digits are your fingers (and toes) then a muscle called 'flexor digitorum' flexes the digits and 'extensor digiti minimi' extends the smallest digit (the little finger). Once you know that 'pollex' is the Latin word for thumb (just as *'hallux'* is for the big toe) then you know what all the muscles that flex, extend, oppose, adduct and abduct the appendage are called ... or would do if it weren't for one, tiny additional wrinkle.

Quite often, there is more than one muscle for doing a particular job and the need arises to differentiate between them. This often involves the use of terms we have already discussed as modifiers. For example the biceps muscle in the arm is not unique, one of the hamstring muscles also has two heads so the former is properly termed 'biceps brachii' and the latter 'biceps femoris' (*femoral* – as in femoral nerve – means 'of the leg'). Similarly, there are two muscles whose primary function is to pronate the arm, turning it so that the palm is faced downwards. Fortunately, they are of quite differing shapes, so one is called 'pronator quadratus' and the other 'pronator teres' – the square and smooth pronators. There are though other modifiers: medial and lateral; superficial and deep; internal and external; superior and inferior which can be added so that many muscles have three or even four parts to their name like *rectus capitis posterior minor* a straight muscle that runs (from the posterior arch of the atlas) to the head (*capitis*, as in capital city) at the back of the body and is smaller than another muscle that is also straight and does much the same thing (the *rectus capitis posterior major* starts off at the axis, which is why it is bigger).

A full list of terms and meanings with examples of named muscles is given in Table 4.5. It is worth taking time to learn these basic building blocks for muscle names; there are only a few dozen yet they combine to make the names of hundreds of muscles.

**Table 4.5** Nomenclature of muscle names

| Shape | Meaning | Example |
| --- | --- | --- |
| Deltoid | Triangular | – |
| Gracilis | Slender | – |
| Lumbrical | Worm-like | Lumbricales |
| Quadratus | Square | Quadratus lumborum |
| Rectus | Straight | Rectus femoris |
| Rhomboid | Rhombus-shaped | – |
| Serratus | Serrated (tooth-like) | Serratus anterior |
| Teres | Smooth | Teres minor |
| Biceps | Two heads | Biceps brachialis |
| Triceps | Three heads | – |
| Quadriceps | Four heads | – |
| Digastric | Two bellies | – |

| **Attachment** | | |
| --- | --- | --- |
| Sternocleidomastoid | From the sternum and clavicle to the mastoid process | – |
| Coracobrachialis | From the coracoid process to the arm | – |

| **Action** | | |
| --- | --- | --- |
| Levator | Elevates | Levator scapula |
| Depressor | Lowers | Depressor septi |
| Extensor | Extends | Extensor carpi radialis |
| Flexor | Flexes | Flexor carpi radialis |
| Abductor | Abducts | Abductor pollicis |
| Adductor | Adducts | Adductor hallucis |
| Opponens | Opposes (movement of thumb to fingers) | Opponens pollicis |
| Constrictor | Constricts | Middle constrictor of pharynx |
| Dilator | Dilates | Dilator pupillae |
| Rotatores | Rotates | – |

| **Modifers** | | |
| --- | --- | --- |
| Anatomical location | e.g. Abdominis* (of the abdomen) | Rectus abdominus |
| Relative location | Superficialis | Flexor digitorum superficialis |
| | Profundus (deep to) | Flexor digitorum profundus |
| | Internal/internus | Internal pterygoid |
| | External/externus | External pterygoid |
| | Middle | Middle scalene |
| | Anterior | Anterior scalene |
| | Posterior | Posterior scalene |
| | Infra (below) | Infraspinatus |
| | Supra (above) | Supraspinatus |
| | Superior | Gemellus superior |
| | Inferior | Gemellus inferior |

*There are numerous other examples: brachii (arm), femoris (leg), oris (mouth), pectoralis (chest) – you should be familiar with these from your knowledge of anatomy; if not, look them up when you encounter them and *become* familiar with them.

## Architecture of skeletal muscle

There is one further way in which muscles can be classified, that is by the shape and direction of their fibres. Although anatomists originally made the categorization based upon appearance, it is important to remember that shape specifies function and, therefore, the architecture of individual muscles has profound implications for its biomechanical properties.

As you will see from Table 4.6, there are a number of variations on three basic themes. Some muscles are strap-like: their fibres run parallel to each other, usually over the whole length of the muscle. The broad tendons are the same width as the muscle itself. These muscles are used when the body needs to exert forces through long distances.

Others are fusiform in appearance with a muscle belly containing unidirectional fibres attached by tendons that are much thinner than the muscle. This allows the contractile force of the muscle to be concentrated into a small area, effectively multiplying its effect.

Another way of doing this is to have the muscle fibres arranged like a feather, lying either side of and attaching to a central tendon. This has the disadvantage that the muscles are no longer pulling in the same direction as the tendon but at an angle, thus only part of the vector of forces contributes to the desired contractile force. However, this is more than compensated for by the increased cross-sectional area of muscle allowed by this arrangement with a resultant increase in power. This power is often further multiplied by the fact that the tendinous attachment of the origin is larger than that of the insertion, which also helps to magnify the pressure exerted on the bone and, with it, the strength of the joint.

## Muscle action

In addition to the multitude of physiological ways in which muscle design meets the requirements of the skeletal frame, there are also biomechanical variations in the manner of muscle action. Most muscles work by **direct action**; that is, the contraction of the muscles fibres pull the tendinous insertions into the bone together, thus moving the joint. There are many examples of this in the body; brachioradialis is a typical example.

By contrast, certain muscles work by **indirect action**. This is best understood by examining the example of a muscle group that works in this manner: the quadriceps. These muscles extend the knee but, in order to 'get round the corner' created by a knee joint that is flexed, the four muscles insert not directly into the tibial tuberosity but instead into a large, sesamoid bone, the patella. This acts as a pulley, sliding between the condyles of the patella and a second tendon then runs from the inferior pole of the patella to anchor the muscle into the tibia.

It is also worth appreciating that there are certain muscles that can move more than one joint. For example, one of the quadriceps, rectus femoris, attaches not to the femur but to the anterior inferior iliac spine and thus crosses the hip joint as well as the knee joint. Although its primary action is still knee flexion, it is also a hip flexor, although quite a weak one owing to the biomechanical disadvantage through which the muscle operates in this capacity. The same is true of sartorious (hip and knee), the long head of the biceps (elbow and shoulder) and many of the hand/foot and wrist/ankle muscles, which cross the elbow and knee respectively. The most extreme example of this multi-joint action is flexor digitorum profundus (we will take the example of the fingers, though the function is duplicated in the toes). This muscle arises from the medial epicondyle of the humerus and attaches into the distal phalanges of the fingers. In doing so, it crosses the elbow, wrist, intercarpal, carpometacarpal, metacarpalphalangeal and distal interphalangeal joints. It can therefore also act as a flexor for all of these joints, even if its primary action is to flex the tips of the fingers.

It is also necessary to appreciate the fact that muscles do not work in isolation; indeed, if they did, the response to a signal from the motor cortex would be a violent, ballistic, uncontrolled contraction that would be functionally useless.

In order for a muscle to move in a smooth, coordinated, functional manner, four groups of muscles must work as a synergistic whole. The role of these muscles is best considered by taking a specific example: flexion of the elbow ... so, which muscles flex the elbow?

Biceps brachialis is the main elbow flexor, and is probably the muscle that sprang immediately to your mind. This is known as the **prime mover** as it is the muscle that does most of the work; however, the biceps muscle does not work alone – there are other muscles that cross the elbow joint and whose actions contribute to or help facilitate elbow flexion ... in fact, in most individuals, there are 10 of them; these muscles are termed **synergists**. **Essential fixators** stabilize adjacent joints, usually by simultaneous contraction of the prime movers and the **antagonists**, muscles that oppose the action of the prime movers and by *eccentric contraction* (gradual relaxation) allow smoothing of the movement, preventing an 'all or nothing' response.

**Table 4.6** Architecture of muscles

| Shape | Appearance |
|---|---|
| **Strap** | |

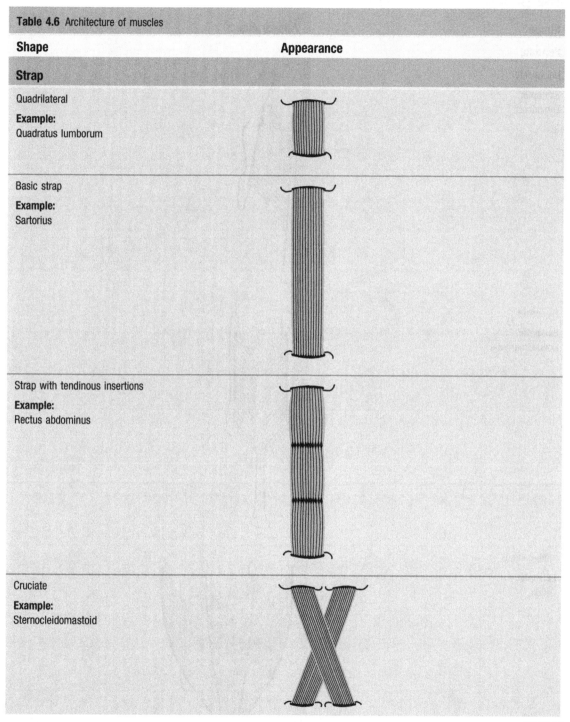

Quadrilateral

**Example:**
Quadratus lumborum

Basic strap

**Example:**
Sartorius

Strap with tendinous insertions

**Example:**
Rectus abdominus

Cruciate

**Example:**
Sternocleidomastoid

*Continued*

**Table 4.6** Architecture of muscles—Cont'd

| Shape | Appearance |
|---|---|
| **Pennate** | |
| Unipennate<br><br>**Example:**<br>Lumbricals | |
| Bipennate<br><br>**Example:**<br>Dorsal interossei | |
| Multi-pennate<br><br>**Example:**<br>Deltoid | |

**Table 4.6** Architecture of muscles—Cont'd

| Shape | Appearance |
|---|---|
| Radial<br>**Example:**<br>Tibialis anterior | |

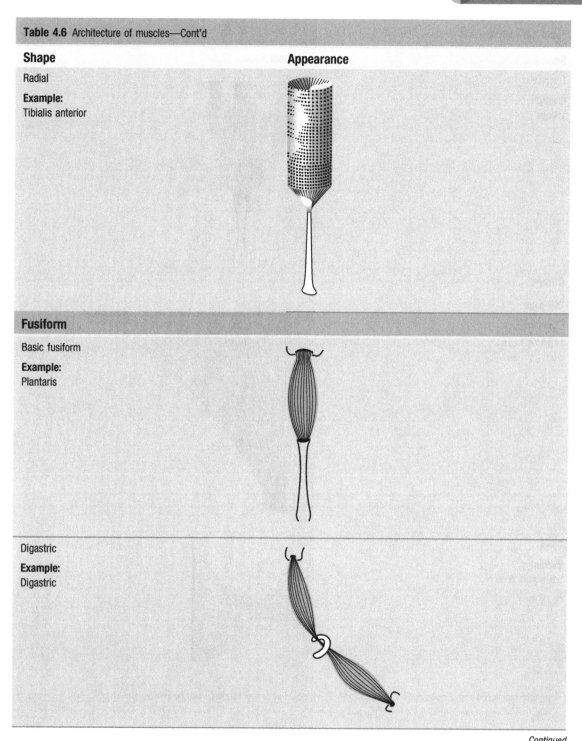

| | |
|---|---|
| **Fusiform** | |
| Basic fusiform<br>**Example:**<br>Plantaris | |
| Digastric<br>**Example:**<br>Digastric | |

*Continued*

**Table 4.6** Architecture of muscles—Cont'd

| Shape | Appearance |
|-------|-----------|
| Tricipital<br><br>**Example:**<br>Triceps | |

**Others**

| | |
|-------|-----------|
| Triangular<br><br>**Example:**<br>Temporalis | |
| Spiral<br><br>**Example:**<br>Latissimus dorsi | |

Illustrations reproduced from *Gray's Anatomy* (online edition), 2004, edited by Susan Standring, with permission from Elsevier.

## CLINICAL FOCUS

The frequently congenitally absent palmaris longus muscles, together with the virtually useless palmaris brevis (whose only known action is to wrinkle the skin of the palm) seem to be a throwback to the days when we used to brachiate … swinging through the branches of primaeval forests. However, if you are in possession of palmaris longus, you should celebrate rather that despair of yourself as an evolutionary throwback; the tendon of the muscle, which is one of the longest in the body, is often sacrificed in surgical procedures where the tendon of another muscle has been ruptured and needs to be reconstructed.

## Learning Outcomes

At the end of this chapter, the student should be able to:
- Describe the types of joints found in the body and the systems of classifications used
- Outline how joint physiology affects biomechanical properties
- Introduce the physiological properties of different muscle types
- Explain the classification of muscle types and the biomechanical consequences of muscle anatomy
- Compare the properties of tendons and ligaments and discuss the neurological and biomechanical consequences of their architecture and anatomical positioning.

## CHECK YOUR EXISTING KNOWLEDGE: ANSWERS

Mark your answers using the guide below to give yourself a score:
  1  A joint with limited movement [3]
  2  They are all types of true suture [4]
  3  a  Complex, compound, diarthrotic synovial bicondylar joint [5]
     b  Simple, diarthrotic synovial ball and socket (spheroidal) joint [5]
     c  Simple, diarthrotic synovial hinge (ginglymus) [5]
     d  Amphiarthroic symphysis (secondary cartilaginous) joint [3]
  4  Sternoclavicular joint *or* 1st metacarpophalangeal joint [3]
  5  You would, by default, make a surgical referral. This is not always appropriate (the patient may not be a suitable candidate for surgery and the outcomes for ligamentous repairs are not the same for each joint), and manual therapy can have a part to play in both treatment and rehabilitation; nevertheless, it should be recognized that surgery is often the treatment of choice. By definition, in a Grade III tear, the body will not be able to repair the damage itself. [4]
  6  Actin and myosin plus adenosine triphosphate (ATP) [3]
  7  a  Named for its attachments (sternum, clavicle, mastoid process) [3]
     b  Named for its action (flexes the finger) plus it is (profundus) deeper than another muscle that also flexes the finger [3]
     c  Named for its shape (rhomboidal) [2]
  8  a  Muscle fibres run obliquely along one side of a tendon [2]
     b  Muscle fibres are parallel and run the length of the muscle between two broad tendons [2]
     c  Muscle belly with curved longitudinal fibres lying between two much thinner tendons [3]

**How to interpret the results:**

46–50: You have a firm grasp of the principles and facts contained in this chapter and should move on to Chapter 5.

36–45: Although you have understood most of the basic principles involved, you need to add some of the finer details that you will require as a manual therapist.

0–35: You need to study this chapter in some detail in order to acquire the necessary grounding needed in future chapters.

If you have scored less than 30 on retesting yourself at the end of studying this chapter, then it could be that you need to augment some of your basic knowledge, particularly anatomy. Presumed knowledge for this chapter includes familiarity with the skeletal system (names and locations of bones); if this is not in place, it might explain why you are having difficulties.

# Bibliography

Allen, R., Schwarz, C. (Eds.), 1998. The Chambers dictionary. Chambers Harrap, Edinburgh.

Beers, M.H., Berkow, R. (Eds.), 1999. In: The Merck manual of diagnosis and therapy, seventeenth ed. Merck, West Point.

Frymann, V.M., 1971. A study of the rhythmic motions of the living cranium. J. Am. Osteopath. Assoc. 70 (9), 928–945.

Green, J.H., Silver, P.H.S., 1981. An introduction to human anatomy. Oxford University Press, Oxford.

Guebert, G.M., Yochum, T.R., Rowe, L.J., 1996. Congenital abnormalities and skeletal variants. In: Yochum, T.R., Rowe, L.J. (Eds.), Essentials of skeletal radiology. Williams & Wilkins, Baltimore, pp. 307–326.

Hamilton, W. (Ed.), 1976. Joints. In: Textbook of human anatomy, second ed. Macmillan, London, p. 35.

Howat, J.M.P., 1999. Cranial motion and cranial categories. In: Chiropractic: anatomy and physiology of sacro occipital technique. Cranial Communication Systems, Oxford, pp. 61–128.

Howat, J.M.P., 1999. Paediatrics. In: Chiropractic: anatomy and physiology of sacro occipital technique. Cranial Communication Systems, Oxford, pp. 201–320.

Koenigsberg, R. (Ed.), 1989. Churchill's illustrated medical dictionary. Churchill Livingstone, New York.

Koo, C.C., Roberts, H.N., 1997. The palmaris longus tendon: another variation in its anatomy. J. Hand Surg. [Br] 22 (1), 138–139.

McGill, S.M., 2007. Lumbar spine stability: mechanism of injury and restabilization. In: Liebenson, C. (Ed.), Rehabilitation of the spine: a practitioner's manual, second ed. Lippincott Williams and Wilkins, Baltimore, pp. 93–111.

Moore, K.L., 1985. Joints. In: Clinically oriented anatomy, second ed. Williams & Wilkins, Baltimore, pp. 33–37.

Pick, M.G., 1999. Accessible sutures of the cranial vault. In: Cranial sutures: analysis, morphology and manipulative strategies. Eastland Press, Seattle, pp. 89–186.

Retzlaff, E.W., Michael, D.K., Roppel, R.M., 1975. Cranial bone mobility. J. Am. Osteopath. Assoc. 74 (9), 869–873.

Schafer, R.C., 1983. Basic neuromuscular considerations. In: Clinical biomechanics: musculoskeletal actions and reactions. Williams and Wilkins, Baltimore, pp. 128–170.

Schauf, C.L., Moffett, D.F., Moffett, S.B., 1990. Skeletal, cardiac and smooth muscle. In: Human physiology: Foundations and frontiers (International Edition). Times Mirror/Mosby College Publishing, St Louis, pp. 284–317.

Standring, S. (Ed.), 2005. Functional anatomy of the musculoskeletal system. In: Gray's anatomy: the anatomical basis of clinical practice. Elsevier, Edinburgh, pp. 83–135.

Thibodeau, G., Patton, K., 2006. Anatomy of the muscular system. In: Anatomy and Physiology, sixth ed. Mosby, Philadelphia, (Chapter 10), e-book.

Thorne, J.O., Collcott, T.C., 1984. Chambers biographical dictionary, Revised ed. W & R Chambers, Edinburgh.

Walther, D.S., 1988. Somatognathic system. In: Applied kinesiology: synopsis. Systems DC, Pueblo, pp. 343–393.

# Chapter Five

5

# The physics of anatomy

## CHAPTER CONTENTS

Check your existing knowledge . . . . . . . 99
Joint movement . . . . . . . . . . . . . . . . . 99
  Introduction . . . . . . . . . . . . . . . . . . . 99
Arthrokinematics . . . . . . . . . . . . . . . . 102
  Roll and glide . . . . . . . . . . . . . . . . . 102
  Spin . . . . . . . . . . . . . . . . . . . . . . . 102
  Circumduction . . . . . . . . . . . . . . . . . 104
Joint features . . . . . . . . . . . . . . . . . 105
  The lower extremity . . . . . . . . . . . . . 105
  The upper extremity . . . . . . . . . . . . . 106

The spine and pelvis . . . . . . . . . . . . . 107
Temporomandibular joint . . . . . . . . . . 115
Posture . . . . . . . . . . . . . . . . . . . . . 116
  Balance . . . . . . . . . . . . . . . . . . . . . 117
  Seated posture . . . . . . . . . . . . . . . . 118
  Recumbent posture . . . . . . . . . . . . . 119
Gait . . . . . . . . . . . . . . . . . . . . . . . . 120
Learning outcomes . . . . . . . . . . . . . . 121
Bibliography . . . . . . . . . . . . . . . . . . . 122

## CHECK YOUR EXISTING KNOWLEDGE

It is highly unlikely that any undergraduate will already have encompassed the material contained in this chapter or considered its consequences with regard to manual therapy.

You should therefore read this chapter in full.

# Joint movement

## Introduction

In Chapter 4, we encountered a wide variety of joint types and also explored some ways in which the basic templates are modified from joint to joint to meet the specific needs of regional biomechanics. Now, we shall explore these variations and the strictures they place on movement in more detail.

Whilst we do this, there are two fundamental principles that we should keep in mind.

### Structure specifies function

There is a reason that joints have evolved to be the shape that they are – remember also that bone is a vibrant, metabolically active, dynamic, constantly changing structure that responds to the physiological and biomechanical stresses placed upon it.

### Stability and mobility are mutually exclusive

If you take, as an example, the shoulder and the hip, both are ball and socket joints and both are moved by similar groups of muscles; unsurprising when you consider man's evolution from quadrupedal

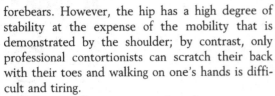

forebears. However, the hip has a high degree of stability at the expense of the mobility that is demonstrated by the shoulder; by contrast, only professional contortionists can scratch their back with their toes and walking on one's hands is difficult and tiring.

Before we begin to consider the movements of individual joints, we should review the global mechanisms that restrict and facilitate movement.

## Muscles

A joint can only be moved in a given direction if there is a muscle that facilitates the action. Although this may seem a self-evident truth, most anatomy teaches only the most common muscles and muscle configurations; there is, in reality, a huge variation in the attachments of even the most standard muscles and many more muscles that are variable, appearing in some individuals and not in others.

This is why some 70% of individuals of European descent can roll their tongues whilst the remainder of the population is incapable of this action. We have already looked at the variability of palmaris longus both in its presence and its attachments; however its variability is by no means unique. Actions such as abduction of the fifth ray is impossible for a significant number of individuals who lack the abductor digiti minimi muscle; 40% of individuals have a psoas minor muscle in addition to the psoas major, which can significantly affect the biomechanics of the thoracolumbar junction; even the biceps brachii – named for its two heads – can frequently lack a second head ... or have up to five of them!

## Ligaments

The image of ligaments acting like a sheet of powerful elastic to limit the motion of a joint and render it stable is one that is frequently presented to the student; in fact, the integral strength of individual ligaments does very little to support most joints. Stability actually comes from the far more powerful muscles and tendons, though the ligaments do have a crucial role to play.

Ligaments have a number of neurological structures embedded within them that fall under the broad heading of **mechanoreceptors**. Stretching of the ligament causes these receptors to be stimulated and send information to the central nervous system.

Some receptors such as *Ruffini end organs* and the receptors found in capsular ligaments and muscle spindles deliver continuous information about the relative position of muscles and joints and are used to facilitate balance, coordination and joint position sense. Other receptors such as Pacinian corpuscles are very much more rapidly adapting and react to stimuli with a sudden burst of high-frequency impulses, which quickly die away even when the stimulus is maintained. These signals are conducted to the postcentral gyrus of the central cortex via large-diameter, myelinated neurons that have high conduction velocities. Association fibres then run to the motor cortex; this means that if the ankle starts to invert signals run very rapidly to the central control systems, which send equally rapid messages to the evertor muscles of the ankle, causing them to contract and maintain the body's balance.

## Kinematic chains

The human body can be regarded mechanically as a series of rigid *members* or *links* (bones), connected by *kinematic pairs* (joints). A **kinematic chain** consists of a series of two or more members connected by a joint.

Functionally, there are two types of chain:

### Open loop chain

If one end of the chain is fixed, then individual kinematic pairs can move independently of each other. Examples of open loop chains in the human body include the upper extremities and the cervical spine/head – if you flex your elbow, it is possible to do so without moving the shoulder, wrist or fingers.

### Closed loop chain

By contrast, if both ends of the chain are fixed, then individual kinematic pairs cannot move independently of each other; by moving one element of the chain, *all* other elements must move to a greater or lesser extent. There are many examples of closed loop chains in the human body including the thoracic spine and ribs; the pelvis; and the bones of the cranium. When both feet are on the ground, the lower extremities and pelvis form a closed loop chain – if you flex your knee, it is not possible to do so without moving both feet, the contralateral knee, both hips and the pelvis and lumbosacral junction.

## CLINICAL FOCUS

The concept of kinematic chains is essential to the understanding of the interrelationship between the joints; without this, treatment will invariably be directed only at the area of symptomatology rather than the possible underlying cause.

This is why foot problems can manifest as low back pain; why sacroiliac dysfunction can cause cervicogenic headaches and why shoulder problems often require assessment of the thoracic and cervical spine, ribs and elbow.

The situation is made yet more complex by the fact that there are several muscles that cross – and therefore can move – more than one joint: biceps (elbow and shoulder); sartorius and rectus femorus (hip and knee); the flexors and extensors of the wrist and ankle, feet and hands; and many of the spinal intrinsic muscles.

Two other muscles that cross multiple spinal segments and can cause associated – and often overlooked – dysfunction are the psoas (which inserts in the crura of the diaphragm and all five lumbar vertebrae, including the annular fibres of the discs, and blends with the fibres of iliacus before inserting into the lesser trochanter of the hip in the groin, crossing as it does so, the sacroiliac joints) and the latissimus dorsi (whose complex attachments can be simplified by picturing the muscle as running from the iliac crest to T6 and thence via the inferior angle of the scapula into the humerus).

## Degrees of freedom

As we have seen previously, all joint motion can be described by rotation about three orthogonal axes ($X$, $Y$ and $Z$) and translation in three orthogonal planes ($XY$, $XZ$, $YZ$). There are therefore three possible rotations and three possible translations; each one of these represents a **degree of freedom**.

For most joints, in the human body, translations are negligible and do not need consideration. Although a few joints do have pure translatory movements, this is usually very limited and almost all gross movement is by rotation alone.

When movement is limited to rotation about one axis, as it is in the phalanges of the fingers and toes, a joint is termed *uniaxial*: that is, it has just one degree of freedom. If independent movement can occur around two axes, it is *biaxial*, with two degrees of freedom. The first carpometacarpal joint is a good example of a biaxial joint: it can flex and extend; it can also adduct and abduct.

The shoulder and hip are both good examples of *triaxial* joints, being able to rotate about all three axes (flexion–extension; abduction–adduction; internal rotation–external rotation). Although these ball and socket joints can rotate about many chosen axes (and, for this reason, they are often termed *multiaxial*), for each position there will still be a maximum of three orthogonal axes, which means that there will still be three degrees of freedom.

As a rule, each class of synovial joint has a set number of degrees of freedom and these are given in Table 5.1. Plane (gliding) joints can translate, although these movements are usually heavily

**Table 5.1** Classification of joints with typical degrees of freedom

| Name (English) | Name (Latin) | Example | Degrees of freedom |
|---|---|---|---|
| Hinge | (Ginglymus) | Interphalangeal joints | 1 (Flexion–extension) |
| Pivot | (Trochoid) | Proximal radio-ulnar joint | 1 (Pronation–supination) |
| Ball & socket | (Spheroidal) | Hip joint | 3 (Flexion–extension; abduction–adduction; internal rotation–external rotation) |
| Saddle | (Sellaris) | 1st metacarpal-phalangeal joint | 2 (Flexion–extension; abduction–adduction) |
| Condyloid | (Ellipsoid) | Radiocarpal joint | 2 (Flexion–extension; abduction–adduction) |
| Bicondylar | (Condylar) | Knee joint (femorotibial) | 2 (Flexion–extension plus a limited amount of rotational movement) |

curtailed by ligamentous attachments. Usually plane joints such as the zygapophyseal, intertarsal and intercarpal joints have two degrees of translational freedom, although some authorities declare joint gapping to represent a third degree of freedom.

## Arthrokinematics

The study of movement occurring intrinsically between the articular surfaces of joints is called **arthrokinematics**. All joint surfaces are either concave or convex (even 'plane' joints are not completely flat) in a reciprocal fashion. The most obvious example of this is the spherical head of the femur sitting in the cup-shaped hemispherical concavity of the acetabulum.

### Roll and glide

So far, we have considered joint movement in terms of pure rotation; of course, although this model is entirely acceptable from a functional standpoint, it does not reflect how joints actually work. If a joint were to rotate and only rotate, it would simply roll out of its socket and dislocate (Fig. 5.1A).

Obviously, this does not happen; instead, a combination of the ligamentous attachments, the line of force of the articular muscles and the lubricating effect of the synovial fluid allow the joint to **roll** and simultaneously **slide** (or *glide*), so that the joint moves in the desired fashion without losing its articular integrity (Fig. 5.1B).

A useful analogy is to consider a car tyre: as the tyre *rolls* it *rotates* along the road. If the surface is made slippery by ice or mud then, when the brakes are applied, the car skids: now it is continuing to travel along the road even though the tyre is stationary; this is *gliding*, which is a *translatory* movement. If the two movements are combined, for instance if the car is attempting to accelerate on ice and the wheels are spinning, then we have a combination of the two movements: the wheel is rotating forwards and translating backwards at an equal rate, the net effect is that the car remains stationary.

### Spin

There is an additional intraarticular motion that we need to consider: **spin**. This is rotary motion of the distal part of the kinematic chain about the longitudinal axis of the proximal part – a concept better understood if visualized (Fig. 5.2).

Spin can occur alone or in conjunction with roll and glide: in pronation–supination of the forearm, it occurs independently; in flexion–extension of

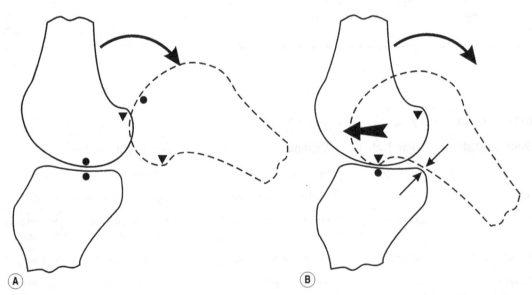

(A)                                                  (B)

**Figure 5.1** • When a joint moves, it must undergo a combination of movements. If we consider a simple hinge (ginglymus) joint, if it were to roll only (A), then it would simply dislocate. Instead, the joint undergoes a combination of roll and slide, which allows the joint surfaces to remain congruent (B).

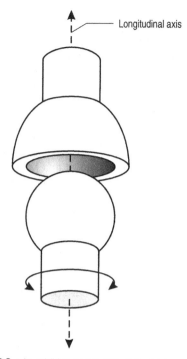

the knee it accompanies roll and glide and, as we shall subsequently discover, plays an important part in the knee's stability.

When roll, glide and spin act together, it can have an interesting effect on joint motion. For example, we can externally rotate the shoulder by the simple action of resting our palm against the thigh and then turning the palm outwards so that it faces forwards; this motion is a combination of roll and glide. We can achieve the same effect by starting in the same position and then flexing the shoulder to 90°, horizontally abducting it by 90° and then adducting it back to our thigh (Fig. 5.3). The translation of the glide component, in conjunction with the rotation of the roll and spin components has caused an external rotation of 90°; the palm is now facing forwards, it is no longer resting against our thigh even though no specific rotation has taken place.

**Figure 5.2** • In addition to roll and glide, joints can also spin; this is the motion seen in internal and external rotation of the abducted shoulder and consists of rotation about the longitudinal axis of the proximal part of the kinematic pair.

### CLINICAL FOCUS

Assessing the 'normal' movement of a joint is an essential tool in the diagnostic armoury of the musculoskeletal clinician – it has a high level of inter- and intra-examiner reliability, particularly in these modern days of sophisticated goniometric measuring devices.

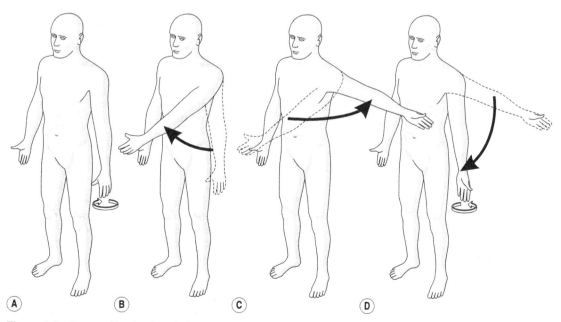

**Figure 5.3** • The combined action of roll spin and glide causes external rotation of the shoulder when it is flexed (A to D), horizontally abducted and adducted.

However, this begs the question of what constitutes normal: a general decline in flexibility of joints occurs with age, although this is much more noticeable in weight-bearing joints than in those of the upper extremity and, throughout life, females have greater flexibility than males.

This means that, say, right cervical rotation of 95° in a 21-year-old female and 55° in an 81-year-old male may both be perfectly normal. It is therefore a much more useful measurement when compared contralaterally (if the pensioner's left cervical rotation was 70°, the right would no longer be regarded as normal) and for assessing outcome measures (does the range of motion equalize following treatment).

It is also important to differentiate between *active* range of motion and *passive* range of motion, which can be an important clinical indicator. For example, patients with shoulder pain often complain that their shoulder starts to hurt at around 80°–90° of abduction; however, when the physician moves their arm passively, no pain is felt. This difference between pain with muscular effort and no pain on passive joint motion strongly suggest a musculotendinous aetiology for the problem, most commonly a rotator cuff impingement syndrome.

# Circumduction

In the same way that roll, spin and glide can be combined to produce new movements, flexion–extension and abduction–adduction can also be combined to produce a new type of movement: **circumduction**.

Circumduction comprises successive flexion, abduction, extension and adduction; it occurs when the distal end of a long bone circumscribes the base of a cone that has its apex at the joint in question, it is the action that we would make if we held our finger at arm's length and used it to draw a circle in the air. Circumduction is also possible in the metacarpophalangeal joints, wrist, elbow, ankle, knee, hips and in the trunk and cervical spine.

## CLINICAL FOCUS

The summative movements of the human body are part of what define us as human: although we have many similarities to other primates, the human skeleton has many distinctive differences to those of chimpanzees, gorillas or other primates. It is also distinct from other humans – *homo sapiens neanderthalensis* had easily recognizable morphological differences: a larger cranial capacity with many other differences in the skull's anatomy; a longer, bowed femur with a shorter tibia and fibula; a more gracile pelvis; wider collar bones and ribs; and larger knee-caps.

These differences, presumed to have arisen from adaptation to living in Northern Eurasia during the last period of glaciation, suggest that Neanderthals would have had different biomechanical features to *homo sapiens sapiens*, modern man. Their thicker bones and shorter levers would have given them greater strength whilst their broad chests and shorter stature gave them a smaller surface area to volume ratio, more efficient at retaining body heat.

However, their joints would have been less flexible, their gait less efficient and their physiology required a high level of protein – Neanderthals were thought to be mainly carnivorous and thus more dependent on hunting for food. They suffered from many of the same conditions as we do today: gum disease, osteomyelitis, bone tumours and degenerative joint disease (osteoarthritis) – their heavier build and more robust morphology with an associated increase in joint loading made them particularly susceptible to this last condition.

One other interesting development in the evolution of human joints is the change in the sacroiliac joint, probably the most common source of low back pain. Although orthopaedic texts frequently suggest that this is as a result of the change from quadrupedal to bipedal status; in fact, it is much more to do with the broadening of the pelvis required for successful parturition of babies with large cranial vaults.

Successful parturition is a far more powerful selective force than locomotive considerations; its effects on reproductive success are immediate and profound. Humans have evolved circular pelvic midplanes to produce an adequate birth canal by modifying pelvic form in order to accentuate the area of the midplane; its original *australopithecine* form would be wholly inadequate by modern requirements.

The morphological changes that were effected between *Australopithecus afarensis* and *Homo sapiens* cannot have reflected improved mechanics: had the long femoral neck and pronounced lateral iliac flare been *retained* in the descendants of

A. afarensis (along with a reduction in *only* the relative interacetabular distance in the pelvis), the mechanical advantage to the abductors in modern humans would now be far greater than it actually is. Therefore, the reduction of these mechanical benefits must have been the selective advantages in increasing the dimensions of the birth canal rather than a response to any change in gait pattern – in other words, our big brains are what give us our bad backs.

# Joint features

Most of our consideration of joints so far has been generalized; however, there are specific joints that have special or unusual features or are of particular clinical interest and, in this section, we shall consider them in turn.

# The lower extremity

As we have already seen, the lower extremity when in normal stance acts as a closed loop kinematic chain with each element interdependent to a greater or lesser degree.

## The foot

As entire books have been written about the foot and an entire profession (podiatry) is dedicated to assessing and treating the pathomechanics of the area, it is self-evident that comprehensive analysis of the area is beyond the scope of this text: a quarter of all the bones in the body are found in the foot. However, there are certain key biomechanical points that need to be grasped if the fundamentals of lower kinematic chain function are to be understood.

The foot can be regarded as two connected closed loop kinematic chains. The forefoot has one longitudinal arch, situated medially, and two transverse arches. The more posterior of these crosses the longitudinal arch to produce the typical biconcave appearance of the posteromedial forefoot; it is this that is reduced in *pes planus* (flat feet). The anterior transverse arch lies underneath the metatarsal phalangeal joints; collapse of this is closely associated with pain in the area: *metatarsalgia*. The forefoot can pronate or supinate (to a limited extent) with respect to the hindfoot (talus and calcaneus).

## CLINICAL FOCUS

Fewer than 1% of feet demonstrate abnormalities at birth; of those that do, the most common are polydactyly (extra toes), syndactyly ('webbed' or fused toes) and talipes equinovarus (club foot). However, by the age of 5 years, 41% of the population has a detectable degree of foot dysfunction and this figure increases to 80% by early adulthood.

Pedal pathomechanics, which in themselves can be caused by aberrant biomechanics elsewhere in the lower kinematic chain, can produce and maintain far-reaching effects and have been associated with pelvic and spinal distortions causing distant somatic and/or visceral disturbances. These will often remain resistant to treatment or quickly return if the problem is left unresolved; treatment traditionally consists of orthotics, which should be custom-made for maximum efficacy, and prescribed exercises.

Although such distortions are often associated with specific conditions such as pes planus, metatarsalgia, *calcaneal heel spurs* and *plantar fasciitis*, the foot can remain asymptomatic if the biomechanical dysfunction is sufficiently compensated for elsewhere.

## Ankle

The unusual feature of the tibiofibulotalar joint is that it is a compound joint in which the tibia, fibula and crural interosseous ligament act together to form a mortice into which the tenon of the talus inserts. It has two degrees of freedom: plantarflexion–dorsiflexion and, more limited, eversion–inversion. It is also unique in the body in that it is the only example of a second order lever.

## Knee

The knee is the largest joint in the body. It is a remarkably stable joint; this ability to bear several times the body's own weight arises from what happens when the joint is fully extended. To understand this, there is a new concept that needs to be introduced, the **close-packed position** (Fig. 5.4). The fit of reciprocal convex–concave surfaces is precise only at one end of the most common excursion of the joint, which is the key feature of the close-packed position. In all other positions the surfaces are not fully congruent, and the joint is said to be *loose-packed*.

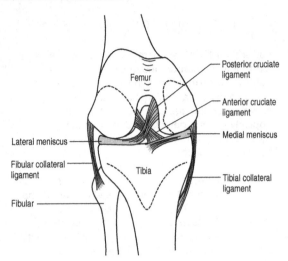

**Figure 5.4 •** The knee.

As the knee approaches full extension, the femur rotates internally with respect to the tibia; the last 10° of extension is accompanied by approximately 6° of rotation. This rotation seats the femoral condyles in the rings of the medial and lateral menisci, also bringing the ligaments to tension.

So stable is this position that the knee cannot be flexed again unless the tibia is externally rotated by the action of the popliteus muscle; hypertonicity in this muscle can significantly disrupt normal knee mechanics and contribute to meniscal damage. Because of the natural valgus deformity of the knee, known as the **Q-angle** (10° in men, 15° in women), the medial meniscus has a higher degree of loading and is more vulnerable to damage and degeneration.

---

### CLINICAL FOCUS

More than any other joint, the knee suffers from a relationship between direct loading and the development of degenerative joint disease. There is virtually a straight-line relationship between increased body mass index and the chances of developing degenerative joint disease; if you are clinically obese, the chances of developing osteoarthritis in the knee is 13.6 times greater than if your body mass index is normal.

Dietary advice therefore plays an important role in the management of knee disorders and should also be a consideration for prophylaxis.

---

### Hip

The hip has, to an extent, been dealt with previously; however, there are several interesting facts associated with the hip. Firstly, the joint is unusual in acting (in certain circumstances) as a first order lever. When the gluteus maximus extends the joint when in a neutral weight-bearing position, the line of action of the muscle (effort) lies between the pivot (the joint) and the load (weight of the leg), creating a rare example in the body of a first class lever.

Because of the length of the angulated femoral neck, so important to our ability to balance, walk and run on two legs, this area has a high degree of loading and is particularly vulnerable to fracture in osteoporosis. A common myth is that sufferers from this condition fracture their hips when they fall; in fact, they tend to fall when their hips fracture, usually as a result of a slight increase in normal axial loading through a stumble or when carrying heavy objects.

## The upper extremity

We have already dealt with several joints in the arm in some detail; however, there are a couple of other wrinkles to the limb that we have not yet covered.

### Wrist

The radiocarpal joint is a compound, complex joint that involves five bones and a fibrocartilage disc. As with its corollary in the lower extremity, the ankle, the joint has two degrees of freedom and allows flexion–extension and abduction–adduction. The nerves and tendon sheaths run through constricted 'tunnels' (carpal tunnel, tunnel of Guyon, radial tunnel), which are prime sites for neural entrapment through degenerative change, acute trauma, congenital abnormalities or repetitive strain.

### Elbow

The elbow, which of course actually comprises three joints: humero-ulnar, humeroradial and radio-ulnar, is also a site for neurological entrapment, most commonly as a consequence of trauma, repetitive strain or muscular abnormalities. It is a common site for ulnar neuropathy and the radial and median nerves can also be entrapped either before or after giving off their major branches, the posterior and anterior interosseous nerves.

## Shoulder

The shoulder is the most complicated joint in the body. It is in fact a complex of three joints (gleno-humeral, acromioclavicular and sternoclavicular) and one articulation (the movement of the scapula across the superior seven ribs). It also contains over two dozen bursae, a similar number of ligaments and is controlled by a dozen or so muscles. Somewhat surprisingly, the whole complex is uniquely controlled by a single nerve root ($C_5$) – every other joint has dual supply; the hip is controlled by three contiguous levels.

We have already discussed the effects of spin in the glenohumeral joint; however, there is another aspect of spin that probably passes unnoticed so automatically does it occur. When we fully abduct our arm, the greater tuberosity of the humerus (into which insert the tendons of supraspinatus, infraspinatus and teres minor) approximates to the acromion process and would, as the arm reaches 90° of abduction, impinge upon these tendinous insertions as they pass through the sub-acromial tunnel.

This does not happen, because the arm automatically spins through 180° of external rotation so that the greater tuberosity is moved out of the way – try performing the action without rotating the arm (use caution!) and see what happens.

## CLINICAL FOCUS

Adhesive capsulitis is the medical term for 'frozen shoulder', although the lay usage of this latter term is often much looser. The condition is rare in people younger than 55 years of age unless they have diabetes and is the result of inflammation, scarring, thickening and shrinkage of the joint capsule, most commonly as the result of a precipitating injury.

It can commonly affect motion around all three orthogonal axes and reduce or eliminate roll, glide and spin. Typically, this will reduce abduction to the point where the only significant component of this motion comes from the scapulothoracic articulation, which is responsible for approximately one-third of this movement. The reduction of abduction to less than 60°with early scapula movement (in a normal shoulder, this does not begin to at least 45°) is almost pathognomoic for adhesive capsulitis.

## The spine and pelvis

The spine and pelvis provide the conduit for the central nervous system and its synaptic connections with its counterparts in the peripheral nervous system. The dura mater anchors into the internal structures of the superior three cervical vertebrae and into the second sacral tubercle; it is also attached to the vertebrae in between by means of small, cruciform *dentate ligaments*.

The spine also acts as a shock absorber, cushioning forces transmitted upwards from the lower limbs and downwards from the body's weight and weight bearing. These forces are absorbed and redistributed by several means:

- The normal curves of the spine:
  - cervical lordosis (35°–45°)
  - thoracic lyphosis (7°–66°, dependent on age and sex)
  - lumbar lordosis (50°–60°)
- The traberculae of the cancellous bone
- The intervertebral discs
- The resting tension of the intrinsic spinal musculature.

The role of the normal spinal curves is to increase the resistance of the spinal column to compressive forces. This resistance can be quantified:

$$R = N_c^2 + 1$$

where $R$ is the resistance to compression and $N_c$ is the number of curves.

This means that a spine with no curves would have a relative resistance of one; a neonate, who has a single full-spine C-curve would have twice the resistance; however, an adult spine with its four curves has *10* times the compressive resistance of a straight column.

 **DICTIONARY DEFINITION**

**LORDOSIS**

From the Greek word *lordos*, meaning 'bent backwards', lordosis refers to the curves of the spine that are convex anteriorly and form the nape of the neck and the small of the back.

**KYPHOSIS**

The reverse of a lordosis is a kyphosis, a curve that is convex posteriorly; the thoracic spine and pelvis ordinarily demonstrate this feature. It comes from the Greek word *kuphos*, meaning 'hunchback'; the medical term for this is hyperkyphosis or, when combined with a lateral curve, kyphoscoliosis.

## SCOLIOSIS

As well as the normal anteroposterior curves of the spine, a significant number of people develop a lateral curve(s) – scoliosis. These are generally defined as C-curves (convex either to the left or right) or S-curves (one curve convex in one direction followed by a second curve convex to the other side). A scoliosis is defined clinically by its range, the upper and lower limits; its angulation, most commonly measured by the Cobb angle (Fig. 5.5); and its apex.

Scoliosis is a symptom rather than a disease; there are over two dozen congenital and acquired causes. The most common of these is juvenile idiopathic scoliosis, which has an incidence of almost 1:20. Considerable controversy exists as to the relative merits and efficacy of management protocols, which most commonly comprise physical therapy, bracing or, in progressive cases with a curve greater that 40°, surgical fixation.

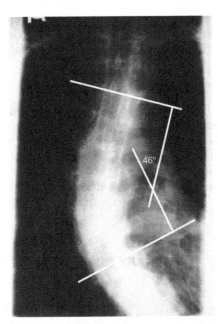

**Figure 5.5 •** Scoliosis can be evaluated using the Cobb (more properly Cobb-Lippman) method. A line is drawn along the superior vertebral end-plate of the most superior, most angulated vertebra. The same is done to the inferior end-plate of the most inferior, most angulated vertebra. Perpendicular lines are then constructed from each of the two lines and their angle of intersection measured.

It is also a highly flexible and mobile (closed loop) kinematic chain, combining both rigidity and flexibility; together with the cranium, it is referred to as the **axial skeleton**. It ordinarily comprises seven cervical, twelve thoracic and five lumbar vertebrae plus five sacral and three coccygeal vertebrae, fused into solid plates though comprising the same embryological template.

## CLINICAL FOCUS

Although the composition of the spinal column and sacrum are often quoted as if they were invariable, in fact up to one-third of the population show variation from this arrangement. Perhaps surprisingly, the prevalence for **transitional segments** is uncertain; various anatomists and radiologists quote the incidence as anywhere between 4% and 34%; there is even disagreement about whether or not there is any correlation between anomalous vertebrae and spinal pain.

A transitional segment is one that does not display the characteristics of the area of the spine with which it is associated. All vertebrae have the same basic template; however, the adaptations for cervical vertebrae (mobility), thoracic spine (rib cage), lumbar spine (stability) and sacrum (pelvic articulation) are very different. This difference is at its least in the junctional areas: occipitocervical, cervicothoracic, thoracolumbar and lumbosacral spine. Regularly, vertebrae in these areas will take on some or all of the characteristics of the adjacent areas.

Patients can appear to have six lumbar vertebrae owing to lumbarization of the first sacral segment, which will often have enlarged transverse processes that can articulate with the sacrum forming **accessory joints**. The reverse can also occur with fusion of the inferior lumbar segment into the sacrum. **Accessory ribs** can appear on the L1 or C7 segments or ribs can be absent from the T1 or T12 vertebrae giving the suggestion of a greater or lesser number of thoracic vertebrae.

The literature has traditionally associated 'cervical ribs' with thoracic outlet compression syndrome – interference with the brachial plexus or associated nerve roots as they travel into, through and out of the thoracic outlet. In fact, although thoracic outlet compression is a fairly common cause of upper limb neuropathy, cervical ribs syndrome is a fairly rare cause; fewer than 2% of cervical ribs are symptomatic in the 2% of patients who have them – functional entrapment between the anterior and medial scalenes, pectoralis minor muscles and first rib is far more common.

## Functional spinal unit

We met with the concept of the functional spinal unit in Chapter 4: two adjacent vertebrae with their shared joints (two paraspinal zygapophyseal, or facet, joints plus the intervertebral disc (absent at C1/2), muscles and ligaments.

Movement of any given functional spinal unit needs to be considered as a whole–it is a closed loop kinematic chain and, as such, all three joints are invariably involved in any movement. The unit also demonstrates the full six degrees of freedom: it can rotate about all three orthogonal axes (flexion–extension, left lateral flexion–right lateral flexion, left rotation–right rotation); however, it can also translate in all three orthogonal planes (anterior–posterior, left–right, compression–distraction).

Although these translatory movements are slight, they are nevertheless important; indeed, without the continual loading and unloading of the disc, the avascular glycoprotein nucleus would not get adequate nutrition.

Because of the interrelationship of the three-joint complex, functional spinal units demonstrate **coupled motion**, that is voluntary, or active, movement in one degree of freedom will create involuntary, or passive, movement in a second degree of freedom. This is most notable – and clinically significant – in the case of lateral flexion and rotation; however, in the lumbar spine, lateral flexion is associated with contralateral rotation, whilst in the cervical spine, it is associated with ipsilateral rotation. Coupled motion is far more restricted in the thoracic spine owing to the presence of the ribs, which articulate via the costovertebral and costotransverse joints. These two joints themselves demonstrate coupled motion on normal respiratory motion.

## Sacroiliac joint

The sacroiliac joint is a one-off that defies classification and whose function – and dysfunction – warrants a textbook in its own right. It is typically described as 'boot-shaped' with the shorter part forming the superior, diarthrodial, synovial portion and the longer, inferior, amphiarthrotic portion being taken up with the *interosseous sacroiliac ligament*. This is a generalization; the joint can demonstrate a significant degree of morphological variability not only between individuals, but in the same individual from left to right.

As with all plane joints there is a slight convexity-concavity of the opposing surface; unlike other plane joints, the adult joint has marked irregularities, which mirror each other across the joint surface. These again vary from individual to individual and from side to side but appear to give the joint – which bears the full weight of the upper body – an added degree of stability, which is assisted by two other ligaments, the *anterior* and *posterior* sacroiliac ligaments. Unlike other plane joints, the sacroiliac joint demonstrates not just sliding and gliding movements but a much larger amount of spin, giving the adult joint some 3°–5° of rotation in the oblique sagittal plane.

The joints form two, closed loop kinematic chains, one with the lumbosacral paraspinal zygapophyseal joints and the other with the pubic symphysis; it demonstrates a degree of coupled motion with both. The joint is also unique in having no intrinsic musculature; movement is passive, the joint rocks backwards and forwards during gait and, to a more subtle extent, during respiration. Functionally, the intermingling of the lumbopelvic musculature with the regional ligaments means that there is some interaction between the joint and the muscles around it; however, this appears to be proprioceptive rather than mechanical.

## Lumbar spine

Although, in recent years, focus has moved away from the disc as a common cause of low back pain, it is still a highly important structure and pathomechanics contribute significantly to dysfunction elsewhere in the spine: loss of disc height and (visco-) elasticity has a dramatic effect on the loci of the three-joint complex's instantaneous axis of rotation.

### Fact File

#### DISC HERNIATION

The usual explanation given to patients regarding disc herniation is that the disc is 'trapping' a nerve; in fact, mechanical compression of neural structures is comparatively uncommon. Instead, the damage to the nerve is mediated by the body's own immune system. Because the nucleus is avascular and is an embryological leftover, when it extrudes into the vascular areas around it, it is not recognized as 'self' and is attacked by white blood cells.

The biochemical fallout from the macrophagic activity damages the Schwann cells surrounding the nerve, lowering its threshold and causing afferent stimuli to the thalamus, which interprets the signal as pain.

The anatomy of the disc is complex; however the key points for a biophysical understanding is that the functional element is the *nucleus pulposus*, a gelatinous mucopolysaccharide matrix, which is over 80% water, with the consistency of toothpaste. The nucleus is a remnant of the embryological notochord and has no vascular or neurological supply of its own, deriving its nutrition from osmosis and hydrostatic pressure from loading and unloading. It is contained by the *annulus fibrosus*, which derives its name from the resemblance of the concentric rings of collagen to the annular rings of trees. These fibres, which inter-cross, run at an angle of approximately 30° from the horizontal; this makes them very good at containing the lateral bulge of a compressed disc but much less able to withstand shearing forces. This is particularly the case when the intervertebral disc is under load and the forces are asymmetrical. The way in which the intervertebral disc responds to loading is shown in Figure 5.6.

## CLINICAL FOCUS

### Cauda equina syndrome

Because the spinal cord stops growing before the spinal canal, the former stops at the L2/3 level. The nerve roots inferior to this travel down the spinal canal before exiting at the appropriate spinal intervertebral foramina. Because of their resemblance to a horse's tail, they are called by this Latin term, *cauda equina*.

A significant posterior disc herniation at any level from L3/4 to L5/S1 can cause compression of these nerves giving the following symptoms:
- Bladder and/or bowel dysfunction, causing voiding or retention
- Severe and often progressive problems in the lower extremities, including loss of or altered sensation between the legs, over the buttocks, the inner thighs and back of the legs (saddle area), and feet/heels
- Pain, numbness, or weakness spreading to one or both legs
- Multiple level radicular symptoms.

The treatment is immediate emergency decompression; surgery within 48 hours leads to a 95% recovery rate. Beyond this there is a significant chance of permanent neurological deficit.

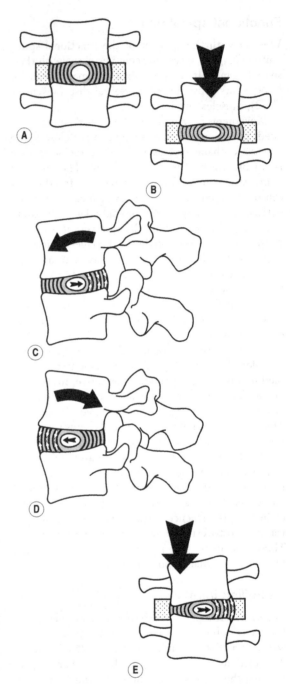

**Figure 5.6** • Disc movement. As an intervertebral disc is loaded, the central nucleus pulposus compresses and the containing annular fibres bulge (A, B). On movement, the annular fibres are again put under regional stress as the nucleus is differentially loaded and bulges unidirectionally. In lumbar flexion, the disc bulges posteriorly (C); in extension, anteriorly (D). In lateral flexion, the disc bulges to the contralateral side (E).

**Table 5.2** Stages of disc herniation and disc degeneration

| | Disc herniation | Disc degeneration |
|---|---|---|
| Grade 0 | Normal | Normal |
| Grade 1 | 'Prodromal disc'<br>• Individual annular fibre tears<br>• Nucleus intact | Mild degeneration<br>• Fibrotic nucleus<br>• Intact disc structure<br>• Uneven vertebral loading |
| Grade 2 | 'Disc protrusion'<br>• Multiple annular fibre tears<br>• Disc is still contained by fibres<br>• Loss of nuclear (and therefore disc) height<br>• Nuclear pressure causes remaining annular fibres to bulge<br>• Possible compromise of neural structures | Moderate degeneration<br>• Nuclear bulging<br>• Vertebral endplate damage<br>• Annular fissuring with disc protrusion/extrusion<br>• Some loss of disc height<br>• Dehydration evident on MRI |
| Grade 3 | 'Disc extrusion'<br>• Nuclear material extrudes from disc<br>• Immune system response with risk of associated damage to neural structures<br>• Sufficiently large posterior extrusion is associated with canal stenosis, cord compression and cauda equina syndrome | Severe degeneration<br>• Marked loss of disc height<br>• Internal collapse of annulus<br>• Endplate disruption<br>• Loss of movement |
| Grade 4 | 'Disc sequestration'<br>• Fragmentation of extruded fragment<br>• If the fragment is free in the spinal canal, it can put pressure on the cord or cauda equina or cause multiple nerve root symptoms | Ankylosis<br>• If the disc and endplates are completely obliterated, osseous fusion of the intervertebral disc space can occur |

Over 95% of all degenerative disc pathology occurs in the inferior three lumbar discs. The average height of a healthy disc is 11.3 mm, although this will decrease by up to 1 mm during the course of a typical day as loading forces water from the disc, which then undergoes viscoelastic compression; this is gradually reversed during sleep. With loss of disc height – in part a natural phenomenon of aging, but also a key component of degenerative disc disease – comes significantly increased loading of the posterior elements and alteration to the biomechanical function of the three-joint complex.

The stages of discal pathologies are detailed in Table 5.2.

 CLINICAL FOCUS

Injury to the lumbar spine is second only to infection in the upper respiratory tract in causing time off work and has a far more serious morbidity.

There is an increasing consensus as to the aetiology of low back pain, which, of course, is a symptom rather than a condition in its own right: there is, therefore, no treatment as such for 'low back pain' and any programme of management should start with an accurate assessment and diagnosis of the specific areas of dysfunction and associated comorbidities.

Over the last 30 years, emphasis has moved away from the disc, osteoarthritis and spondylolysis as the be all and end all of low back pain; instead, paraspinal zygapophyseal and sacroiliac joints with their supporting ligaments are seen as the prime instigators with associated myofascial pain syndromes as sources of secondary pain.

Treatment protocols have also changed radically. After several decades in which up to 40% of patients would be worsened by surgery, surgery is now considered a treatment of last resort and has been removed from the hands of general orthopaedic surgeons and placed with teams of specialist surgeons from both neurological and orthopaedic backgrounds. Pain clinics too have changed; fewer than one in three patients would derive benefit from the 'learn to live with it' approach aimed at pain control. Now many such clinics focus on the patient's biopsychosocial status rather than pain levels alone and use multidisciplinary management.

This change in approach is reflected in guidelines for the management of low back pain. Twenty years ago, physiotherapy was considered a token gesture before restorative surgery, and chiropractic and osteopathy a form of voodoo ritual to be avoided at all costs; today, spinal manipulative therapy is considered the gold standard in treatment of many types of low back pain and recent evidence shows that, if this treatment is followed up with coordinated rehabilitative exercise, patients fare even better.

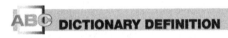 **DICTIONARY DEFINITION**

**SPONDYLOLYSIS**

Originating from two Greek words *spondylos*, meaning 'vertebra' and *lysis*, meaning to cut, a spondylolysis is an interruption of the pars interarticularis, the osseous column that supports the inferior and superior aspects of the paraspinal zygapophyseal joints. The lesions, which can be unilateral or bilateral, appear to be the non-union of paediatric stress fractures and the consequence of bipedal weight bearing.

They occur predominantly (90%) at L5 and, although most are stable, they can be associated with anterior translation of the vertebra (*spondylolisthesis*) or, occasionally, posterior translation (*retrolisthesis*).

The orientation of the lumbar facet joints in the sagittal (XY) plane means that they have considerably more flexion–extension than they do movements about the other two orthogonal axes (Table 5.3).

## Thoracic spine

Motion in the thoracic spine is restricted by the ribs (Table 5.4); however not all ribs are equal, there are three distinct regions within the thoracic spine and the differences between them affect local kinematics and biomechanics.

**Table 5.3** Approximate segmental lumbar spine ranges of motion in degrees

| Spinal level | Flexion–extension | Lateral flexion | Rotation |
|---|---|---|---|
| T12/L1 | 12 | 8 | 2 |
| L1/2 | 12 | 8 | 2 |
| L2/3 | 14 | 7 | 3 |
| L3/4 | 15 | 8 | 2 |
| L4/5 | 17 | 6 | 2 |
| L5/S1 | 20 | 3 | 5 |
| Total | 90 | 32 | 16 |

**Table 5.4** Approximate segmental ranges of motion for the thoracic spine in degrees

| | Flexion–extension | Lateral flexion | Rotation |
|---|---|---|---|
| C7/T1 | 9 | 4 | 8 |
| T1/2 | 4 | 5 | 9 |
| T2/3 | 4 | 5 | 8 |
| T3/4 | 4 | 5 | 8 |
| T4/5 | 4 | 5 | 8 |
| T5/6 | 4 | 5 | 8 |
| T6/7 | 5 | 5 | 8 |
| T7/8 | 6 | 5 | 8 |
| T8/9 | 6 | 5 | 7 |
| T9/10 | 6 | 5 | 3 |
| T10/11 | 9 | 6 | 2 |
| T11/12 | 12 | 9 | 2 |
| T12/L1 | 12 | 8 | 2 |
| Total | 85 | 72 | 57 |

The first seven ribs are **true ribs**. They have four articulations: posteriorly, the costotransverse and costovertebral joints; anteriorly, the costochondral joints, articulating with the rib cartilage. This, in turn, articulates with the breastbone via the cost-osternal joint. By contrast, the eighth, ninth and tenth ribs (the **false ribs**) communicate with the common costal cartilage, which, in turn, communicates with either the seventh costal cartilage or, occasionally, independently with xiphisternum. The eleventh and twelfth ribs are **floating ribs,** which have no anterior articular attachments; in 5–8% of patients, the tenth ribs also 'float'. Fractures of these ribs are often unstable and can cause puncturing of adjacent organs – the kidneys are particularly vulnerable in this regard.

## Cervical spine

The uppermost area of the spine is by far the most mobile (Table 5.5) and, when considered with the cranium, forms an open-loop kinematic chain. As ever, this increased mobility comes at a price – the cervical spine is the most vulnerable to trauma, as any whiplash victim will tell you.

The most atypical part of the spine is the superior two vertebrae, also the only two to have individual names: the atlas and the axis. The former derives its name from the Greek Titan, Atlas (as do the Atlas Mountains), who bore the Earth upon his shoulders (apart from one brief stint when Heracles took over); the latter from the amount of rotation afforded by the joint between the axis and atlas, which accounts for almost half of all cervical rotation – four times as much as any other joint (Fig. 5.7).

The two vertebrae are also alone in having no intervertebral discs. The axis forms a ring that has just two articulations superiorly (the atlanto-occipital joints). Inferiorly, it does have a three joint complex but it is one that is unique to the functional spinal unit. In addition to the two posterior zygapophyseal joints (atlanto-axial joints), there is, in place of the intervertebral disc, a pivot joint comprising the odontoid process (dens) of the axis, which is bounded by the anterior arch of the atlas and its transverse ligament.

The musculature of the upper cervical segments is also distinct from the pattern of the intrinsic muscles followed elsewhere in the spine (the suboccipital muscles are important clinically as a potential cause of headache) and the biomechanics are also modified by the dural attachments discussed earlier. This area of the spine is regarded as being of key importance to spinal manipulators, in particular chiropractors; indeed, there is at least one entire technique based on adjusting the C1 vertebra and no other!

## CLINICAL FOCUS

Whiplash is of course much more than simply neck pain. From the mid-1990s, the term **whiplash-associated disorders** has been used to describe the range of biomechanical, neurological, physiological and psychological sequelae to road traffic accidents and similar traumas.

Although neck pain is the commonest symptom, thoracic and rib pain (75%); low back pain (50%); headache (45%); arm pain (32%); temporomandibular dysfunction (7%); sleep disturbance (5%); and avoidance phobias (3%) are all recognized co-morbidities that can complicate management of the condition, which presents to physical therapists on a daily basis.

With regard to the ubiquitous cervical component of the injury, the mechanism of acceleration–deceleration injury is complex and has yet to be fully understood. There are, however, a number of key learning points that need to be understood.

Most injuries are reported after rear or, to a lesser extent, side impact injuries: an important component in this is that such injuries are often unguarded – the victims do not know that the impact is coming. Although bracing against impact increases the likelihood of ligamentous or osseous compromise, at lower speeds, this mechanism often guards against serious injury.

**Table 5.5** Approximate segmental ranges of motion for the cervical spine in degrees

|  | Flexion–extension | Lateral flexion | Rotation |
|---|---|---|---|
| C0/C1 | 13 | 8 | 0 |
| C1/2 | 10 | 0 | 47 |
| C2/3 | 8 | 10 | 9 |
| C3/4 | 13 | 11 | 11 |
| C4/5 | 12 | 11 | 12 |
| C5/6 | 17 | 8 | 10 |
| C6/7 | 16 | 7 | 9 |
| C7/T1 | 9 | 4 | 8 |
| **Total** | **98** | **59** | **105** |

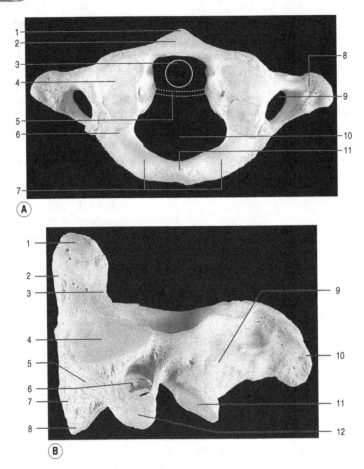

**Figure 5.7** • (A) The atlas from above. 1. Anterior tubercle. 2. Anterior arch. 3. Outline of dens. 4. Superior articular facet, on lateral mass (bipartile facet in this specimen). 5. Outline of transverse ligament. 6. Groove for vertebral artery and C1 (beneath bony overhang from lateral mass here). 7. Posterior arch. 8. Transverse process. 9. Foramen transversarium. 10. Vertebral foramen. 11 Posterior tubercle. (B) The axis from the side. 1. Dens – attachment of alar ligament. 2. Facet for anterior arch of atlas. 3. Groove for transverse ligament of atlas. 4. Superior articular facet. 5. Lateral mass. 6. Divergent foramen transversum. 7. Body. 8. Ventral lip of body. 9. Lamina. 10. Spinous process. 11. Inferior articular facet. 12. Transverse process. The protuberence of the dens (B) is contained by the anterior arch of the atlas anteriorly and the transverse ligament posteriorly forming a pivot joint. This arrangement affords almost four times the amount of rotation of any other functional spinal unit. Reproduced from Standring, S, ed 2005 Gray's anatomy, 39e (online edition), with permission from Elsevier.

Rear impact injury is the more complicated scenario as the victim interacts not only with the colliding vehicle but with their own seat and headrest. In order to simplify our understanding, we can assume that the standard three-point seat belt immobilizes the torso (of course, the asymmetrical restrain does not do this and causes a rotary component that frequently damages the paraspinal zygapophyseal and costal joints of the thoracic spine and sacroiliac joints) and that injuries below this level are due to forced translatory motion.

The cervicothoracic junction, cervical spine and cranium then act as a three-member open-loop kinematic chain (Fig. 5.8). The impact of the collision, which most usually happens when the victim is stationary with their foot on the brake, causes the seat to be thrust forward along with the pinioned trunk. However, the neck and shoulder are free of this restraint and do not move in relation to this. The effect on the individual is that their spine and cranium are translated posteriorly (actually their torso is being translated anteriorly but the motion is relative). However, these structures have only a limited ability to translate and the momentum is converted instead into rotation of the cervical spine. When this reaches the end of its range of motion, the cranium continues to move like a hinged or 'double' pendulum.

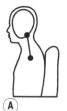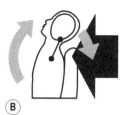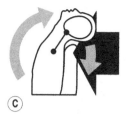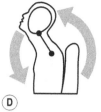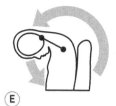

(A)  (B)  (C)  (D)  (E)

**Figure 5.8** • Rear impact whiplash. The driver starts in neutral (A). The rear impact imparts a relative posterior translation to the head and neck (B), and also a moment of inertia that is expressed as 'ramping'. When the cervical spine has reached the limit of its extension, the cranium continues to move, pivoting around the upper cervical complex (C). Once the transfer of momentum from the impacting vehicle is complete, the pinioned torso undergoes deceleration causing a relative anterior translation then rotation of the head and still hyperextended cranium (D). Once the cervical spine is fully extended the cranium moves from hyperextension to hyperflexion, the same effect as a whip (E).

The situation is further complicated by the **ramping** force of the collision. As the impact is below the victim's centre of gravity, there will be pivoting about the line of force of impact. This moment of inertia is curtailed by the restraint of the seat and seatbelt and the momentum is converted into superior translation along the seat back, elevating the victim, often by several inches. This has the effect of converting a headrest from being a restraint into a pivot, over which the cervical spine can hyperextend, localizing and intensifying the forces.

A key component in determining the nature of the injuries sustained is the speed of the accident. Injuries have been shown to occur at speeds as low as 4 mph; however, at these speeds, the damage is more likely to be to muscle fibres and tendons, which sustain damage as they contract to resist the sudden and unexpected movement. At higher speeds (>25 mph), the body does not have time to react to the initial, extending impact but does have time to try to resist the subsequent anterior motion. These injuries commonly present with impaction damage to the paraspinal zygapophyseal joints, extension damage to anterior ligamentous and tendinous structures and tearing of the posterior muscle fibres.

At higher speeds still (>50 mph), all motion tends to be entirely passive and primary injury to muscles is far less, although secondary problems do develop owing to derangement of mechanoreceptors in the damaged joint capsules, annular fibres, ligaments and tendons.

## Temporomandibular joint

One of the most overlooked joints in the body, the temporomandibular joint (TMJ) is a common source of pain: temporomandibular disorder (TMD) affects a significant percentage of the population to a greater or lesser extent and often benefits from multidisciplinary management from manual physicians and dental or orthodontic practitioners.

Even more importantly, it can demonstrate a high degree of comorbidity and appears to be a not infrequent aetiological factor in headache, neck pain, late whiplash and low back pain; certainly, the TMJ has a close anatomical interrelationship with the cervical spine and a major functional role within the orthognathic system as a whole: the dentition, mandible and axial skeleton. It is also thought to be the joint with the greatest density of proprioceptive nerve endings and, as such, is involved in head-righting mechanisms, coordination and balance.

The movement of the joint – and, indeed, its pathomechanics – is highly complicated and the subject of entire books. Depending on the sophistication of the anatomical text, you may variously see it described as anything from a simple hinge joint to a complex, compound bicondylar joint. From our standpoint, we need to understand that the joint has several components: the articulation itself takes place between the mandible and a shallow, concave socket within the temporal bone (Fig. 5.9); there is also a bony process, the *coronoid process*, which serves as an anchor point for the temporalis muscle, one of the five *muscles of mastication* that move the jaw.

The joint also has an articular disc within it, which can pivot and slide enabling the joint to undergo two separate motions. In the initial stages of opening, the joint acts like a simple hinge; however, once it reaches approximately two-thirds of full opening, it ceases rotary movement and undergoes an anterior translation for the final third. You can feel this change of motion by putting your fingers over the condyles of the joint (immediately

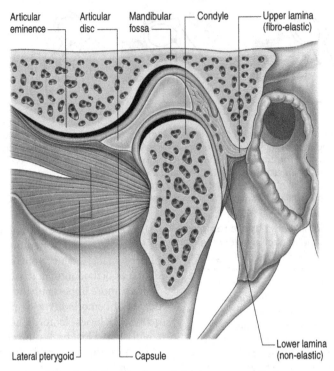

Articular eminence — Articular disc — Mandibular fossa — Condyle — Upper lamina (fibro-elastic)

Lateral pterygoid — Capsule — Lower lamina (non-elastic)

**Figure 5.9** • Sagittal section through the temporomandibular joint. Reproduced from Standring, S, ed 2005 Gray's anatomy, 39e (online edition), with permission from Elsevier.

in front of the ears) and slowly open and close your mouth; if you have damage to your articular disc, the change may be accompanied by a popping or clicking sound.

As part of an holistic examination of a patient, or re-examination of a patient who is failing to respond to normal treatment protocols, it is important to evaluate TMJ gait and range of motion and dentition and to palpate the muscles of mastication for evidence of hypertonicity, asymmetry or myofascial trigger points.

# Posture

For around 2 000 000 years, the *Homo* genus has been walking upright; our invariable bipedal stance differentiates us from all other species – other primates alternate between bipedal and quadrupedal posture, as do bears (*Ursus*), the only other plantigrade mammals. This arrangement has obvious advantages: not only does it increase our visual range but it gives us the freedom to use our opposing thumbs to make tools.

 **DICTIONARY DEFINITION**

### PLANTIGRADE

Plantigrade animals walk on the soles (or plantar surfaces) of their feet; primates and bears the only mammals to do so, the remainder walk on modified toe structures and are therefore digitigrade.

A two-footed posture comes at a price however; we are much less stable than our four-footed friends, just as a motorcycle is inherently less stable than a car. From the standpoint of a physicist, there are two reasons for this instability and both relate to the body's centre of gravity. Any symmetrical structure is only stable so long as its centre of gravity is located above the area transcribed by its contact points with the ground, the locus of stability (Fig. 5.10). You can demonstrate this on yourself: stand with your feet together, then lean sideways, keeping your body straight. As your centre of gravity (remember, it is located anterior to the second sacral tubercle) moves past the outside of your foot,

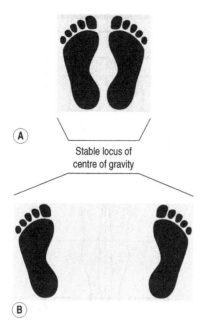

Stable locus of
centre of gravity

**Figure 5.10** • Bipedal stance is only stable if the centre of gravity is above the area transcribed by the feet, the locus of stability. If the feet are together (**A**), this area is smaller when compared to a wide-footed stance (**B**), which is inherently more stable.

you should be able to feel your muscles start to tense; the system is no longer inherently stable and requires external forces to anchor it. As you lean a little further, your body's strength is no longer sufficient to overcome the moment of inertia being created by the force of gravity and you will fall (or, more probably, take a corrective step to reposition your stance to that the centre of gravity again lies within the rectangle described by your feet).

If you repeat the experiment with your feet apart, you will find that you are a lot more stable, the body has to move a lot further before the centre of gravity reaches an unstable position. This is reflected in everyday intuitive behaviour, if we want to brace ourselves against impact, we adopt a wide-footed stance.

The second factor that affects our stability is the distance between the ground and our centre of gravity; again, this is much larger than in quadrupedal animals. The greater the distance, the less movement is required to bring the centre of gravity outside the locus of stability; again, this is reflected in everyday activity – when we brace, we also tend to crouch thus lowering our centre of gravity. If you repeat the previous experiment, you will find that

you can bend further with your legs crouching than with your legs straight.

## Balance

It is tempting to think of standing posture as a static thing – after all, when someone is standing, they are, by definition, not moving. However, in order to maintain balance, the body is in a constant state of flux both neurologically and physiologically. Four main mechanisms are involved in maintaining balance:

### Plantar pressure receptors

The soles of the feet contain a rich array of proprioceptors. When position shifts so that the pressure is greater in the forefeet, the body responds by increasing the tone in the dorsiflexors and inhibiting the plantarflexors in order to bring the body back to neutral. Similar righting mechanisms exist to correct posterior and lateral sway.

### Visual system

When an image on the retina moves, the brain is capable of determining whether the object itself is moving, whether the eyeball is moving or whether the head is moving – or any combination thereof. The importance of the visual system in maintaining balance can be demonstrated by comparing the ease of balancing on one foot with the eyes open and then closed.

### Tonic neck reflexes

This ability is facilitated by *tonic neck reflexes*, the proprioceptive ability to coordinate head and eye position: notice how your visual field remains vertical even when you tilt your head from side to side.

### Vestibular system

The **semicircular canals** provide information as to the angular acceleration of the head around each of the orthogonal axes whilst the *saccule* and *utricle*, collectively known as the **otolith organs,** sense linear motion and gravity.

The input from these sensory arrays is coordinated by the cerebellum, so that sway usually consists of micro-motion; this becomes much more visually obvious when one or more of the systems are impaired, as can happen with peripheral neuropathy, loss of vision or inner ear pathology such as Ménière's disease.

A postural evaluation should play a central part in the physical examination of any patient. Asymmetry can give an array of clinical information about biomechanical and neurological dysfunction in both the axial skeleton and extremities.

Understanding the subtleties and significance of postural variations only comes from undergraduate training reinforced by clinical experience. Such understanding begins with an appreciation of what constitutes 'normal' posture; this is best done using a postural analyser, which can be as simple as a basic plumb line.

Viewing the patient from behind (Fig. 5.11) anatomical markers should normally be symmetrical from left to right, although it is normal for the shoulder to be lower on the side of handedness. As well as looking for left to right differences, it is also important to look for anterior to posterior deviation, which can supply information about pelvic derangement and rotary scoliosis amongst other conditions.

Lateral assessment can give key information of relative muscle strength and tightness (Fig. 5.12). The key alignment points are detailed in Table 5.6.

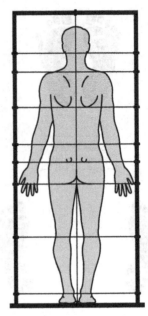

**Figure 5.11** • A postural analyzer can be used in order to mensurate postural deviations. Elasticated level-lines can be used to determine inequality of height in key anatomical markers: the acromion and mastoid processes, inferior angle of the scapulae, waist line, posterior superior iliac spines, gluteal folds, popliteal creases and malleoli.

# Seated posture

Of course, we do not spend the whole of our lives standing; increasingly, people spend more and more time sitting in front of televisions, computers and games consoles (with a concomitant increase in neck and shoulder pain, repetitive strain injury and low back conditions). Sitting appears to be a very much more stable position than standing: the area of contact is increased and is only just below the centre of gravity (this will move superiorly when sitting as the legs, which are now in contact, no longer contribute to the centre of gravity).

In fact, it is chair design that makes sitting stable; if we try to balance on the primary point of contact,

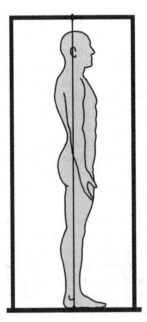

**Figure 5.12** • Using a plumb line to assess posture (see Table 5.6).

**Table 5.6** Key alignment points for assessing anteroposterior posture

- Earlobe
- Slightly posterior to mastoid process
- Odontoid process*
- Middle of shoulder joint
- Midpoint of anterior border of T2*
- Midpoint of anterior border of T12*
- Anterior to S2*
- Slightly posterior to axis of hip joint
- Slightly posterior to patella
- Slightly anterior to lateral malleolus

*These structures are only visible radiologically, although their position can be estimated using surface anatomy.

the ischial tuberosities (try perching on a narrow swing), you will quickly see that the anterior positioning of the legs moves the centre of gravity anteriorly (try sticking out your legs in front of you and see what happened to your balance; similarly, tuck them underneath the swing and you will find the balance improves significantly).

It is the additional support that the conventional chair gives to the thighs and back that makes sitting so much more stable than standing, adding to the base of support (chair seat) and removing a degree of freedom (the chair back). The ideal sitting position is detailed in Table 5.7; unfortunately, this is seldom achieved: many modern seats are too soft, low, deep, short or long or they have a backward slope. Furthermore, it is common for individuals to 'slump' in their seats resulting in the centre of gravity being placed behind the ischial tuberosities and resulting in lumbar lordotic reversal,

**Table 5.7** Ideal seated posture

- Ischial tuberosities provide major base of support
- Upper thighs add to sitting base
- Absence of pressure to popliteal fossa
- Lumbar spine held in neutral or slight flexion
- Thoracic spine supported by backrest inclined slightly backward from vertical
- Hips positioned slightly above knees
- Weight of legs supported by feet (using footrest if required)

ligamentous strain and posterior bulging of the intervertebral discs.

## Recumbent posture

Of course, even more than standing or sitting, we spend on average 7.5 hours each day (or night) lying down; this is known as **recumbent posture**. The pull of gravity in this case is through each segment of the body that is in contact with the supporting surface; obviously, if the surface gives sufficiently at the pressure points, the remainder of the body will be brought into contact with the supporting surface, whilst allowing its longitudinal axis to remain in neutral.

 CLINICAL FOCUS

There is much controversy and disagreement about what constitutes an ideal sleeping posture; indeed, what might be the ideal posture for one **somatotype** could well prove unsuitable for another. There are certain rules that can be generalized: by and large, sleeping on one's stomach is less desirable; the cervical spine must be kept in rotation for prolonged periods and, in the obese patient, pressure is put on the abdomen and diaphragm and there can be alteration to spinal curves.

Although sleeping on one's back has always been put forward as the most desirable position, it also predisposes towards snoring and sleep apnoea and, depending on the characteristics of the mattress and the weight distribution of the individual, can aggravate certain spinal conditions.

A recumbent side posture will often aggravate shoulder conditions and thoracic outlet conditions. Because of the tendency to bend the upper leg in order to increase stability, side posture can also adversely affect pathologies in which there is hemipelvic asymmetry, such as sacroiliac joint syndrome (or help alleviate them).

In any position, the rule about keeping their body's longitudinal axis in neutral holds and this will affect the choice of pillow: prone, often no pillow will be required; supine, and the depth of pillow will be influenced by the give of the mattress and the natural lordosis of the individual; lying on the side, and the ideal pillow depth will be determined by the give of the mattress and the breadth of the shoulders.

## DICTIONARY DEFINITION

### SOMATOTYPE

As well as the genetically determined variation in gender and height, there is also individual variation in body shape and composition, the *somatotype*. This affects both musculature and biomechanical function: there are three somatotypes and most people are a mixture, although certain traits can predominate.

- Ectomorphs: thin body and face, long neck ('beanpoles')
- Mesomorphs: large head, broad shoulders, heavily muscled with little subcutaneous fat ('athletic')
- Endomorphs: round head and abdomen, high subcutaneous fat ('roly-poly').

# Gait

More than anything else, the hunter-gatherer *Homo sapiens* evolved to walk; clinically, this is reflected in that many types of low back syndromes will be improved by walking and worsened by sitting. In the former case, forces are being divided between the hips and sacroiliac joints and loading is dynamic and transient; in the latter, all the forces are static and transmitted through the sacroiliac joints alone.

Much clinical information can be gleaned from assessment of gait and this can be done quantitatively (Fig. 5.13) as well as qualitatively. As with posture, this process starts with an understanding of what constitutes 'normal' gait.

Obviously, when we are walking, the process is cyclical. If we consider this from the standpoint of the right foot, there are a number of distinct phases that can be identified (obviously, the left foot is working reciprocally); these are detailed in Figure 5.14. In bipedal gait, one foot is always in contact with the ground and, for part of the time, both feet are in contact, the 'double stance' phase.

There is considerable weight transference during the gait cycle, the heel strike is slightly lateral, whilst toe-off is predominantly on the medial first ray. There is also weight transfer from left to right and anterior to posterior. To compensate for this,

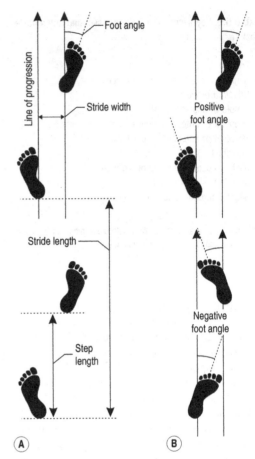

**Figure 5.13** • Various features of gait can be measured and therefore quantitatively assessed. These include step and stride length, stride width (A) and foot angle (B).

the left arm swings posteriorly as the right leg moves anteriorly, and anteriorly as the leg moves posteriorly. There is a similar relationship between right arm and left leg. This action is hardwired into most individuals, starting with the cross-crawl reflex as a child; so much so that, if the right leg is positioned posteriorly, the left latissimus dorsi muscle, the primary extensor of the arm, will be neurologically inhibited and appear weak compared to the neutral or leg advanced position.

In addition to the movements described above, the body's centre of gravity also moves inferiorly when the stance is open and superiorly when the stance is closed. There are many disorders of gait with many aetiologies; some of the more commonly encountered are detailed in Table 5.8.

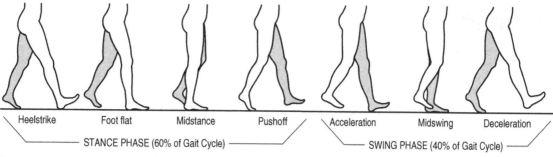

Heelstrike   Foot flat   Midstance   Pushoff   Acceleration   Midswing   Deceleration

STANCE PHASE (60% of Gait Cycle) ⎯⎯⎯   SWING PHASE (40% of Gait Cycle) ⎯⎯

**Figure 5.14** • The different phases of the gait cycle.

**Table 5.8** Some of the more commonly encountered pathological gaits

| Name | Description | Associated condition(s) |
|---|---|---|
| Cerebellar ataxia | Drunken gait ± trunk ataxia | Cerebellar dysfunction |
| Sensory ataxia | Stamping gait (increased impact to compensate for diminished proprioception) | Peripheral neuropathy |
| Hemiplegic gait | Leg held in forced extension with plantarflexion; anterior motion is by circumduction | Spasticity following cerebrovascular accident |
| Scissor gait | As above but with both legs | Multiple sclerosis<br>Spinal stenosis |
| High-stepping gait | Flaccid paralysis of dorsiflexors results in high knee lift and forced foot strike | Peroneal nerve palsy |
| Waddling gait | Extreme weakness of thigh and hip muscles compensated for by posterior weight carriage | Muscular dystrophy |
| Fenestration | Stooped forwards, fast paced | Parkinson's disease |
| Antalgic gait: lower extremity | Limping or hobbling, favouring the uninjured limb | Numerous traumatic and degenerative conditions |
| Antalgic gait: spine | Lateral lean<br><br>Anterior lean<br>Exaggerated hip motion | Indicative of space-occupying lesion, most commonly intervertebral disc herniation<br>Common in paraspinal zygapophyseal joint injury<br>Sacroiliac joint syndrome |

## Learning Outcomes

On completion of this chapter, the reader should fully understand:
• The relationship between joint structure and joint function
• The workings of open and closed loop kinematic chains and their biomechanical implications
• The concept and application of a joint's degree of freedom
• Joint roll, glide and spin and their interrelationship
• The arthrokinetics and principal features of the spine, pelvis and extremities
• The assessment and mechanics of posture and gait

# Bibliography

Allen, R., Schwarz, C. (Eds.), 1998. The Chambers dictionary. Chambers Harrap, Edinburgh.

Asaki, S., Sekikawa, M., Kim, Y.T., 2006. Sensory innervation of temporomandibular joint disk. J. Orthop. Surg. (Hong Kong) 14 (1), 3–8.

Barnes, C.J., Van Steyn, S.J., Fischer, R.A., 2001. The effects of age, sex, and shoulder dominance on range of motion of the shoulder. J. Shoulder Elbow Surg. 10, 242–246.

Barrack, R.L., Munn, B.G., 2000. Effects of knee ligament injury and reconstruction on proprioception. In: Lephart, S.M., Fu, F.H. (Eds.), Proprioception and neuromuscular control in joint stability. Human Kinetics, pp. 197–209.

Beers, M.H., Berkow, R. (Eds.), 1999. In: The Merck manual of diagnosis and therapy, seventeenth ed. Merck, West Point, PA.

Bell, R.D., Hoshizaki, T.B., 1981. Relationships of age and sex with range of motion of seventeen joint actions in humans. Can. J. Appl. Sport Sci. 6 (4), 202–206.

Bergman, T.F., 1994. Mechanisms for control of head movement. In: Curl, D.D., (Ed.), Chiropractic approach to head pain. Williams & Wilkins, Baltimore, pp. 74–83.

Bowen, V., Cassidy, J.D., 1981. Macroscopic and microscopic anatomy of the sacroiliac joint from embryonic life until the eighth decade. Spine 6, 620–628.

Bramble, D.M., Lieberman, D.E., 2004. Endurance running and the evolution of Homo. Nature 432, 345–352.

Caldwell, W.E., Moloy, H.C., 1933. Anatomical variations in the female pelvis and their effect in labor with a suggested classification. Am. J. Obstet. Gynecol. 26, 479–505.

Cartmill, M., Schmitt, D., 1997. The effect of pelvic width on pelvic rotation during bipedalism in modern and fossil hominids. Am. J. Phys. Anthropol. 24, S49.

Cassidy, J.D., Lopes, A.A., Yong Hing, K., 1992. The immediate effect of manipulation versus mobilisation on pain and range of motion in the cervical spine: a randomised controlled trial. J. Manipulative Physiol. Ther. 15, 570–575.

Chapman, S., Nakielny, R., 1990. The Spine. In: Aids to radiological differential diagnosis, second ed. Ballière Tindall, Philadelphia, pp. 52–76.

Clarkson, H.M., 2005. Principles and methods. In: Joint motion and function assessment: a research-based practical guide. Lippincott Williams and Wilkins, Baltimore, pp. 3–30.

Class, O., 1994. Critical appraisal of the literature in juvenile idiopathic scoliosis. European Journal of Chiropractic 42 (3), 69–76.

Coggon, D., Reading, I., Croft, P., et al., 2001. Knee osteoarthritis and obesity. Int. J. Obes. Relat. Metab. Disord. 25 (5), 622–627.

Croft, P.R., Macfarlane, G.J., Papageorgiou, A.C., Thomas, E., Silman, A.J., 1998. Outcome of low back pain in general practice: a prospective study. BMJ 316, 1356–1359.

Darby, S.A., Cramer, G.D., 1994. Pain generators and pain pathways of the head and neck. In: Curl, D.D. (Ed.), Chiropractic approach to head pain. Williams and Wilkins, Baltimore, pp. 55–73.

Van Deursen, D.J., Everett, T., 2005. Biomechanics of human movement. In: Trew, M., Everett, T. (Eds.), Human movement: an introductory text, fourth ed. Churchill Livingstone, Edinburgh, pp. 37–68.

Delport, E.G., Cucuzzella, T.R., Kim, N., et al., 2006. Lumbosacral transitional vertebrae: incidence in a consecutive patient series. Pain Physician 9 (1), 53–56.

Elster, A.D., 1989. Bertolotti's syndrome revisited. Transitional vertebrae of the lumbar spine. Spine 14 (12), 1373–1377.

Fechtel, S.G., Gatterman, M.I., Panzer, D.M., Postural complex 1990. In: Gatterman, M.I. (Ed.), Chiropractic management of spine related disorders. Williams and Wilkins, Baltimore, pp. 285–282.

Fenton, J., Phykitt, D.E., 2004. Thoracic spine anatomic considerations. In:

DiGiovanna, E.L., Schiowitz, S., Dowling, D.J. (Eds.), An osteopathic approach to diagnosis and treatment, third ed. Lippincott Williams & Wilkins, Baltimore, pp. 175–179.

Fredriksson, K., Alfredsson, L., Ahlberg, G., et al., 2002. Work environment and neck and shoulder pain: the influence of exposure time. Results from a population based case-control study. Occup. Environ. Med. 59 (3), 182–188.

Freeman, M.D., Nordhoff, L.S., 2005. Crash speeds and injury risk: epidemiological and forensic consideration. In: Nordhoff Jr., L.S. (Ed.), Motor vehicle collision injuries: biomechanics, diagnosis and management, second ed. Jones and Bartlett, Boston, pp. 363–390.

Gatterman, M.I., 1990. Basic kinesiological and biomechanical principles applied to the spine. In: Gatterman, M.I. (Ed.), Chiropractic management of spine related disorders. Williams and Wilkins, Baltimore, pp. 22–36.

Ghalayini, S.R.A., Board, T.N., Srinivasan, M.S., 2007. Anatomic variations in the long head of biceps: contribution to shoulder dysfunction. Arthroscopy 23, 1012–1018.

Green, J.H., Silver, P.H.S., 1981. In: An introduction to human anatomy. Oxford University Press, Oxford.

Greenstein, G., 1994. Functional anatomy and biomechanics of the cervical spine. In: Curl, D.D. (Ed.), Chiropractic approach to head pain. Williams & Wilkins, Baltimore, pp. 96–120.

Guebert, G.M., Yochum, T.R., Rowe, L.J., 1996. Congenital abnormalities and skeletal variants. In: Yochum, T.R., Rowe, L.J., (Eds.), Essentials of skeletal radiology. Williams and Wilkins, Baltimore, pp. 307–326.

Hamilton, W. (Ed.), 1976. Joints. In: Textbook of human anatomy, second ed. Exeter, A Wheaton, pp. 35.

Harvey, E., Burton, A.K., Moffett, J.K., et al., 2003. Spinal manipulation for low-back pain: a treatment package agreed to by the UK chiropractic, osteopathy and physiotherapy professional associations. Man. Ther. 8 (1), 46–51.

Hindle, A., 2005. Function of the upper limb. In: Trew, M., Everett, T. (Eds.), Human movement: an introductory text, fourth ed. Churchill Livingstone, Edinburgh, pp. 193–202.

Hinson, R., Zeng, Z.B., 1999. Epidural attachments in the upper cervical spine. Abstracts from the 19th Annual Upper Cervical Spine conference, November 21–22 1998. Chiropr. Res. J. 6, 21–22.

Hodges, S., 2000. Human evolution: a start for population genomics. Nature 408 (6813), 652–653.

Howat, J.M.P., 1999. Cranial motion and cranial categories. In: Chiropractic: anatomy and physiology of sacro occipital technique. Cranial Communication Systems, Oxford, 61–128.

Jayne, N., Hatfield, N., 2006. The newborn at risk: congenital disorder. In: Introductory maternity and pediatric nursing: basis of human movement in health and disease. Lippincott Williams and Wilkins, Baltimore, pp. 512–552.

Kinzel, G.L., Gutkowski, L.J., 1983. Joint models, degrees of freedom, and anatomical motion measurement. J. Biomech. Eng. 105, 55–62.

Kirkaldy-Willis, W.H., 1983. The site and nature of the lesion. In: Managing low back pain. Churchill Livingstone, New York, pp. 91–108.

Koenigsberg, R. (Ed.), 1989. Churchill's illustrated medical dictionary. Churchill Livingstone, New York.

Koo, C.C., Roberts, H.N., 1997. The palmaris longus tendon: another variation in its anatomy. J. Hand Surg. [Br] 22 (1), 138–139.

Lovejoy, C., 2004. The natural history of human gait and posture. Part 1. Spine and pelvis. Gait Posture 21, 95–112.

Luoma, K., Vehmas, T., Raininko, R., et al., 2004. Lumbosacral transitional vertebra: relation to disc degeneration and low back pain. Spine 15, 29 (2), 200–205.

Meade, T.W., Frank, A.O., 1990. Low back pain: comparison of chiropractic and hospital outpatient treatment. BMJ 300 (6741), 1723.

Meade, T.W., 1999. Patients were more satisfied with chiropractic than other treatments for low back pain. BMJ 319 (7201), 57.

Meade, T.W., Dyer, S., Browne, W., et al., 1990. Low back pain of mechanical origin: randomised comparison of chiropractic and hospital outpatient treatment. BMJ 300 (6737), 1431–1437.

Meade, T.W., Dyer, S., Browne, W., et al., 1995. Randomised comparison of chiropractic and hospital outpatient management for low back pain: results from extended follow up. BMJ 311 (7001), 349–351.

Mitchell, B.S., Humphreys, B.K., O'Sullivan, E., 1998. Attachments of the ligamentum nuchae to cervical posterior spinal dura and the lateral part of the occipital bone. J. Manipulative Physiol. Ther. 21 (3), 145–148.

Miura, C., Hida, W., Miki, H., et al., 1992. Effects of posture on flow-volume curves during normocapnia and hypercapnia in patients with obstructive sleep apnoea 47 (7), 524–528.

Moore, A., Petty, N.J., 2005. Function of the spine. In: Trew, M., Everett, T. (Eds.), Human movement: an introductory text, fourth ed. Churchill Livingstone, Edinburgh, pp. 203–224.

Moore, K.L., 1985. Joints. In: Clinically oriented anatomy, second ed. Williams and Wilkins, Baltimore, pp. 33–37.

National Institute for Health and Clinical Excellence. 2006. Non-rigid stabilisation procedures for the treatment of low back pain, Intervention procedure guidance 186. NHS: June.

Niosi, C.A., Oxland, T.R., 2004. Degenerative mechanics of the lumbar spine. Spine J. 4, S202–S208.

Nordhoff, L.S., 2005. Injury biomechanics in motor vehicle collisions: overview of issues relevant to the clinician. In: Nordhoff Jr., L.S. (Ed.), Motor vehicle collision injuries: biomechanics, diagnosis and management, second ed. Jones and Bartlett, Boston, pp. 391–426.

Nordhoff, L.S., Underhill, M.L., Murphy, D., 2005. Diagnosis of common crash injuries and sequela. In: Nordhoff Jr., L.S. (Ed.), Motor vehicle collision injuries: biomechanics, diagnosis and management, second ed. Jones and Bartlett, Boston, pp. 41–130.

North American Spine Society. 2006. Whiplash and whiplash associated disorders, Online. Available: www. spine.org.

Okeson, J.P., 2008. Functional neuroanatomy and physiology of the masticatory system. In: Management of temporomandibular disorders and occlusion, sixth ed. Elsevier, St Louis, pp. 25–57.

Okeson, J.P., 2008. Signs and symptoms of temporomandibular disorders. In: Management of temporomandibular disorders and occlusion, sixth ed. Elsevier, St Louis, pp. 164–215.

Otani, K., Konno, S., Kikuchi, S., 2001. Lumbosacral transitional vertebrae and nerve-root symptoms. J. Bone Joint Surg. Br. 83 (8), 1137–1140.

Pavlov, P., Roebroeks, W., Svendsen, J.I., 2004. The Pleistocene colonization of northeastern Europe: a report on recent research. J. Hum. Evol. 47 (1–2): 3–17.

Prentice, W.E., 2001. Joint mobilization and traction techniques in rehabilitation. In: Prentice, W.E., Voight, M.L. (Eds.), Techniques in musculoskeletal rehabilitation. McGraw-Hill Professional, Colombus, pp. 235–258.

Raunest, J., Sager, M., Bürgener, E., 1996. Proprioceptive mechanisms in the cruciate ligaments: an electromyographic study on reflex activity in the thigh muscles. J. Trauma 41, 375–406.

Riemann, B.L., Myers, J.B., Stone, D.A., et al., 2003. Effect of lateral ankle ligament proprioception alteration on single leg stance stability [H-13b free communication/slide ankle instability]. Med. Sci. Sports Exerc. 35, S1–S357.

Rogala, E.J., Drummond, D.S., Gurr, J., 1978. Scoliosis: incidence and natural history. A prospective epidemiological study. J. Bone Joint Surg. 60, 173–176.

Rowe, L.J., Yochum, T.R., 1987. Measurements in skeletal radiology. In: Yochum, T.R., Rowe, L.J. (Eds.), Essential of skeletal radiology, vol I. Williams and Wilkins, Baltimore, pp. 169–224.

Rowe, L.J., Yochum, T.R., 1987. Scoliosis. In: Yochum, T.R., Rowe, L.J. (Eds.), Essential of skeletal radiology, vol I. Williams & Wilkins, Baltimore, pp. 225–242.

Royal College of General Practitioners. 2001. Principal recommendations linked to evidence: manipulation. In:

Clinical guidelines: Low back pain. Royal College of General Practitioners, London.

Schafer, R.C., 1983. Clinical biomechanics of the spine and pelvis. In: Clinical biomechanics: musculoskeletal actions and reactions. Williams and Wilkins, Baltimore, pp. 171–494.

Schafer, R.C., 1983. Clinical biomechanics of the extremities. In: Clinical biomechanics: musculoskeletal actions and reactions. Williams and Wilkins, Baltimore, pp. 495–603.

Schiowitz, S., 2004. Lumbar anatomical considerations. In: DiGiovanna, E.L., Schiowitz, S., Dowling, D.J. (Eds.), An osteopathic approach to diagnosis and treatment, third ed. Lippincott Williams and Wilkins, Baltimore, pp. 233–236.

Schiowitz, S., 2004. Pelvic and sacral anatomical considerations. In: DiGiovanna, E.L., Schiowitz, S., Dowling, D.J. (Eds.), An osteopathic approach to diagnosis and treatment, third ed. Lippincott Williams and Wilkins, Baltimore, pp. 285–292.

Schiowitz, S., Fenton, J., 2004. Cervical anatomic considerations. In: DiGiovanna, E.L., Schiowitz, S., Dowling, D.J. (Eds.), An osteopathic approach to diagnosis and treatment, third ed. Lippincott Williams and Wilkins, Baltimore, pp. 125–129.

Schiowitz, S., DiGiovanna, E.L., DiGiovanna, J.A., 2004. Gait and postural considerations. In: DiGiovanna, E.L., Schiowitz, S., Dowling, D.J. (Eds.), An osteopathic approach to diagnosis and treatment, third ed. Lippincott Williams and Wilkins, Baltimore, pp. 293–30.

Schiowitz, S., DiGiovanna, E.L., Brous, N., 2004. General anatomical considerations. In: DiGiovanna, E.L., Schiowitz, S., Dowling, D.J. (Eds.), An osteopathic approach to diagnosis and treatment, third ed. Lippincott Williams and Wilkins, Baltimore, pp. 24–36.

Smellie, S., 2003. The limitations of a standard workstation for its user population. Clinical Chiropractic 6, 101–108.

Spitzer, W.O., Skovron, M.L., Salmi, L. R., et al., 1995. Scientific monograph of the Quebec Task Force on Whiplash Associated Disorders:
redefining whiplash and its management. Spine 20, 8S.

Squires, B., Gargan, M.F., Bannister, G. C., 1996. Soft tissue injuries of the cervical spine: 15-year follow-up. J. Bone Joint Surg. 86, 955–957.

Standring, S. (Ed.), 2005. Functional anatomy of the musculoskeletal system. In: Gray's Anatomy: the anatomical basis of clinical practice. Elsevier, Edinburgh, pp. 83–135.

Standring, S. (Ed.), 2005. Palmaris longus. In: Gray's anatomy: the anatomical basis of clinical practice. Elsevier, Edinburgh. Online. Available: www.graysanatomyonline. com 18th October 2008, 14:25 BST.

Standring, S. (Ed.), 2005. Psoas major. In: Gray's anatomy: the anatomical basis of clinical practice. Elsevier, Edinburgh. Online. Available: www. graysanatomyonline.com 18 October 2008, 21:10 BST.

Standring, S. (Ed.), 2005. Psoas minor. In: Gray's anatomy: the anatomical basis of clinical practice. Elsevier, Edinburgh. Online. Available: www. graysanatomyonline.com 18 October 2008, 14:25 BST.

Stemper, B.D., Yoganandan, N., Pintar, F.A., 2003. Kinetics of the head-neck complex in low-speed rear impact. Biomed. Sci. Instrum. 39, 245–250.

Stemper, B.D., Yoganandan, N., Pintar, F.A., 2004. Gender- and region-dependent local facet joint kinematics in rear impact: implications in whiplash injury. Spine 29 (16), 1764–1771.

Stewart, J.P.R., Erskine, C.A., 1979. An experimental analysis of injuries to the menisci of the knee joint. Int. Orthop. 3, 9–12.

Storm, C., Wänman, A., 2006. Temporomandibular disorders, headaches, and cervical pain among females in a Sami population. Acta Odontol. Scand. 64 (5), 319–325.

Tague, R.G., Lovejoy, C.O., 1986. The obstetric pelvis of A L288-1 (Lucy). J. Hum. Evol. 15, 237–273.

Talbot, L., 2003. Failed back surgery syndrome. BMJ 327, 985–986.

Thibodeau, G., Patton, K., 2006. Anatomy of the muscular system. In: Anatomy and Physiology, sixth ed. Mosby, Philadelphia (Chapter 10) (ebook).
Thorne, J.O., Collcott, T.C., 1984. Chambers biographical dictionary, revised edition. W & R Chambers, Edinburgh.

Tini, P.G., Wieser, C., Zinn, W.M., 1977. The transitional vertebra of the lumbosacral spine: its radiological classification, incidence, prevalence and clinical significance. Rheumatol. Rehabil. 16, 180–185.

Travell, J.G., Simons, D.G., 1992. Low back and pelvis. In: Myofascial pain and dysfunction, vol 2. Williams and Wilkins, Baltimore.

Trew, M., 2005. Function of the lower limb. In: Trew, M., Everett, T. (Eds.), Human movement: an introductory text, fourth ed. Churchill Livingstone, Edinburgh, pp. 172–192.

Trew, M., Everett, T., 2005. Measuring and evaluating human movement. In: Human Movement: An introductory text, fourth ed. Churchill Livingstone, Edinburgh, pp. 143–160.

UK BEAM Trial Team. 2004. United Kingdom back pain exercise and manipulation (UK BEAM) randomised trial: effectiveness of physical treatments for back pain in primary care. BMJ 329, 1377.

Visscher, C., Hofman, N., Mes, C., et al., 2005. Is temporomandibular pain in chronic whiplash-associated disorders part of a more widespread pain syndrome? Clin. J. Pain 21 (4), 353–357.

Waddell, G.I., 1995. Modern management of spinal disorders. J. Manipulative Physiol. Ther. 18, 590–596.

Walters, I.P., 1994. Craniofacial orthopedics and head pain. In: Curl, D.D. (Ed.), Chiropractic approach to head pain. Williams and Wilkins, Baltimore, pp. 304–326.

Wiesinger, B., Malker, H., Englund, E., et al., 2007. Back pain in relation to musculoskeletal disorders in the jaw-face: a matched case-control study. Pain 131 (3), 311–319.

Yochum, T.R., Rowe, L.J. (Eds.), 1987. The natural history of spondylosis and spondylolisthesis. In: Essential of skeletal radiology, vol I. Williams and Wilkins, Baltimore, pp. 243–272.

# Chapter Six

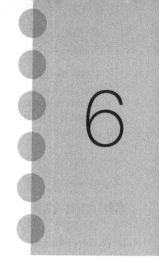

6

# Atomic structure

## CHAPTER CONTENTS

Check your existing knowledge . . . . . . . . 125
Atomic theory . . . . . . . . . . . . . . . . . . 126
  The Thomson atom . . . . . . . . . . . . . . 127
  The Rutherford atom . . . . . . . . . . . . . 127
  Isotopes . . . . . . . . . . . . . . . . . . . . . 129
  Intra-atomic forces . . . . . . . . . . . . . . 131
  Wave theory . . . . . . . . . . . . . . . . . . 133
  Quantum mechanics . . . . . . . . . . . . . 133
  The Bohr atom . . . . . . . . . . . . . . . . 135
Electrons and electron shells . . . . . . . . 136
  The photoelectric effect . . . . . . . . . . . 136
  Electron shells . . . . . . . . . . . . . . . . . 137

Intramolecular bonding . . . . . . . . . . . . 143
  Ionic bonding . . . . . . . . . . . . . . . . . . 144
  Covalent bonding . . . . . . . . . . . . . . . 144
  The water molecule . . . . . . . . . . . . . . 145
Intermolecular bonding . . . . . . . . . . . . 147
  Van der Waals bonds . . . . . . . . . . . . 148
Learning outcomes . . . . . . . . . . . . . . . 148
Check your existing knowledge:
answers . . . . . . . . . . . . . . . . . . . . . . 148
Bibliography . . . . . . . . . . . . . . . . . . . 149

## CHECK YOUR EXISTING KNOWLEDGE

1 Define the following terms:
  a Isotope
  b Nucleon
  c Mass number
  d Atomic number
  e Ion

2 Why don't the nuclei of atoms fly apart?

3 What are Young's fringes?

4 An electron has an energy of 500 $eV$ and mass $9 \times 10^{-31}$ kg. If Planck's constant is $6.6 \times 10^{-34}$ Js, what is the electron's wavelength?

5 How many electrons are there in:
  a A closed $M$ shell?
  b The ground state of hydrogen?
  c A filled $s$ sub-orbital?
  d A sodium ion?
  e The $2p$ sub-orbital of $_8O$?

6 State Einstein's photoelectric equation

7  Write the quantum electron structure for $_{18}$A (argon)
8  Hund's rule gives rise to what physical property of some Group VIIIb elements (you may wish to refer to the periodic table, Fig. 6.1)
9  What is a hydrogen bond?
10  Why is the bond angle in a water molecule 104.5°and not 90°?

# Atomic theory

It is important to realize at the outset that the descriptions of atoms and atomic particles that you will encounter here and in other texts are merely models designed to help us understand how atoms behave and interact. As with any model, there is a degree of simplification – in the case of atomic modelling, this simplification is often so gross that the model bears no relationship to reality. Atoms are, pretty much, incomprehensible things: you can't see them, even with the most powerful

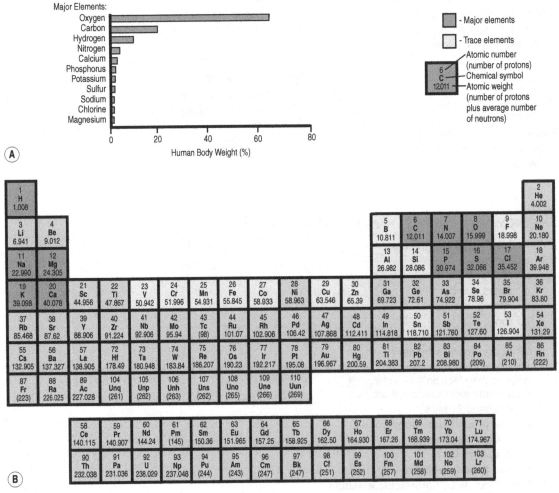

**Figure 6.1** • The periodic table B showing the major elements that occur in the body and their relative contribution to body mass A. Note the chemicals with similar properties occur (for example, F, Cl, Br, I, At or Cu, Ag, Au) in the same column. Reproduced from Thibodeau and Patton 2006 with permission from Elsevier.

microscopes (you will learn why in Chapter 8); you can't taste them, feel them, hear them; you can't touch them, merely the fields that surround them.

All that we know about atoms is inferred from indirect experimental observation or mathematical models. At the atomic level, we sometimes have to leave common sense behind and deal with concepts such as particles being in two places at the same time, particles behaving as waves and waves behaving as particles. This is why we have models; there are times when too much knowledge simply confuses the picture. You often don't need to think of an electron as a three-dimensional, standing probability wave (thankfully) and it is much easier – and more useful – to picture a billiard ball whizzing about and bumping into other billiard balls . . . just so long as you always remember that electrons aren't actually billiard balls.

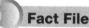

## Fact File

### THE THOMPSON PRIZES

It is somewhat ironic that one of the founders of nuclear physics, J.J. Thomson, was awarded the Nobel Prize for physics in 1906 for discovering there were particles called electrons. His son, George, became the only son of a Nobel Laureate to also win a Nobel Prize when, in 1937, he proved that electrons were (also) waves.

In order to comprehend the different forms of atomic models, and realize when it is appropriate – and inappropriate – to use them, it is useful to understand how they developed and evolved.

For centuries, man struggled to understand how matter was constructed, whether from discrete, uniform particles in differing proportions or from mixtures of fundamental 'elements': earth, water, fire and air. By the 19th century, as we have already seen, science was becoming a respectable, disciplined field and its practitioners had begun to understand the difference between certain types of substances. Most importantly, they discovered that **mixtures**, such as air, could be separated into their constituent parts whilst **compounds** were chemically combined and, by using chemistry, could be broken down into other, simpler substances. However, beyond a certain point, it was no longer possible to chemically decompose a substance and these fundamental substances were known as **elements**.

Therefore, for example, air is composed of a *mixture* of gases, which are not chemically combined. One of these gases is carbon dioxide, a *compound* whose molecule consists of two *elements*, carbon and oxygen. It was generally accepted that these elements consisted of what was then considered a fundamental particle, the atom, and that the atoms for each element must somehow be uniquely different . . . but how?

## The Thomson atom

With J.J. Thomson's 1898 discovery of electrons, and the realization that all atoms contained these particles, scientists had their first insight into the structure of the atoms. They knew that atoms were electrically neutral; therefore, there must be a positive charge balancing the negative charge of the electrons. This led to the 'Thomson' model of the atoms – also called the 'plum-pudding' model. In this scenario, the spherical atom of positively charged matter has electrons studded into it, like raisins in a plum, or Christmas, pudding (Fig. 6.2).

## The Rutherford atom

Thomson's proposal fitted the bill nicely for 13 years until a minor experiment by a couple of (then) minor scientists showed it to be impossible and, in doing so, for ever upset the laws of classical physics. It was an experiment that almost never happened. Hans Geiger was a visiting research fellow working under the direction of the God-like Ernest Rutherford at the University of Manchester.

## Fact File

### HANS GEIGER

Geiger's work on atomic theory is largely forgotten: credit is almost invariably ascribed to Rutherford or, occasionally and more appropriately, to Marsden. Instead, Geiger ended up with eponymous immortality by having a radiation detector named after him, despite the fact that the actual work was done by Müller, after whom the more correctly and completely termed Geiger-Müller counter is also named, though is now almost always shortened, rather unfairly, to 'Geiger counter'.

Thomson atomic model

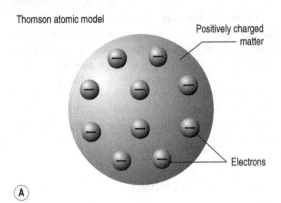

Positively charged matter

Electrons

(A)

Rutherford atomic model

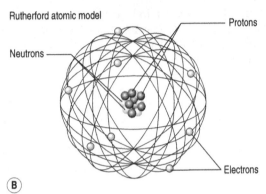

Protons

Neutrons

Electrons

(B)

Bohr atomic model

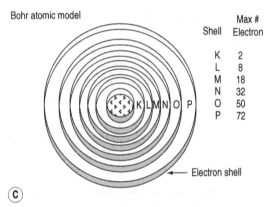

| Shell | Max # Electron |
|-------|----------------|
| K | 2 |
| L | 8 |
| M | 18 |
| N | 32 |
| O | 50 |
| P | 72 |

Electron shell

(C)

**Figure 6.2** ● The development of atomic theories. (A) The Thomson or 'plum pudding' model in which electrons are embedded in a diffuse, positively charged matrix. (B) The Rutherford model: electrons are orbiting separately around a small, dense positively charged nucleus (in defiance of classical electrostatic theory). (C) The Bohr model of the atom. Electrons orbit at intervals that support standing waves that are integral multiples of their de Broglie wavelength. Each shell consists of a number of sub-orbitals (s, p, d, f etc.), each of which has a discrete energy value associated with it. This model, which utilizes quantum mechanics rather than classical physical theory, is widely accepted and utilized today.

For some time, it had been known that α-particles could be slightly deflected when fired at thin sheets of metal foil. This was entirely consistent with the Thomson model of the electron with weak electric forces being exerted on the passing α-particles by the uniformly distributed charges of the 'plum pudding' atoms.

## ABC DICTIONARY DEFINITION

### ALPHA PARTICLES

α-particles are helium nuclei (two protons plus two neutrons), which have a positive charge twice that of a single electron. We shall encounter them in detail in Chapter 8; for the moment, this level of detail will suffice.

To measure for large deflections was a ridiculous waste of time, there was no way in which a thin piece of gold foil could deflect relatively heavy α-particles; it was 'make-work' for Ernest Marsden, a rather unpromising PhD student.

To everyone's surprise, and no little incredulity, Marsden found large deviations. Geiger flatly refused to believe his results and, when he was finally convinced, Rutherford – after whom the experiment is usually named – refused to believe Geiger. When Marsden was sent back to repeat the experiment yet again, he had the idea of placing the detectors on the 'wrong' side of the metal foil. He found that, not only were α-particles being deflected through large angles, but some were even being scattered in a backward direction.

Rutherford described this as 'the equivalent of firing a 15" artillery shell at a piece of tissue paper and watching the shell bounce back at you'. He sent Marsden back to repeat the experiment once more, this time supervising it himself. Marsden got his PhD with what must still be the most important postgraduate thesis of all time. Sadly, Marsden, like 7 million other young men of his generation, was killed in World War 1 and history was never able to judge whether he was a genius or merely serendipitous. Rutherford's great contribution was to deduce, correctly, how such a thing could have happened.

He realized that the only model that could account for the α-particles' extraordinary behaviour was if the positive charge was all concentrated into a small, tightly bound, dense nucleus with the electrons more diffusely dispersed at a distance (Fig. 6.2). This alone could account for the findings: it would mean that much of apparently solid objects was empty space, which was why most of the α-particles passed through the foil without deviation. The light, widely separated electrons had little influence on the passage of the incoming particles but if they came within the electric field of the large, positive charge of the nucleus, they could be deflected or even repelled (Fig. 6.3).

In fact, it transpires that 99.999999% of matter is empty space; if the nucleus of a hydrogen atom is represented by a thumb-tack stuck in the middle of a football field, then the electron would be lurking somewhere in the furthest, uppermost row of seats in the surrounding stadium. In Rutherford's model, the electric field intensity of the gold atomic nucleus is 100 000 000 times that of the Thomson model.

Geiger and Marsden went on to show that foils of different metals would deflect α-particles in differing amounts and that, from this, they could estimate the nuclear charge, which always turned out to be an exact multiple of the charge of an electron ($e$), though positive rather than negative ($+e$). For gold foil, they found that the nuclear charge was $+79e$. As this charge was unique for each material, elements became defined by the number of protons in their nucleus, the **atomic number (Z)**.

## Isotopes

It quickly became apparent that a proton and a hydrogen **ion** were identical and that the majority of the atom's mass (99.9995%) resided in the nucleus. There were, however, two problems with Rutherford's proposed nuclear model. The first was that it didn't account for **isotopes**. Isotopes are differing forms of an element; they have the same chemical properties but the mass of their atomic nuclei varies. For example, hydrogen has three isotopes, the common variety that we have just discussed with an atomic mass of approximately one proton; deuterium, which accounts for approximately 0.015% of all hydrogen and has an atomic mass equivalent to two protons; and the much rarer ($1:10^{-15}$) tritium, which has a third 'proton-mass' (Fig. 6.4). The isotopes all have the same chemical properties – you can make $H_2O$ using deuterium or tritium; this is so-called 'heavy water'– but different **atomic mass numbers (A)**, 1 for hydrogen, 2 for deuterium and 3 for tritium.

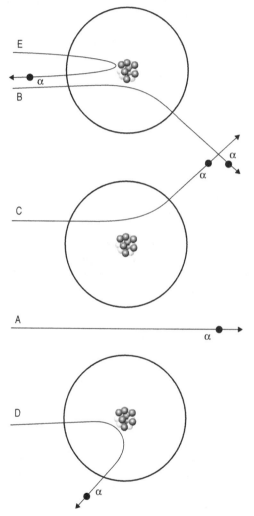

**Figure 6.3** • Marsden's classical experiment in which α-particles were fired at a thin gold foil. Although most α-particles travelled straight through the foil without being altered in their path (**A**), many showed significant deviation (**B, C**) or even reflection (**D, E**) in a manner that was inconsistent with the then prevalent Thomson model of the atom. It was this experiment and its unexpected results that led Rutherford to develop a new atomic model in which electrons orbited a positively charged nucleus.

**ABC DICTIONARY DEFINITION**

**ION**

An ion is an atom from which an electron or electrons has been removed or added so that it bears a charge, which will always be a multiple of $\pm e$.

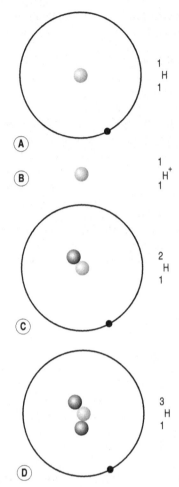

$$
\begin{array}{cc}
\text{(A)} & {}^{1}_{1}\text{H} \\
\text{(B)} & {}^{1}_{1}\text{H}^{+} \\
\text{(C)} & {}^{2}_{1}\text{H} \\
\text{(D)} & {}^{3}_{1}\text{H}
\end{array}
$$

**Figure 6.4** • Different forms of the element hydrogen (H). The figures to the left of the element's abbreviated form represent the mass number (superiorly), equivalent to the combined number of protons and neutrons in the nucleus (nucleon count), and the atomic number (proton count). The latter is unique to each element, hence it is the same for each isotope of hydrogen shown here. The mass number rises as the nucleon count increases. Hydrogen in its commonest form, ${}^{1}\text{H}$, consists of a single proton (A); deuterium ${}^{2}\text{H}$ has an additional neutron (C) while the much rarer tritium ${}^{3}\text{H}$ nucleus comprises a proton and two neutrons (D). If the atom loses an electron(s) (or gains one or more), it is no longer electro-neutral and becomes an ion (B).

Perhaps the isotope that has the greatest public awareness is carbon-14. Carbon, which has six protons ($Z = 6$), normally has an atomic mass number of 12; however, it also exists in a form where $A = 14$. Conveniently, this form is radioactive and decays slowly back into carbon-12. By finding the ratio of carbon-12 to carbon-14, scientists are able to calculate the approximate age of organic materials, all of which contain large numbers of carbon atoms.

It is also the carbon atom that forms the basis for the definition of the **mole**, which, as we learned in Chapter 1, is one of the seven fundamental SI units (Table 1.1). You may recall that the mole was defined as the amount of a given substance that contains as many elementary entities as there are atoms in 0.012 kilogram of carbon-12.

One mole of carbon-12 contains $6.022\ 52 \times 10^{23}$ carbon atoms, a number known as **Avogadro's constant**, in honour of Amedeo Avogadro, an Italian mathematical physicist who demonstrated that, at constant temperature and pressure, identical volumes of different gases contain the same number of particles.

A mole of *any* substance – be it composed of atoms, molecules, ions, electrons, photons etc. – also contains this number of entities. However, the mass of $6.022\ 52 \times 10^{23}$ carbon atoms does not equal 12 g exactly. This is because the sample will not consist of purely '12A-carbon'; two other isotopes of carbon also exist. We have already mentioned '14A-carbon', which is radioactive and so will ultimately decay back into a stable isotope but there is also '13A-carbon', which comprises 1.1% of all naturally occurring carbon. So the mass of $6.022\ 52 \times 10^{23}$ carbon atoms is actually 12.011 g. This is known as the **atomic weight** of carbon.

In the 1870s, Dmitri Mendeleev, a Russian chemist, found that, if he arranged chemical elements in order of increasing atomic weight, certain elements with similar properties – for example fluorine, chlorine, iodine and bromine – occurred periodically at regular and predictable intervals. He also spotted that there were obvious gaps in the table and was able to make predictions as to the chemical properties of the missing elements. As his predictions came to be realized, the Periodic Table (Fig. 6.1) became a standard reference tool for all scientists.

Meanwhile, the solution to Rutherford's isotope problem came with the proposal of the **neutron,** an uncharged nuclear particle that can be regarded as a combined proton and electron. Thus, the neutron contributes to the atomic mass number but has no influence on the atomic number, which is a function of the proton count only. An element (X) can, therefore, be written in terms of its proton (Z) and **nucleon** (A) count, with, if appropriate, its ionic charge:

$${}^{A}_{Z}\text{X}$$

The three isotopes of carbon we discussed become $^{12}_6C$ (six protons and six neutrons), $^{13}_6C$ (six protons and seven neutrons) and $^{14}_6C$ (six protons and eight neutrons). Examples of some of the elements that we have discussed, and others that you are likely to commonly encounter, are given in Table 6.1.

 **DICTIONARY DEFINITION**

**NUCLEON**

A nucleon is any particle found in a nucleus: for our purposes, protons and neutrons.

## Intra-atomic forces

Returning again to Rutherford's model, there was, as has been already intimated, a second problem. Today, we are so accepting of this basic model of the atom that we are seemingly blind to this fundamental flaw. According to the laws of classical physics – and these were the only physical laws there were in 1909 – Rutherford's atom should, of course, instantly fly apart. The compressed positive forces of the nuclear protons would, as like charges, repel. This process would be aided by the attraction to the oppositely charged orbiting electrons – assuming a way could be found to limit the mutual repulsion of the electrons themselves.

Electrostatically, Rutherford's atom makes no sense at all; even if it did, Newton's laws of motion and Coulomb's law of electric force would preclude an electron from being able to maintain a stable orbit in the way that the planets travel around the mutually attractive sun – instead it would rapidly spiral inwards and collide with the nucleus.

 **DICTIONARY DEFINITION**

**COULOMB'S LAW**

Coulomb's law of electrostatic force states that the size of the attraction or repulsion is directly proportional to the size of the charges ($Q_1$ and $Q_2$) and obeys the inverse square law with regard to separation ($r$):

$$F \propto Q_1Q_2/r^2$$

The solution to this seeming paradox came in two parts. Scientists had to wait until the 1930s for confirmation of the **weak nuclear force**, which, it was proposed, could overcome the electromagnetic repulsion of the positive protons – at least, up to a point. As the size of the nucleus, and its charge, grew, the element became increasingly unstable, and thus increasingly subject to rapid radioactive decay. Eventually, it reached a point where it was not physically possible to force protons together, the electromagnetic repulsion overwhelming the weak nuclear attraction.

 **Fact File**

**ELECTROWEAK FORCE**

Today, we understand that weak nuclear force and electromagnetism are simply manifestations of the same basic force (now called the electroweak force), just as Maxwell showed 150 years ago that electricity and magnetism were intrinsically associated.

This means that the heaviest, naturally occurring element is uranium, which has a **half-life** of 4.5 billion years. Beyond that, elements have to be synthesized but even the most stable isotopes have half-lives of only a few minutes or less. In fact, elements up to $Z = 112$ have been synthesized, by which time the half-life has reduced to fractions of seconds only.

 **DICTIONARY DEFINITION**

**HALF-LIFE**

The concept of half-life is dealt with more fully in Chapter 8; for now, it is enough to know that it is the time required for 50% of a given quantity of an element to decay radioactively. Of the remaining 50%, half will again decay in the period of the half-life, leaving quarter of the original sample . . . and so on.

There was less of a wait for the solution to the problem of the orbiting electron. In 1914, Niels Bohr proposed a radical new theory that led to the development of quantum mechanics. In order to understand the principles of his idea, we need to firstly understand a little bit about waves and about something to which we have already alluded: **wave-particle duality**.

**Table 6.1** Some common elements, their isomer nomenclature and comments

| Element (Z) | Nomenclature of common (>1%), natural isotopes | Comment |
|---|---|---|
| Hydrogen (1) | $^{1}_{1}H$, $^{2}_{1}H$, (protinium), (deuterium)*, $^{3}_{1}H$ (tritium)* | Ubiquitous in animal tissue, the element that facilitates magnetic resonance imaging |
| Helium (2) | $^{4}_{2}He$ | Nucleus is an $\alpha$-particle $^{4}_{2}He^{2+}$ |
| Carbon (6) | $^{12}_{6}C$, $^{13}_{6}C$, $^{14}_{6}C$* | Carbon dating (see above). The backbone of organic molecules |
| Nitrogen (7) | $^{14}_{7}H$ | Main component of air. Component of all proteins and DNA |
| Oxygen (8) | $^{16}_{8}O$ | Essential for cellular respiration |
| Sodium (11) | $^{23}_{11}Na$ | $Na^{+}$ ion is essential in cell membrane transport |
| Magnesium (12) | $^{24}_{12}Mg$, $^{25}_{12}Mg$, $^{26}_{12}Mg$ | Catalyst for enzyme reactions in carbohydrate metabolism |
| Aluminium (13) | $^{27}_{13}Al$ | Used for x-ray filters and step-wedges |
| Chlorine (17) | $^{35}_{17}Cl$ | $Cl^{-}$ ion is essential in cell membrane transport |
| Potassium (19) | $^{39}_{19}K$, $^{41}_{19}K$ | Man-made isotopes used in medicine |
| Calcium (20) | $^{40}_{20}Ca$, $^{44}_{20}Ca$ | Major component of bones and teeth; $Ca^{2+}$ triggers muscle contraction |
| Iron (26) | $^{54}_{26}Fe$, $^{56}_{26}Fe$, $^{57}_{26}Fe$ | Critical component of haemoglobin |
| Cobalt (27) | $^{59}_{27}Co$ | Man-made isotopes used in medicine |
| Copper (29) | $^{63}_{29}Cu$, $^{65}_{29}Cu$ | Key enzymatic component. Used for x-ray filters and anodes/targets |
| Zinc (30) | $^{64}_{30}Zn$, $^{66}_{30}Zn$, $^{67}_{30}Zn$, $^{68}_{30}Zn$ | Key enzymatic component |
| Tin (50) | $^{116}_{50}Sn$, $^{116}_{50}Sn$, $^{116}_{50}Sn$ | Used for x-ray filters |
| Iodine (53) | $^{127}_{53}I$ | Component of thyroid hormone. Radioactive, synthesized $^{131}_{53}I$ used investigatively and therapeutically |
| Barium (56) | $^{134}_{56}Ba$, $^{135}_{56}Ba$, $^{136}_{56}Ba$, $^{137}_{56}Ba$, $^{138}_{56}Ba$ | Radio-opaque medium used in radiographic examination of the gastrointestinal tract |
| Gadolinium (64) | $^{154}_{64}Gd$, $^{155}_{64}Gd$, $^{158}_{64}Gd$, $^{160}_{64}Gd$ | Commonest contrast agent for musculoskeletal MRI |
| Tungsten (74) | $^{182}_{74}W$, $^{183}_{74}W$, $^{184}_{74}W$, $^{186}_{74}W$ | x-ray machine filament |
| Gold (79) | $^{197}_{79}Au$ | Used in treatment of rheumatoid arthritis. Was the original foil used by Geiger and Marsden |
| Mercury (80) | $^{198}_{80}Hg$, $^{199}_{80}Hg$, $^{200}_{80}Hg$, $^{201}_{80}Hg$, $^{202}_{80}Hg$, $^{203}_{80}Hg$ | Used in traditional thermometers |
| Lead (82) | $^{204}_{82}Pb$, $^{206}_{82}Pb$, $^{207}_{82}Pb$, $^{208}_{82}Pb$ | Used for x-ray and other radiation shielding |
| Radon (86) | $^{222}_{86}Rn$ | Synthetic isotopes used in radiotherapy |
| Radium (88) | $^{226}_{88}Rd$, $^{228}_{88}Rd$, $^{224}_{88}Rd$ | Synthetic isotopes used in radiotherapy |

*Not occurring at > 1% but listed because of inclusion in discussion above.

# Wave theory

Waves are a way of transmitting energy through a medium. It is a common misconception that the medium itself moves; in fact, only the wave moves, transmitting the energy as it does so, whilst the medium oscillates or vibrates about a fixed position. So, in the case of a wave travelling across an ocean, although the wave moves forwards, the individual water molecules merely move up (the crest) and down (the following trough). However, when the wave reaches the shelving beach, it runs out of medium in which to travel and momentum causes the wave to fall over forwards (or break). It is this frequently observed phenomenon that causes people to intuitively think of the water itself travelling forwards rather than the wave.

Waves have a number of properties that solid objects lack. They can be **refracted**, or bent, as they pass from one medium to another; they can also be **defracted**. We are all familiar with the circular ripple effect causing by dropping a pebble into smooth water. If a linear wave front hits a narrow slit, it will pass through the slit and radiate outwards as if the slit were a new point source (Fig. 6.5). If there are a number of such slits in a row, the individual peaks

and troughs will interact; coincidental peaks and troughs cancelling each other, coincidental peaks and coincidental troughs reinforcing each other (Fig. 6.5C).

This accounts for a phenomenon known to sailors, the tidal race – patches of sea often found off headlands or near river estuaries where two tidal streams, moving in different directions, interact to produce an area of choppy water. It is also observed in light where these **interference patterns** will produce successive areas of light (reinforcement) and dark (cancellation). These diffraction patterns are known as **Young's fringes**.

So, we apparently have a clear differentiation between waves, such as light or those we see in a ripple tank, which will diffract through narrow slits, and solid objects, such as billiard balls, that pass through narrow slits without any change to their direction. If life were that simple, we wouldn't need quantum mechanics.

# Quantum mechanics

There are a number of experiments that defy this classical understanding of waves and particles. If a

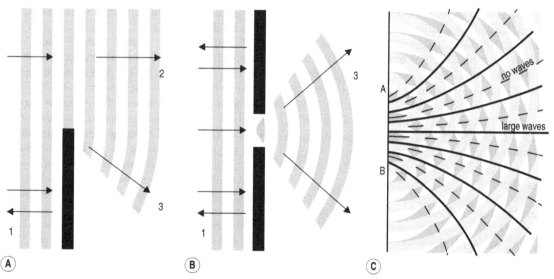

**Figure 6.5** • When a wave front meets an obstruction such as a promontory (A) the part of the wave hitting the barrier will reflect (1) and the remainder of the wave will continue onwards (2). However, the part of the wave intersecting the end of the promontory will radiate outwards as if from a new point source (3). This gives the effect of a rounded wave appearing to 'bend' around the corner. A similar phenomenon occurs when the wave front hits a narrow slit (B); it passes through the slit and radiates outwards as if from a new point source. When the peaks and troughs from adjacent slits interfere (C), they can reinforce or cancel each other. This gives rise to distinctive patterns – with light waves, these areas of light (peak–peak/trough–trough = reinforcement) and dark (peak–trough/trough–peak = cancellation) are known as Young's fringes.

'water-wheel' with alternate polished and black sails is placed in a vacuum, not only will it turn, but it is possible to detect the difference in momentum change

(= force) when the light is absorbed (*mc*) or reflected (*2mc*). This phenomenon is known as **radiation pressure** – surely though, we have already learnt momentum is a property of particles with mass, not of *waves*.

The corollary was the disturbing observation in 1927 by G. P. Thomson – son of J. J. – that it was perfectly possible to diffract electrons, despite the fact that they were apparently particles. In 1905, Einstein had already shown that light needed to be considered as discrete bundles of energy, which he termed **photons**, rather than as classical waves. By the time of Thomson's experiment, Louis de Broglie had already developed a relationship between de Broglie (pronounced 'der broy') wavelength ($\lambda$) and momentum (*mv*):

$$\lambda_{dB} = h/mv$$

where $h$ is a value known as **Planck's constant** ($6.6 \times 10^{-34}$ Js). (By contrast, the energy of a photon is $hf$, where $f$ is the frequency of the light.)

We can further illustrate this point by plugging some values into this equation. If we take an electron that has been accelerated through an electrical potential difference of 100 volts, it will have an energy of 100 eV. 1 eV = $1.6 \times 10^{-19}$ J; therefore the electron has an energy of $1.6 \times 10^{-17}$ J. Once

we also know that the mass of an electron is $9.1 \times 10^{-31}$ kg, then we can calculate its velocity:

$$E = \tfrac{1}{2}mv^2$$

Therefore:

$$v = \sqrt{2E/m} = \sqrt{(2 \times 1.6 \times 10^{-17}/9.1 \times 10^{-31})}$$
$$= 5.9 \times 10^6 \, ms^{-1}$$

We also know that:

$$\lambda_{dB} = h/mv$$
$$= \sqrt{6.6 \times 10^{-34}/9.1 \times 10^{-31} \times 5.9 \times 10^6}$$
$$= 1.2 \times 10^{-10} m.$$

This is not dissimilar to the wavelength of x-rays and about the same as the interatomic distance in solids, which is why electron microscopes can 'see' things that conventional light microscopes cannot.

By contrast something large, like a charging buffalo – mass around 1500 kg; velocity, say, 10 ms$^{-1}$ – will have a de Broglie wavelength of $10^{-30}$ m, so short as to demonstrate no wave tendencies at non-relativistic speeds. Certainly, it would be unwise to assume that it would diffract around you at the moment of impact.

Of course, saying that a particle such as an electron (or indeed a proton, neutron, α-particle, β-particle etc.) can behave like a wave doesn't answer the question: what sort of wave? Obviously, this 'mass-wave' is not part of the electromagnetic spectrum. Rather, it is regarded as being the probability of the particle being in a given point at the same time. In the case of the buffalo, the chances of it actually being anywhere other than where classical physics predicts are so unimaginably small as to make being struck by lightning twice on the same day a worrying probability.

This concept of a 'probability wave' can lead to some rather bizarre behaviour. If, instead of a beam of light, single photons are sequentially released through a diffraction grating, common sense would dictate that they would pass straight through; there is nothing for them to interfere with, so no fringes can form. Fringes do form. The only possible conclusion is that the diffraction pattern is due to the *probability* of a photon going to a particular point. The same thing occurs when you fire a single photon at a half-silvered mirror, which allows 50% of light to travel straight through whilst reflecting the other half. Logic would dictate that there is a 50% chance of the light travelling straight through the mirror and a 50% chance of it being reflected. One or the other, heads or tails – but not both. In fact, incredibly, both do happen; the photon can be in two places at once because it is a probability wave and there are equal chances of either event having happened.

We actually see the effects of quantum mechanics every day without realizing it – next time you look at your television or computer screen you should perhaps realize how intellectually challenging, seemingly nonsensical and fascinating the image that you are viewing really is.

There is one more feature of waves of which you need to be aware, fortunately lying in the intuitively reconcilable world of classical physics! We have already seen how the peaks and troughs of waves can interfere with each other. If the waves are in a fixed string – as they are in a stringed musical instrument – reflection occurs at both ends and, if the wavelength is an exact divisor of the string length (i.e. 1, ½, ⅓ etc.) a system of nodes and antinodes is set up (Fig. 6.6). The string, therefore, has a series of permitted modes in which it can vibrate at a natural frequency. Other modes will not allow support of this **resonance** and thus standing waves will not occur.

## The Bohr atom

The concept of a charging buffalo acting as a compressed probability wave front may well be conceptually intriguing; likewise, understanding the physics behind the beauty of a sustained note from a Stradivarius may be interesting – but what has it to do with atomic theory?

Enter Niels Bohr, Nobel Prize winner, genius and all-round nice guy (Fig. 6.7). He used quantum theory to develop a model of the atom that persists to this day. In the Bohr atom, there are a finite number of permitted electron orbits. These equate to those circumferences ($2\pi r_n$, where $r_n$ is the radius of the orbit containing $n$ wavelengths) that can support

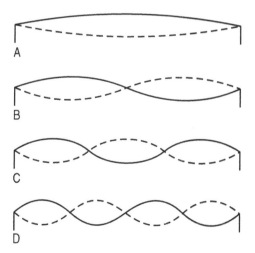

**Figure 6.6** ● Standing wave modes. Resonance will occur when the length of a string, $L$, is an exact multiple of the wavelength, $\lambda$, of the vibration. This allows a standing wave with a set number of nodes and antinodes to be perpetuated. In A, $L = \lambda$; In B, $L = 2\lambda$; In C, $L = 3\lambda$; In D, $L = 4\lambda$ and so on indefinitely.

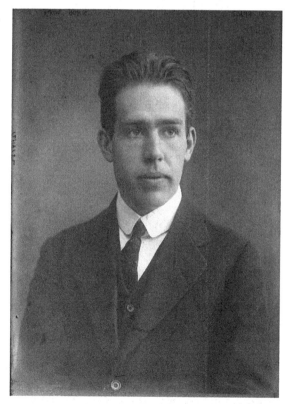

**Figure 6.7** ● Niels Bohr (1885–1962), the founding father of quantum mechanics.

an integral number of de Broglie wavelengths, $n\lambda$. The various permitted orbits involve different electron energies; these energies are inversely proportional to the orbit radius, $r_n$. The energy levels of the hydrogen electron are shown in Figure 6.8. When the electron is in the energy level $n = 1$, it is said to be in its **ground state**, if it is at a higher level $(n > 1)$, then it is an **excited state**; however, if it is given enough energy $(5.4 \times 10^{-19}$ J$)$ to completely escape the atom $(n = \infty)$, the atom becomes an ion and the electron is said to have become a **free electron**, as it is no longer associated with any energy level. This figure of $5.4 \times 10^{-19}$ J is therefore known as the **ionizing energy**.

> ### Fact File
>
> #### NIELS BOHR
>
> The father of quantum mechanics – for which he won his laureate in 1922 – Bohr was one of the most influential, yet perhaps least heralded, physicists of all time – a true genius to rank with Newton and Einstein though much more able and willing to build what was a new science by collaboration rather than isolated intellectualism. His life was also less secluded; a Jew and fierce resistor of the Nazi occupation of his native Denmark, he was forced to make a daring escape to Sweden from where he was rescued by a British snatch squad. He spent much of the remainder of his life working against nuclear proliferation and campaigning for peace.

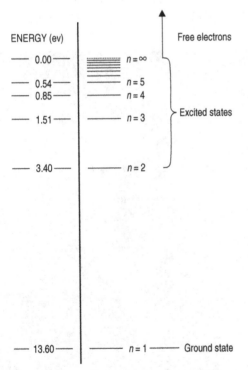

Figure 6.8 • The energy levels in which a hydrogen electron can exist according to quantum theory. To be stable, it must exist at the lowest possible energy state $(n = 1)$, known as its ground state. If it receives external energy from collision with a photon, it can be temporarily elevated to a higher, excited state. If the energy is sufficient $(> 5.4 \times 10^{-19}$ J$)$, it can escape the atom altogether becoming a free electron. The atom then becomes a positively charged ion, known as a cation (negatively charged ions are also known as anions).

## Electrons and electron shells

### The photoelectric effect

As we saw above, light comes in discrete particles called photons, each with an amount of energy that is proportional to its frequency (by now, hopefully, thinking of things as being both waves and particles is no longer making your brain curl up at the corners and smoke). When light (or other electromagnetic radiation) shines onto a metal surface, it can cause electrons to be emitted. Whether this happens or not depends on whether the frequency of the light is greater than the **threshold frequency, $f_0$,** which corresponds to the energy $(E = hf)$ required to ionize the atom. However, because – as we shall see later – other factors can influence the amount of energy required to liberate electrons from a given surface, the energy required per electron is known as the **work function, $\Phi$,** of the surface.

It is worth noting that this effect is not dependent on the intensity of the light, this merely determines the *number* of electrons that will be emitted; more ionizing photons, more electrons but only if the photons have sufficient energy in the first place. Any 'spare' energy above and beyond the ionizing energy is reflected in the kinetic energy of the free electron as stated in **Einstein's photoelectric equation:**

**Kinetic energy = photon energy − work function**

$$\tfrac{1}{2}mv^2 = hf - \Phi$$

# Electron shells

Of course, not all photons have sufficient energy to ionize; if their energy is less than the threshold frequency, the electron with which they collide will remain bound to the atom. However, it will be enough to excite the electron into a higher quantum shell. Such an arrangement is unstable, and the electron will quickly ($\sim 10^{-8}$ s) drop back into its ground state, discarding its energy as a photon. So the effect works both ways, but we already know that the quantum shells all have discrete energy values so, whenever an electron drops from a higher shell to a lower one, the energy of the photon must be equal to the *difference* in the energies associated with the two shells.

As there are only a finite number of permutations, the light emitted by a single element, when diffracted, must have a distinct and limited spectrum. The first such spectrum had already been identified by Johann Balmer who, in 1885, analyzed light from the sun (which is predominantly atomic hydrogen) and found a series of six lines. It was these lines (and others, discovered 1906–1924, lying in the infrared and ultraviolet region), which Bohr calculated corresponded to transitions between specific electron shells (Fig. 6.9).

These shells (n = 1, 2, 3 etc.) are referred to by a series of letters, starting with $K$ (Table 6.2) and there are very strict laws as to how many electrons can exist in each shell. These laws were formulated when improvements in spectroscopy showed that the 'lines' that had been identified for each atom actually consisted of a tight grouping of very fine lines, suggesting the existence of sub-levels within each electron shell.

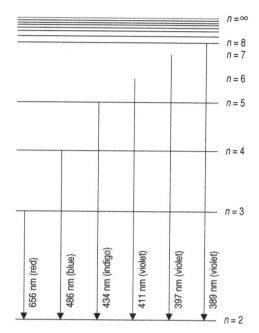

**Figure 6.9** • The Balmer series of visible spectral lines from the hydrogen atom. Each line represents the energy (inversely proportional to the wavelength) of the photon released during transition from a higher energy level to the n = 2 level (the spectral lines representing transitions to the ground state, n = 1 – known as the Lyman series – lie in the ultraviolet part of the electromagnetic spectrum).

**Table 6.2** Nomenclature of electron shells

| $n =$ | 1 | 2 | 3 | 4 | 5 | 6... |
|---|---|---|---|---|---|---|
|  | K | L | M | N | O | P... |

## Electron sub-levels

These sub-levels, known as the **azimuthal quantum number**, $l$, relate to the probability of finding an electron in a certain volume of space: this needn't concern us, but we do need to be familiar with the nomenclature that it generates.

The $l$ value begins at 0 and increases in integral increments up to $(n - 1)$. The number of electrons that can be accommodated in each level is given by the formula $2(2l + 1)$.

> **So, if $n = 1$, $l = 0$ and the number of electrons in this level $= 2(2l + 1) = 2$**
>
> **When $n = 2$, $l = 1$ and the maximum electron count is $2 \times (2 + 1) = 6$**

**Table 6.3** Nomenclature of electron sub-shells (azimuthal quantum numbers)

| $l =$ | 0 | 1 | 2 | 3 | 4 |
|---|---|---|---|---|---|
| Referred to as | s | p | d | f | g |
| Max. electron occupation $2(2l + 1)$ | 2 | 6 | 10 | 14 | 18 |

You can use this formula to check the values in Table 6.3, where you will note the quantum numbers are referred to by letters.

The other law governing the distribution of electrons is that, in the ground state, higher energy level shells will always fill before the lower ones. Therefore, the *s* sub-level will always fill before the *p* sub-level, which, in turn, will fill before the *d* sub-level and so on. This means that no two electrons can ever have the same combination of quantum numbers; this is known as the **Pauli exclusion principle**, after Wolfgang Pauli who identified it in 1925.

Thus, for every element, we can write a unique quantum code that defines the element in its stable, ground state as surely as the number of protons in the nucleus.

For example:

- Hydrogen ($Z = 1$) is written as $1s^1$
- Helium ($Z = 2$) is written as $1s^2$ (thus completing the $K$ shell)
- Lithium ($Z = 3$) is written as $1s^2 2s^1$
- Neon ($Z = 10$) is written as $1s^2 2s^1 2p^6$ (completing the $L$ shell)
- Sodium ($Z = 11$) is written as $1s^2 2s^2 2p^6 3s^1$
- Argon ($Z = 18$) is written as $1s^2 2s^2 2p^6 3s^2 3p^6$
- Krypton ($Z = 36$) is written as $1s^2 2s^2 2p^6 3s^2 3p^6 3d^{10}\, 4s^2 4p^6$.

You will see from this, that there is one further slight complication that we need to consider. In the first two shells, it is true that *all* the sub-levels of one shell will fill before *any* of the sub-levels of the next shell. When a shell is full, it is said to be closed. In the first two shells, closure coincides with the inert gases.

However, with the outer shells, there are two factors that complicate the order in which electrons fill the various sub-levels. Firstly, as can be seen in Figure 6.8, the *difference* in the binding energies between the outer quantum levels starts to decrease quite significantly (they are subject to the inverse square law) and there is overlap between the lower energy sub-level(s) of one shell and the higher energy levels of the next (Fig. 6.10). The first manifestation of this is in the transition from the inert gas argon ($_{18}$A), which has only eight electrons in its $M$ shell (corresponding to complete *s* and *p* sub-levels) to potassium ($_{19}$K) whose outermost electron is in a $4s$ sub-level rather than a $3d$ sub-level. The $3d$ sub-level does not fill, thus closing the $M$ shell, until copper ($_{29}$Cu). The order is which the sub-levels fill is:

1s,2s,2p,3s,3p,4s,3d,4p,5s,4d,5p,6s,4f, 5d,6p,7s,6d

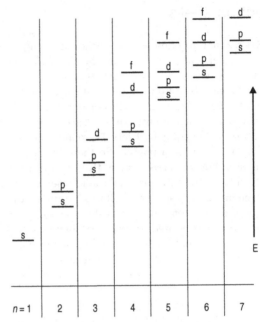

**Figure 6.10** • The energy states (not to scale) of sub-levels within different orbitals. With the higher quantum levels, the higher energy sub-levels of an outer shell can have a greater binding energy than the lower energy sub-levels of an inner shell and so the former will fill before the latter. This effect is first noted with potassium.

This can be seen in the complete listing of all the elements and their electron structure is detailed in Table 6.4. The second factor that can cause anomalies in the quantum structure of an atom's electrons is an effect known as **electron shielding**.

As the number of electrons in the inner shells builds, it creates a barrier of negative, repulsive charge that counters the effect of the increasingly distant, positive attractive force of the protons in the nucleus. This means that the binding energy associated with each sub-level is not fixed but will vary from element to element (or on the individual element's level of excitation) depending on the effect of electron shielding.

The effect is best noted in the configuration of the electrons in chromium ($_{24}$Cr) and copper ($_{29}$Cu). In both of these elements, an additional $3d$ electron is present at the expense of a vacancy in a previously filled $4s$ sub-level; the additional $4s$ electrons have 'tipped the scales' so that very similar binding energy of the $3d$ sub-level is now greater than that of the $4s$ sub-level.

These effects also explain a number of features of the periodic table (Fig. 6.1). The chemistry of

**Table 6.4** Electron configuration of the elements

| | | K | L | L | M | M | M | N | N | N | N | O | O | O | O | P | P | P | Q |
|---|---|---|---|---|---|---|---|---|---|---|---|---|---|---|---|---|---|---|---|
| Z | | 1s | 2s | 2p | 3s | 3p | 3d | 4s | 4p | 4d | 4f | 5s | 5p | 5d | 5f | 6s | 6p | 6d | 7s |
| 1 | H | 1 | | | | | | | | | | | | | | | | | |
| 2 | He | 2 | | | | | | | | | | | | | | | | | |
| 3 | Li | 2 | 1 | | | | | | | | | | | | | | | | |
| 4 | Be | 2 | 2 | | | | | | | | | | | | | | | | |
| 5 | B | 2 | 2 | 1 | | | | | | | | | | | | | | | |
| 6 | C | 2 | 2 | 2 | | | | | | | | | | | | | | | |
| 7 | N | 2 | 2 | 3 | | | | | | | | | | | | | | | |
| 8 | O | 2 | 2 | 4 | | | | | | | | | | | | | | | |
| 9 | F | 2 | 2 | 5 | | | | | | | | | | | | | | | |
| 10 | Ne | 2 | 2 | 6 | | | | | | | | | | | | | | | |
| 11 | Na | 2 | 2 | 6 | 1 | | | | | | | | | | | | | | |
| 12 | Mg | 2 | 2 | 6 | 2 | | | | | | | | | | | | | | |
| 13 | Al | 2 | 2 | 6 | 2 | 1 | | | | | | | | | | | | | |
| 14 | Si | 2 | 2 | 6 | 2 | 2 | | | | | | | | | | | | | |
| 15 | P | 2 | 2 | 6 | 2 | 3 | | | | | | | | | | | | | |
| 16 | S | 2 | 2 | 6 | 2 | 4 | | | | | | | | | | | | | |
| 17 | Cl | 2 | 2 | 6 | 2 | 5 | | | | | | | | | | | | | |
| 18 | A | 2 | 2 | 6 | 2 | 6 | | | | | | | | | | | | | |
| 19 | K | 2 | 2 | 6 | 2 | 6 | | 1 | | | | | | | | | | | |
| 20 | Ca | 2 | 2 | 6 | 2 | 6 | | 2 | | | | | | | | | | | |
| 21 | Sc | 2 | 2 | 6 | 2 | 6 | 1 | 2 | | | | | | | | | | | |
| 22 | Ti | 2 | 2 | 6 | 2 | 6 | 2 | 2 | | | | | | | | | | | |
| 23 | V | 2 | 2 | 6 | 2 | 6 | 3 | 2 | | | | | | | | | | | |
| 24 | Cr | 2 | 2 | 6 | 2 | 6 | 4 | 1 | | | | | | | | | | | |
| 25 | Mn | 2 | 2 | 6 | 2 | 6 | 5 | 2 | | | | | | | | | | | |
| 26 | Fe | 2 | 2 | 6 | 2 | 6 | 6 | 2 | | | | | | | | | | | |
| 27 | Co | 2 | 2 | 6 | 2 | 6 | 7 | 2 | | | | | | | | | | | |
| 28 | Ni | 2 | 2 | 6 | 2 | 6 | 8 | 2 | | | | | | | | | | | |
| 29 | Cu | 2 | 2 | 6 | 2 | 6 | 10 | 1 | | | | | | | | | | | |
| 30 | Zn | 2 | 2 | 6 | 2 | 6 | 10 | 2 | | | | | | | | | | | |

*Continued*

**Table 6.4** Electron configuration of the elements—Cont'd

| | | K | L | L | M | M | M | N | N | N | N | O | O | O | O | P | P | P | Q |
|---|---|---|---|---|---|---|---|---|---|---|---|---|---|---|---|---|---|---|---|
| 31 | Ga | 2 | 2 | 6 | 2 | 6 | 10 | 2 | 1 | | | | | | | | | | |
| 32 | Ge | 2 | 2 | 6 | 2 | 6 | 10 | 2 | 2 | | | | | | | | | | |
| 33 | As | 2 | 2 | 6 | 2 | 6 | 10 | 2 | 3 | | | | | | | | | | |
| 34 | Se | 2 | 2 | 6 | 2 | 6 | 10 | 2 | 4 | | | | | | | | | | |
| 35 | Br | 2 | 2 | 6 | 2 | 6 | 10 | 2 | 5 | | | | | | | | | | |
| 36 | Kr | 2 | 2 | 6 | 2 | 6 | 10 | 2 | 6 | | | | | | | | | | |
| 37 | Rb | 2 | 2 | 6 | 2 | 6 | 10 | 2 | 6 | | | 1 | | | | | | | |
| 38 | Sr | 2 | 2 | 6 | 2 | 6 | 10 | 2 | 6 | | | 2 | | | | | | | |
| 39 | Y | 2 | 2 | 6 | 2 | 6 | 10 | 2 | 6 | 1 | | 2 | | | | | | | |
| 40 | Zr | 2 | 2 | 6 | 2 | 6 | 10 | 2 | 6 | 2 | | 2 | | | | | | | |
| 41 | Nb | 2 | 2 | 6 | 2 | 6 | 10 | 2 | 6 | 3 | | 1 | | | | | | | |
| 42 | Mo | 2 | 2 | 6 | 2 | 6 | 10 | 2 | 6 | 4 | | 1 | | | | | | | |
| 43 | Tc | 2 | 2 | 6 | 2 | 6 | 10 | 2 | 6 | 5 | | 2 | | | | | | | |
| 44 | Ru | 2 | 2 | 6 | 2 | 6 | 10 | 2 | 6 | 6 | | 1 | | | | | | | |
| 45 | Rh | 2 | 2 | 6 | 2 | 6 | 10 | 2 | 6 | 7 | | 1 | | | | | | | |
| 46 | Pd | 2 | 2 | 6 | 2 | 6 | 10 | 2 | 6 | 8 | | | | | | | | | |
| 47 | Ag | 2 | 2 | 6 | 2 | 6 | 10 | 2 | 6 | 10 | | 1 | | | | | | | |
| 48 | Cd | 2 | 2 | 6 | 2 | 6 | 10 | 2 | 6 | 10 | | 2 | | | | | | | |
| 49 | In | 2 | 2 | 6 | 2 | 6 | 10 | 2 | 6 | 10 | | 2 | 1 | | | | | | |
| 50 | Sn | 2 | 2 | 6 | 2 | 6 | 10 | 2 | 6 | 10 | | 2 | 2 | | | | | | |
| 51 | Sb | 2 | 2 | 6 | 2 | 6 | 10 | 2 | 6 | 10 | | 2 | 3 | | | | | | |
| 52 | Te | 2 | 2 | 6 | 2 | 6 | 10 | 2 | 6 | 10 | | 2 | 4 | | | | | | |
| 53 | I | 2 | 2 | 6 | 2 | 6 | 10 | 2 | 6 | 10 | | 2 | 5 | | | | | | |
| 54 | Xe | 2 | 2 | 6 | 2 | 6 | 10 | 2 | 6 | 10 | | 2 | 6 | | | | | | |
| 55 | Cs | 2 | 2 | 6 | 2 | 6 | 10 | 2 | 6 | 10 | | 2 | 6 | | | 1 | | | |
| 56 | Ba | 2 | 2 | 6 | 2 | 6 | 10 | 2 | 6 | 10 | | 2 | 6 | | | 2 | | | |
| 57 | La | 2 | 2 | 6 | 2 | 6 | 10 | 2 | 6 | 10 | | 2 | 6 | 1 | | 2 | | | |
| 58 | Ce | 2 | 2 | 6 | 2 | 6 | 10 | 2 | 6 | 10 | 2 | 2 | 6 | | | 2 | | | |
| 59 | Pr | 2 | 2 | 6 | 2 | 6 | 10 | 2 | 6 | 10 | 3 | 2 | 6 | | | 2 | | | |
| 60 | Nd | 2 | 2 | 6 | 2 | 6 | 10 | 2 | 6 | 10 | 4 | 2 | 6 | | | 2 | | | |
| 61 | Pm | 2 | 2 | 6 | 2 | 6 | 10 | 2 | 6 | 10 | 5 | 2 | 6 | | | 2 | | | |
| 62 | Sm | 2 | 2 | 6 | 2 | 6 | 10 | 2 | 6 | 10 | 6 | 2 | 6 | | | 2 | | | |

**Table 6.4** Electron configuration of the elements—Cont'd

| | | K | L | L | M | M | M | N | N | N | N | O | O | O | O | P | P | P | Q |
|---|---|---|---|---|---|---|---|---|---|---|---|---|---|---|---|---|---|---|---|
| 63 | Eu | 2 | 2 | 6 | 2 | 6 | 10 | 2 | 6 | 10 | 7 | 2 | 6 | | | 2 | | | |
| 64 | Gd | 2 | 2 | 6 | 2 | 6 | 10 | 2 | 6 | 10 | 7 | 2 | 6 | 1 | | 2 | | | |
| 65 | Tb | 2 | 2 | 6 | 2 | 6 | 10 | 2 | 6 | 10 | 9 | 2 | 6 | | | 2 | | | |
| 66 | Dy | 2 | 2 | 6 | 2 | 6 | 10 | 2 | 6 | 10 | 10 | 2 | 6 | | | 2 | | | |
| 67 | Ho | 2 | 2 | 6 | 2 | 6 | 10 | 2 | 6 | 10 | 11 | 2 | 6 | | | 2 | | | |
| 68 | Er | 2 | 2 | 6 | 2 | 6 | 10 | 2 | 6 | 10 | 12 | 2 | 6 | | | 2 | | | |
| 69 | Tm | 2 | 2 | 6 | 2 | 6 | 10 | 2 | 6 | 10 | 13 | 2 | 6 | | | 2 | | | |
| 70 | Yb | 2 | 2 | 6 | 2 | 6 | 10 | 2 | 6 | 10 | 14 | 2 | 6 | | | 2 | | | |
| 71 | Lu | 2 | 2 | 6 | 2 | 6 | 10 | 2 | 6 | 10 | 14 | 2 | 6 | 1 | | 2 | | | |
| 72 | Hf | 2 | 2 | 6 | 2 | 6 | 10 | 2 | 6 | 10 | 14 | 2 | 6 | 2 | | 2 | | | |
| 73 | Ta | 2 | 2 | 6 | 2 | 6 | 10 | 2 | 6 | 10 | 14 | 2 | 6 | 3 | | 2 | | | |
| 74 | W | 2 | 2 | 6 | 2 | 6 | 10 | 2 | 6 | 10 | 14 | 2 | 6 | 4 | | 2 | | | |
| 75 | Re | 2 | 2 | 6 | 2 | 6 | 10 | 2 | 6 | 10 | 14 | 2 | 6 | 5 | | 2 | | | |
| 76 | Os | 2 | 2 | 6 | 2 | 6 | 10 | 2 | 6 | 10 | 14 | 2 | 6 | 6 | | 2 | | | |
| 77 | Ir | 2 | 2 | 6 | 2 | 6 | 10 | 2 | 6 | 10 | 14 | 2 | 6 | 7 | | 2 | | | |
| 78 | Pt | 2 | 2 | 6 | 2 | 6 | 10 | 2 | 6 | 10 | 14 | 2 | 6 | 9 | | 1 | | | |
| 79 | Au | 2 | 2 | 6 | 2 | 6 | 10 | 2 | 6 | 10 | 14 | 2 | 6 | 10 | | 1 | | | |
| 80 | Hg | 2 | 2 | 6 | 2 | 6 | 10 | 2 | 6 | 10 | 14 | 2 | 6 | 10 | | 2 | | | |
| 81 | Tl | 2 | 2 | 6 | 2 | 6 | 10 | 2 | 6 | 10 | 14 | 2 | 6 | 10 | | 2 | 1 | | |
| 82 | Pb | 2 | 2 | 6 | 2 | 6 | 10 | 2 | 6 | 10 | 14 | 2 | 6 | 10 | | 2 | 2 | | |
| 83 | Bi | 2 | 2 | 6 | 2 | 6 | 10 | 2 | 6 | 10 | 14 | 2 | 6 | 10 | | 2 | 3 | | |
| 84 | Po | 2 | 2 | 6 | 2 | 6 | 10 | 2 | 6 | 10 | 14 | 2 | 6 | 10 | | 2 | 4 | | |
| 85 | At | 2 | 2 | 6 | 2 | 6 | 10 | 2 | 6 | 10 | 14 | 2 | 6 | 10 | | 2 | 5 | | |
| 86 | Rn | 2 | 2 | 6 | 2 | 6 | 10 | 2 | 6 | 10 | 14 | 2 | 6 | 10 | | 2 | 6 | | |
| 87 | Fr | 2 | 2 | 6 | 2 | 6 | 10 | 2 | 6 | 10 | 14 | 2 | 6 | 10 | | 2 | 6 | | 1 |
| 88 | Ra | 2 | 2 | 6 | 2 | 6 | 10 | 2 | 6 | 10 | 14 | 2 | 6 | 10 | | 2 | 6 | | 2 |
| 89 | Ac | 2 | 2 | 6 | 2 | 6 | 10 | 2 | 6 | 10 | 14 | 2 | 6 | 10 | | 2 | 6 | 1 | 2 |
| 90 | Th | 2 | 2 | 6 | 2 | 6 | 10 | 2 | 6 | 10 | 14 | 2 | 6 | 10 | | 2 | 6 | 2 | 2 |
| 91 | Pa | 2 | 2 | 6 | 2 | 6 | 10 | 2 | 6 | 10 | 14 | 2 | 6 | 10 | 2 | 2 | 6 | 1 | 2 |
| 92 | U | 2 | 2 | 6 | 2 | 6 | 10 | 2 | 6 | 10 | 14 | 2 | 6 | 10 | 3 | 2 | 6 | 1 | 2 |
| 93 | Np | 2 | 2 | 6 | 2 | 6 | 10 | 2 | 6 | 10 | 14 | 2 | 6 | 10 | 4 | 2 | 6 | 1 | 2 |

*Continued*

**Table 6.4** Electron configuration of the elements—Cont'd

| | | K | L | L | M | M | M | N | N | N | N | O | O | O | O | P | P | P | Q |
|---|---|---|---|---|---|---|---|---|---|---|---|---|---|---|---|---|---|---|---|
| 94 | Pu | 2 | 2 | 6 | 2 | 6 | 10 | 2 | 6 | 10 | 14 | 2 | 6 | 10 | 5 | 2 | 6 | 1 | 2 |
| 95 | Am | 2 | 2 | 6 | 2 | 6 | 10 | 2 | 6 | 10 | 14 | 2 | 6 | 10 | 6 | 2 | 6 | 1 | 2 |
| 96 | Cm | 2 | 2 | 6 | 2 | 6 | 10 | 2 | 6 | 10 | 14 | 2 | 6 | 10 | 7 | 2 | 6 | 1 | 2 |
| 97 | Bk | 2 | 2 | 6 | 2 | 6 | 10 | 2 | 6 | 10 | 14 | 2 | 6 | 10 | 8 | 2 | 6 | 1 | 2 |
| 98 | Cf | 2 | 2 | 6 | 2 | 6 | 10 | 2 | 6 | 10 | 14 | 2 | 6 | 10 | 10 | 2 | 6 | | 2 |
| 99 | E | 2 | 2 | 6 | 2 | 6 | 10 | 2 | 6 | 10 | 14 | 2 | 6 | 10 | 11 | 2 | 6 | | 2 |
| 100 | Fm | 2 | 2 | 6 | 2 | 6 | 10 | 2 | 6 | 10 | 14 | 2 | 6 | 10 | 12 | 2 | 6 | | 2 |
| 101 | Md | 2 | 2 | 6 | 2 | 6 | 10 | 2 | 6 | 10 | 14 | 2 | 6 | 10 | 13 | 2 | 6 | | 2 |
| 102 | No | 2 | 2 | 6 | 2 | 6 | 10 | 2 | 6 | 10 | 14 | 2 | 6 | 10 | 14 | 2 | 6 | | 2 |
| 103 | Lw | 2 | 2 | 6 | 2 | 6 | 10 | 2 | 6 | 10 | 14 | 2 | 6 | 10 | 14 | 2 | 6 | 1 | 2 |

Group I ($ns^1$) and Group II ($ns^2$) is characterized by the outer s-electrons and the elements, all of which are metallic, are collectively referred to as the **s-block**. Strong similarities exist between all these elements, with the differences explained in terms of the relative sizes of the atoms or their ionic charge (Group I ions are monopositive; Group II, dipositive).

Groups III to 0 contain elements whose chemistry is determined by electrons of the p sub-level and are therefore known as the **p-block** elements. Group 0 elements, the noble gases, have unique properties and are almost totally unreactive, attributable to their stable electronic structures consisting of closed shells.

The elements of periods 4, 5 and 6 have their chemistry governed by electrons of the d sub-levels and are known as **d-block** or **transition metals** elements. Within the 6th period lie the lanthanides; all have remarkably similar chemical properties, which are easy to understand on the basis of their electron sequence.

All of the lanthanides have the same $5s^2 5p^6 6s^2$ configurations but also have incomplete 4f sub-levels. The sequential addition of these 4f electrons has virtually no effect on the chemical properties of the lanthanide elements, which are determined by the outer electrons.

Similarly, in the 7th period lie the actinides, the series of 15 radioactive elements from actinium ($_{89}$Ac) to lawrencium ($_{103}$Lr). All of the actinides have a $6s^2 6p^2 7s^2$ configuration and differ only in the number and arrangement of their 5f and 6d electrons, which, again, have little influence on chemical properties.

There is one other feature of the quantum arrangement of electrons that contributes to their physical and chemical properties and that is the electron's spin. Like nearly all fundamental particles, electrons spin. When a charged particle spins, it generates a magnetic field: north and south poles, much like the spinning, iron-cored planet Earth. Thus, there are two configurations in which electrons can lie – north pole upwards or south pole upwards. There is a very specific way in which the differently spinning electrons fill a sub-level, such that the maximum possible number of electrons are unpaired (Fig. 6.11). This is known as **Hund's Rule**. The ferromagnetic properties of the 4th period Group VIIIb elements, iron, cobalt and nickel, are due to this phenomenon; the 3d sub-levels are only partly occupied by unpaired electrons with parallel spins, which do not cancel each other out, giving the atom a large magnetic moment.

## Fact File

### LANTHANIDES

The series of 15 metallic elements from lanthanum ($_{57}$La) to lutetium ($_{71}$Lu) are collectively known as the lanthanides, although they are more commonly referred to as 'rare earth' elements. This is a misnomer as the term 'earth' applies to the oxide rather than to the metal itself; many are also now known to be quite common in nature.

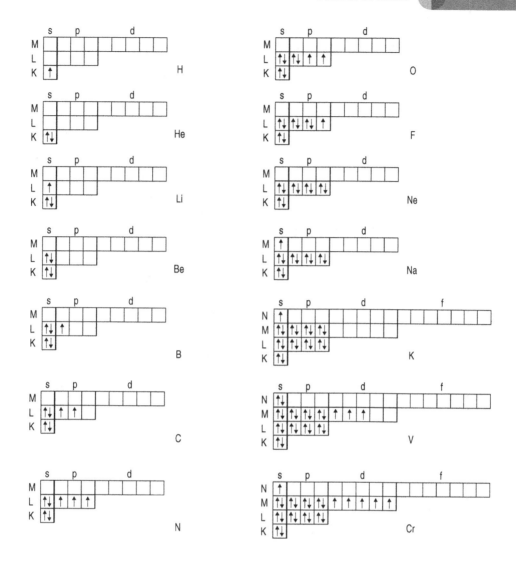

**Figure 6.11** ● The electron quantum and spin configurations for selected elements.

As we shall see below, Hund's Rule also has an application in the formation of certain types of bonding found when individual atoms join together to form molecules.

## Intramolecular bonding

Quantum theory does not just apply to atoms, it also can be used to explain chemical bonding between atoms to form **molecules**. We have mentioned molecules previously, but without defining them: a molecule is a stable, cohesive arrangement of two or more atoms to form the smallest fundamental unit of a chemical compound; that is, the smallest unit that can have independent existence and take part in chemical reactions. By 'stable', we mean that the molecule must require additional energy from an external source in order to reduce to its constituent atoms once more.

Atoms can aggregate into molecules in two basic ways: either by **ionic** (or *electrovalent*) bonding or by the formation of **covalent** bonds. Let us start by considering what happens when two atoms are brought close together. In many cases, nothing will happen; no molecule will form. When the electron structures of two atoms overlap, they become a single system. According to Pauli's exclusion principle, no two electrons within a single system can exist in the same energy state. If some of the interacting electrons are forced into higher energy states than those that they inhabited when they were in separate atoms, the system will (probably) have much more energy than before and, therefore, be unstable. In order to avoid this, the electrons will flee from each other to avoid the formation of a single system. This asymmetrical distribution exposes the positive nuclei to each other, leading to repulsive forces that force the atoms apart.

## Ionic bonding

We have already seen how positive ions can form by removing the outer electrons; this can most easily be done when there are single electrons in an $s$ sub-level (Group I), though Group II elements are also quite adept at forming $X^{2+}$ ions. Some elements, such as aluminium, can form triply charged positive ions. Such elements are known as **electropositive** elements. It is worth noting that, with the

formation of a positive ion, the electron structure reverts to that of an inert gas with a correspondingly smaller ionic diameter than the original atom, having discarded its outer shell.

By contrast, the ionic radii of **electronegative** elements remain unchanged. Most common negatively charged ions are halogens, all of which have five electrons in their outer $p$ sub-orbitals and form singly charged ions ($Cl^-$, $I^-$ etc.). They readily accept additional electrons to close the sub-level and, thus, once again take on the electron formation of an inert gas meaning the resultant combination has a high degree of stability (Fig. 6.12). Most ionic combinations form not just individual molecules but complex crystal structures.

## Covalent bonding

The second way in which atoms can bond is to share electrons by overlapping their adjacent electron orbitals. The simplest – and commonest – such example is the hydrogen molecule, $H_2$ (Fig. 6.13). This can form without violating the exclusion principle, providing the two electrons have non-parallel spins. The electrons interact with both nuclei so that both appear to possess two electrons,

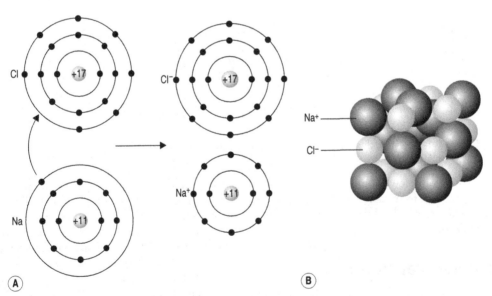

**(A)**   **(B)**

**Figure 6.12** • Ionic bonding in sodium chloride (NaCl). Sodium readily gives up its single $s$-electron, forming a system with a closed $L$ shell. The electron is readily accepted by chlorine, which already has five $p$-level electrons, thus closing its sub-orbital (**A**). The ionic attraction between the $Na^+$ ion and the $Cl^-$ ion allows the compound the form a stable crystalline structure (**B**).

H₂ molecule

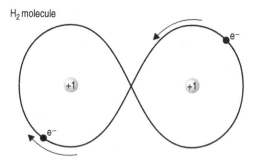

**Figure 6.13** • The simplest molecule is formed by two hydrogen atoms which share their electrons, closing their 1s orbitals.

thus closing the K shell and forming a highly stable system.

Covalent bonds can be extremely stable and need not be formed between atoms of different elements. The structure of diamond, a form of carbon that is the hardest known substance, is due to a central carbon atom sharing each of its four outer $(2s^2 2p^2)$ electrons with another carbon atom, which, in turn, is sharing with four other atoms giving each atom an effectively closed L shell.

Electrons, being negatively charged, have a tendency to repel each other and they will therefore usually orientate themselves in order to be as far apart as possible, thus establishing an electrostatic equilibrium. This means that the bonds between the atoms of a molecule form fixed angles. The three commonest are demonstrated in Figure 6.14; however, some molecules do not conform to these standard arrangements, and most predominant amongst these is water.

## The water molecule

Perhaps because water is so abundant, we take it for granted without ever stopping to consider how truly remarkable a chemical it is. We have all heard the phrase that 'water is essential for life'. This is not just a reflection of the dependency we have upon it as a species – we can live without food for weeks, but without water we die within a few days – but rather a reflection of its unique chemical and physical properties, all of which can be explained in terms of its molecular bonding.

Firstly, let us consider some of these properties with which we are all so familiar that we have probably forgotten how unusual and unlikely they really are. Firstly, there is the fact that water is a liquid in the range of temperatures that we typically experience in the majority of the Earth's environments. Both its melting and boiling points (273K and 373K respectively) are actually far, far higher than might be expected in comparison with anomalous compounds such as ammonia, $NH_3$ (195K, 240K), or hydrogen sulphide, $H_2S$ (191K, 213K).

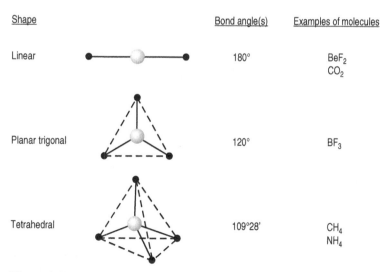

| Shape | | Bond angle(s) | Examples of molecules |
|---|---|---|---|
| Linear | | 180° | $BeF_2$ $CO_2$ |
| Planar trigonal | | 120° | $BF_3$ |
| Tetrahedral | | 109°28' | $CH_4$ $NH_4$ |

**Figure 6.14** • Common types of covalent bonding.

Water is also highly unusual in that its solid form (ice) is less dense that its liquid form. This means that ice floats and that the compressive forces found in the bottom of the ocean do not cause water to solidify as they would with most other chemical compounds: water reaches its maximum density at 4K above its freezing point.

In addition, water is a uniquely powerful solvent and many of the body's physiological systems – blood, lymph, digestion – consist of aqueous solutions. Water also carries, dissolved in it, many of the nutrients and trace elements needed by plants and marine organisms.

So, what is the reason for this extraordinary behaviour? Much of it has to do with the shape of the water molecule (Fig. 6.15), which, in turn, is governed by the way in which its atoms combine. The oxygen atom has six electrons in its outer (L) shell ($1s^2 2s^2 2p^4$). In order to obey the laws of electromagnetic repulsion and magnetic spin, the electrons in each sub-level arrange themselves in very specific, predictable patterns. In the case of the p-orbital electrons, the three pairs align themselves along the orthogonal x, y and z axis; those electrons with positive spin (north pole upwards) can be regarded as occupying the positive axes; those with negative spin (south pole upwards), the negative

axes. In fact the three electron pairs are often referred to as $p_x$, $p_y$ and $p_z$.

So this immediately explains why water is not a simple linear shape as might at first be expected. Its $p_x$ electrons are paired and therefore it is the unpaired $p_y$ and $p_z$ electrons that are shared with hydrogen electrons to form a closed shell. These electrons must lie at 90° to each other, due to the orientation of the axes that define them, so you would now expect the O–H bonds to lie at right angles to each other ... still not quite the case.

The reason for the 104.5° angle is the quite powerful proton–proton repulsion of the two hydrogen nuclei, and this angle represents a balance between these electrostatic forces and those governing the distribution of p-shell electrons. However, this *intramolecular* balance leads to an *extra*-molecular imbalance – at one 'end' of the molecule (the oxygen end), there are two unshared electron pairs; at the other, two minimally shielded hydrogen nuclei. This means that one end of the molecule has a negative charge, the other, an equal but opposite positive one. The water molecule is said to be **polar**, as are many molecules with covalent hydrogen bonds. Substances whose molecules are polar are going to interact – either attracting or repelling other polar molecules, depending on orientation.

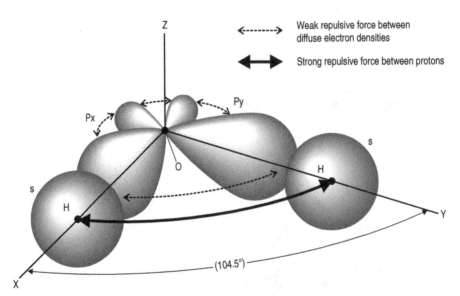

**Figure 6.15** • The shape of the water molecule, which has a profound effect on its chemical and physical properties, is due to the orientation of the p-orbital electrons in the oxygen and the repulsion of the hydrogen nuclei.

These electrostatic forces have a profound effect on their biochemical properties and the physiological consequences.

 CLINICAL FOCUS

The importance of water in multiple life processes can be best appreciated by considering the effect of its unique and unusual chemical and physical properties on human physiology.

Normal **cellular function** requires the presence of many chemical substances. Many of these compounds are quite large and must be broken into smaller and more reactive particles (ions) in order that reactions can take place. As we have seen, the polar nature of water encourages ionization of substances in solution and water molecules will surround any molecule that has an electrical charge making it a powerful solvent. The fact that so many substances dissolve in water is of utmost importance in the life process.

The critical role that water plays as a solvent permits the **transportation** of many essential materials within the body. For example, by dissolving food substances in blood, water enables these materials to enter and leave the blood capillaries in the digestive organs and eventually enter cells in every area of the body. In turn, waste products are transported to excretory organs.

Another important function of water stems from the fact that it has a high **specific heat**, meaning that it both absorbs and gives up heat slowly. This means that the body, with its large water content, can resist sudden changes in temperature, helping it to maintain thermal homeostasis. This ability to lose and gain large amounts of heat with little change in temperature allows body heat produced, for example, by the contraction of muscles during exercise, to be transported by blood to the body surface and radiated into the environment with minimal change in core temperature.

At this point, the body benefits from water's high **heat of vaporization**, another important physical quality. This characteristic is a measure of the amount of energy required to change a liquid to its gaseous form. With water, a large amount of energy is required in order to break the many hydrogen bonds that hold adjacent water molecules together in the liquid state. Thus, when sweat evaporates from the skin, it carries with it large amounts of excess heat, making it a very efficient coolant.

Of course, water does more than just act as a solvent, produce ionization, and facilitate chemical reactions. It also has essential roles of its own, playing a key part in such processes as cell permeability, active transport of materials, secretion, membrane potential and lubrication, to name a few. As a physician, it is important to understand the remarkable impact such an apparently simple molecule can make on the physiology of every organism we encounter.

# Intermolecular bonding

Let us first consider the effects of these forces, known as **hydrogen bonds**, on water molecules themselves. The attraction of the hydrogen atoms to the non-bonding electron pairs of the oxygen atom form temporary associations between molecules, which continually break and reform. These associations are stronger than in ice, which is highly structured but more loosely bound, explaining why the liquid form of water is denser than the solid. It also requires much more kinetic energy to allow a water molecule to overcome these bonds as it becomes steam, explaining the higher boiling point compared to analogous but non-polar molecules that were discussed above. This hydrogen bonding also accounts for water's higher than expected viscosity and its very high surface tension – without which, we would not be able to breathe!

It also explains why water is such a good solvent. If an ionic compound – let us remain with our previous example of sodium chloride – is placed in water, it will of course dissolve. This is because the polar water molecules reduce the electrostatic attraction between the positive sodium and negative chlorine ions, helping to pull the ions apart. Once separated, the sodium ions attract the unbonded electron pairs of the oxygen atoms, the chlorine atoms the hydrogen nuclei. These ions become surrounded by water molecules; this, in effect, disperses their charge over a much larger structure and prevents any significant recombination. The ions are said to be **hydrated**.

Hydrogen bonds do not just act between water molecules, they occur between most **organic compounds**, those in which one or more carbon atoms are linked covalently to atom(s) of other elements, most commonly hydrogen, oxygen and nitrogen. The hydrogen bonds significantly influence the shape of such molecules; often a long molecule will loop back to form a hydrogen bond with itself. This is crucial to the physiological processes of life where shape specifies function.

The formation of hydrogen bonds between different organic compounds can also alter the shape and, with it, the function of the respective compounds. This is the principle behind such fundamental physiological processes as oxygen carrying in haemoglobin, gene replication and the unfolding of sections of DNA (gene expression) that leads to the manufacture of proteins.

## Van der Waals bonds

There is one further type of bonding of which we should be aware. Van der Waals forces (pronounced 'van-der-Vawls' after the Dutch physicist who won the Nobel Prize in 1910 for his work on influence of the interaction that now bears his name) are weak electrostatic forces that exist between neutral (i.e. non-polar) particles. They are very short-range compared with hydrogen bonds: rather than obeying the inverse square law, the attractive forces diminish with the inverse of the seventh power – if you double the separation, the attraction, already weak, decreases by a factor of 49; treble it and it is effectively negated at less than of its original value. Van der Waals forces are only of significance when particles are immediately adjacent.

They can arise from three sources. Firstly, as we have already seen, the arrangement of electron spin-pairs in their sub-orbitals can lead to fixed distortion of the distribution of electrons. This means that one area of the electron shell is always slightly more negative and the opposite side will be relatively positive. These atoms will tend to align their charges, resulting in a net attraction.

These imbalances also tend to temporarily distort the distribution of electrons in adjacent atoms and molecules, creating short-term imbalances that can, nevertheless, induce temporary attractive forces and induce further changes in neighbouring particles. Finally, the fact that electrons are in constant motion, both between and within shells, means that instantaneous imbalances can occur: at any one moment, part of the shell will have an excess of negative charge and part will have a deficiency. As before, these imbalances will trigger distortions in the electrons of adjacent particles. Although these imbalances are transient in the extreme ($\sim 10^{-9}$ s), they are sufficiently long-lived to have a significant influence of the behaviour of substances particularly when there is an absence of other forms of interaction, such as in the inert gases. Without van der Waals forces, it would not be possible for these substances, and other non-polar gases such as chlorine ($Cl_2$), methane ($CH_4$) and carbon dioxide ($CO_2$), to form solids under compression.

### Learning Outcomes

If you have understood the contents of this chapter, you should now understand:
- The development of atomic theory, and the contribution of various models to our current understanding of the structure of atoms
- The concept of waves and classical wave mechanics and be able to compare this to the concept of wave-particle duality
- How electrons behave within the overall atomic structure and how this behaviour affects the physical and chemical properties of different substances
- The different types of molecule, their means of formation and the relationship to the quantum behaviour of electrons
- The way in which molecules interact and be able to explain this in terms of their structure.

## CHECK YOUR EXISTING KNOWLEDGE: ANSWERS

1 a Two or more different forms of the same element, differing in their mass numbers owing to differing numbers of neutrons in their nuclei
  b A particle found in the nucleus of an atom (a proton or neutron)
  c The sum of the nucleons for a given isotope
  d The number of protons in an atomic nucleus
  e A charged particle consisting of an atom (or molecule) that has lost or gained electron(s)

2 The weak nuclear force (electroweak force) overcomes the electrostatic repulsion of the protons

3 A diffraction pattern caused by the interference of light waves passing through a series of slits

4 $\lambda = h/mv. E = \frac{1}{2}mv^2$
   $200\,eV = 200 \times (1.6 \times 10^{-19}\,J) = 3.2 \times 10^{-17}\,J = \frac{1}{2} \times 9.1 \times 10^{-31} \times v^2$
   Therefore $v = \sqrt{7} \times 10^{13} = 8.3 \times 10^6\,ms^{-1}$
   Therefore $\lambda = (6.6 \times 10^{-34})/(9.1 \times 10^{-31})\,(8.3 \times 10^6) = 8.7 \times 10^{-11}\,m$

5 a. 18; b 1; c 2; d 10; e 4

6 The kinetic energy of a free electron = photon energy − work function
   $\frac{1}{2}mv^2 = hf\Phi$

7 Argon: $1s^2 2s^2 2p^6 3s^2 3p^6$

8 Ferromagnetism.

9 The attraction between molecules whose polarity is due to an asymmetrical distribution of partially shielded hydrogen nuclei.

10 Owing to the mutual repulsion of the hydrogen atoms within the molecule (if you can explain why it's 104.5° and not 180°, you can *definitely* move straight to the next chapter).

Marking: The concepts that are presented in this chapter are wide ranging and an essential prerequisite to those in the chapters that follow. Do not proceed unless you got *all* the answers right. If you got fewer than two questions wrong, it is acceptable to browse the text until you discover the source of your error and remedy it; otherwise, study the chapter in its entirety.

# Bibliography

Allison, W., 2006. Magnetism and magnetic resonance. In: Fundamental physics for probing and imaging. Oxford University Press, Oxford, pp. 21–54.

Allison, W., 2006. Mechanical waves and properties of matter. In: Fundamental physics for probing and imaging. Oxford University Press, Oxford, pp. 85–130.

Alonso, M., Finn, E.J., 1980. Atoms with one electron. In: Fundamental university physics volume III: quantum and statistical physics. Addison-Wesley, Reading, Mass (Chapter 2), pp. 53–108.

Alonso, M., Finn, E.J., 1980. Atoms with many electrons. In: Fundamental university physics volume III: quantum and statistical physics. Addison-Wesley, Reading, Mass (Chapter 3), pp. 150–182.

Beiser, A., 1973. Atomic structure. In: Concepts of modern physics, second ed. McGraw-Hill Kogakusha, Tokyo (Chapter 4), pp. 101–138.

Beiser, A., 1973. Quantum mechanics. In: Concepts of modern physics, second ed. McGraw-Hill Kogakusha, Tokyo (Chapter 5), pp. 139–172.

Beiser, A., 1973. The atomic nucleus. In: Concepts of modern physics, second ed. McGraw-Hill Kogakusha, Tokyo (Chapter 5), pp. 361–430.

Daintith, J., Deeson, E. (Eds.), 1983. Dictionary of physics. Charles Letts, London.

DeVries, R., Manne, A., 2003. Cervical MRI. Part I: a basic overview. Clinical Chiropractic 6, 137–143.

Encyclopædia Britannica, Avogardo, Amedeo, from Encyclopædia Britannica, 2006. Ultimate Reference Suite DVD July 24, 2007.

Encyclopædia Britannica, Bohr, Niels, from Encyclopædia Britannica, 2006. Ultimate Reference Suite DVD July 25, 2007.

Encyclopædia Britannica, Young, Thomas, from Encyclopædia Britannica, 2006. Ultimate Reference Suite DVD July 24, 2007.

EnvironmentalChemistry.com, Periodic table of elements. Online. Available: www. Environmentalchemistry. com/yogi/periodic 22 Jun 2007, 18:54 BST.

Garood, J.R., 1979. Nuclear and quantum physics. In: GCE A-level physics. Intercontinental Book

Productions, Maidenhead, pp. 276–314.

Garood, J.R., 1979. Oscillations and waves. In: GCE A-level physics. Intercontinental Book Productions, Maidenhead, pp. 111–139.

Geiger, H., Marsden, E., 1909. On a diffuse reflection of the α-particle. Proceedings of the Royal Society Series A 82, 495–500.

Geiger, H., Marsden, E., 1913. The laws of deflexion of α particles through large angles. Philosophical Magazine April, Series 6, 25(148). Online. Available: dbhs.wvusd.k12.ca.us/ webdocs/Chem-History/ GeigerMarsden-1913/ GeigerMarsden-1913 html 20 June 2007, 14:52 BST.

Hay, G.A., Hughes, D., 1983. Thermionic emission and x-ray tubes. In: First-year physics for radiographers. Ballière Tindall, London (Chapter 11), pp. 161–198.

Helms, C.A., 2005. Lumbar spine: disc disease and stenosis. In: Fundamentals of skeletal radiology, third ed. (Chapter 11), pp. 195–206.

Johnson, K., 1986. Nuclear physics. In: GCSE Physics for you, revised ed.

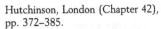
Hutchinson, London (Chapter 42), pp. 372–385.

Magnetic Resonance- Technology Information Portal>Contrast Agents, Online. Available: www.mr-tip.com 22 Jun 2007, 16:57 BST.

Mott, N.F., 1972. Standing waves and the quantization of energy. In: Elementary quantum mechanics. London Wykeham Publication, London (Chapter 5), pp. 37–46.

Murray, P.R.S., 1987. Electronic structure and atomic orbitals. In: Advanced chemistry. Pan, London (Chapter 3), pp. 55–64.

Thibodeau, G., Patton, K., 2006. The chemical basis of life. In: Anatomy and physiology, sixth ed. E-book. Elsevier, Philadelphia (Chapter 2). Online. Available: www.elsevier.com.

Thorne, J.O., Collocott, T.C. (Eds.), 1984. Chambers biographical dictionary. Chambers, Edinburgh.

# Chapter Seven

7

# Electricity and magnetism

## CHAPTER CONTENTS

Check your existing knowledge . . . . . . . . 151
Introduction . . . . . . . . . . . . . . . . . . 152
Electromagnetism . . . . . . . . . . . . . . . . 153
Electrostatics . . . . . . . . . . . . . . . 154
Electric potential . . . . . . . . . . . . . . . 155
Conductors and insulators . . . . . . . . . . 156
  Superconductors . . . . . . . . . . . . . . . 156
  Conductors . . . . . . . . . . . . . . . . . 156
  Insulators . . . . . . . . . . . . . . . . . . 156
  Semiconductors . . . . . . . . . . . . . . . 157
Electrodynamics . . . . . . . . . . . . . . 158
  Circuit diagrams . . . . . . . . . . . . . . 158
  Current . . . . . . . . . . . . . . . . . . . 158
  Electrical power . . . . . . . . . . . . . . . 160

Electronics . . . . . . . . . . . . . . . . . . 161
  Resistors . . . . . . . . . . . . . . . . . . 161
  Thermistors . . . . . . . . . . . . . . . . . 161
  Capacitors . . . . . . . . . . . . . . . . . 162
  Diodes . . . . . . . . . . . . . . . . . . . 165
Systems . . . . . . . . . . . . . . . . . . . 165
Magnetism . . . . . . . . . . . . . . . . . . 168
Electromagnetic induction . . . . . . . . . . 168
The transformer . . . . . . . . . . . . . . . 169
Electricity in the home and clinic . . . . . . . 171
Learning outcomes . . . . . . . . . . . . . . 175
Check your existing knowledge: answers . . 175
Bibliography . . . . . . . . . . . . . . . . . 177

## CHECK YOUR EXISTING KNOWLEDGE

1  Two equal positive charges are separated by a distance, $d$.
   a  Will they attract or repel each other?
   b  What happens to the force between them if their separation is halved?
   c  What happens to the force between them if one charge is doubled and the other halved?
2  What is the total resistance in the circuits shown below?

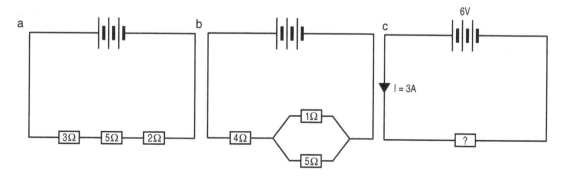

3 An electric kettle has a power rating of 3 kW.
   a   If it is plugged into a circuit with a voltage of 120 V, what current will flow?
   b   What is the resistance of the filament?
   c   What is the most appropriate standard fuse to use in the plug?
4 What is:
   a   A thermistor?
   b   A diode?
   c   A transducer?
   d   A linear amplifier?
5 What is the total capacitance in the circuits shown below?

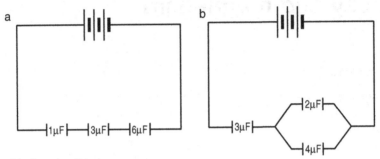

6 What is the output in the circuit below:

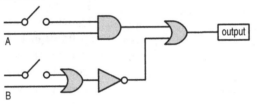

   a   When A is open and B closed?
   b   When B is open and A closed?
   c   When both A and B are open?
   d   When both A and B are closed?
7 A transformer has a primary voltage of 100 V and 100 turns. What is the output voltage:
   a   If the secondary circuit has 10 turns?
   b   If the secondary circuit has 500 turns?
8 Name three ways of increasing the output from a dynamo

# Introduction

Knowledge of electricity and magnetism has been with us for centuries: the Greeks knew that, if you rubbed amber against fur, you could generate static electricity; indeed, their word for amber, 'elektron', was the word used by the 16th century physicist, William Gilbert, to describe the way in which amber and other objects capable of becoming electrostatically charged could attract and repel other objects. This, in turn, gave rise to the English words 'electric' and 'electricity'.

Gilbert, who published his ideas in 1600, three years before his death at the age of 63, in the work *De Magnete, Magneticisque Corporibus, et de Magno Magnete Tellure* ('On the Magnet, Magnetic Bodies, and the Great Magnet of the Earth'), was also the first person to suggest that electricity and magnetism might be different manifestations of the same fundamental force. Magnetism had also been known to the ancient Greeks; its first practical application was the navigational compass, but it would not be until the 19th century that the laws of electricity and magnetism would be quantified and unified.

Until 1800, when Alessandro Volta succeeded in making a battery using plates of zinc and silver interspersed with damp cardboard, the study of electricity had been confined to **electrostatics**, the physics of static charges. Pioneering physicists such as Priestly, Coulomb, Poisson and Faraday had succeeded in showing that both static electricity and magnetism followed the same inverse square law as gravity; in this case known as **Coulomb's Law**.

## Fact File

### ALESSANDRO VOLTA

Volta had actually made his name by discovering and isolating the gas methane. It was his friendship with Luigi Galvani – famous for the 'Galvanic effect' of contracting the muscles of (dead) frogs by the application of copper and silver plates – that kindled his interest in the subject of electricity. The battery was subsequently developed almost by accident; because of the serendipitous happenstance, the volt was named after him.

## Fact File

### COULOMB'S LAW 2

You will recall that Coulomb's Law was defined in the previous chapter: the electric force between two charged masses is proportional to the size of the two charges and inversely proportional to the square of the distance between them.

Despite its attribution to Coulomb, this relationship was actually first described by Joseph Priestly; proved quantitatively by Henry Cavendish and John Robinson, neither of whom bothered to publish their work; and confirmed experimentally by Michael Faraday. Such are the vagaries of eponymic immortality in the world of physics.

# Electromagnetism

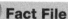

Electricity remained a scientific oddity until the development of the wire telegraph in the late 1830s, which started the revolution in communication – suddenly, it was possible to send messages across continents in minutes rather than weeks.

## Fact File

### TELEGRAPH

The invention of the telegraph, and the code which it utilized for its messages, is commonly credited to Samuel Morse. In fact, William Cooke and Charles Wheatstone patented and built the first telegraph in 1836 on a stretch of the Great Western Railway in England fully 8 years before Morse (who was actually an artist rather than an inventor or scientist) – even the code of dots and dashes was developed in the main by his business partner, Alfred Vail.

Despite the increasing practical applications of electricity, its true nature remained a mystery for another 30 years when the Scottish physicist James Clerk Maxwell described the first element of the 'Holy Grail' of physics, the Unified Field Theory, when he successfully demonstrated that electricity and magnetism were merely different manifestations of the same fundamental force.

Although the two forces seem quite distinct on a mundane level, and are governed by different equations, it is a remarkable fact that a changing electric field will create a magnetic field and, conversely, a changing magnetic field will generate an electric field – the principle on which the dynamo that powers bicycle lights works.

 **DICTIONARY DEFINITION**

**UNIFIED FIELD THEORY**

The theory that, in particle physics, all fundamental forces and the relationships between the elementary particles can be described with a single theoretical framework. Electricity, magnetism and the weak nuclear force have been successfully unified and the theory has been established to add the strong nuclear force, though experimental evidence is beyond the capabilities of current particle accelerators. The extremely weak, long-range force of gravity remains beyond attempts to bring it within the fold.

 CLINICAL FOCUS

This relationship between electrical and magnetic fields has an important implication for the physician. We have seen in previous chapters that many of the particles that comprise the human body have a charge associated with them and that certain particles, including protons, have spin.

As protons have a positive charge and are spinning, this means they must also have a magnetic field associated with them: effectively a 'north pole' and a 'south pole', just like a miniature Earth, which, in turn, has a magnetic field generated by its spinning iron core. By contrast, the moon – which has no such core and is no longer spinning – has no magnetic field.

This means that, if you were to put them in a strong magnetic field, the protons' magnetic fields would all line up the same way. When the field is switched off, the protons would revert to their original state, emitting photons as they do. All you would need to do is set up a ring of photon detectors and you could build up an accurate three-dimensional picture of the concentrations of protons in the sample being imaged.

Fortunately, the body is replete with free protons – hydrogen ions. Indeed, with its ubiquitous presence in organic and water molecules, hydrogen is easily the most common atom (and ion) found in our bodies and the principle that has just been described is that behind the working of an MRI (magnetic resonance imaging) machine (of which more in Chapter 9).

Maxwell also showed that electric and magnetic fields travel together through space as waves of electromagnetic radiation, with the changing fields mutually sustaining each other. Examples of such waves are radio and television signals, microwaves, infrared rays, visible light, ultraviolet light, x-rays, and gamma rays. In Maxwell's time, all waves were thought to need a medium to propagate them and, in the absence of any tangible medium to support light and radio waves (which could obviously travel in the vacuum of space), the 'ether' was proposed as the intangible medium of propagation. It was Maxwell who showed that electromagnetic waves required no medium.

All of these waves travel at the same speed, the velocity of light (roughly $3 \times 10^8$ ms$^{-1}$). They differ from each other only in the frequency at which their electric and magnetic fields oscillate; prior to Maxwell, many of these phenomena (or those that had by then been discovered) were regarded as being unrelated.

In this chapter, we will be looking at electricity and magnetism; electromagnetism is explored in depth in Chapter 8.

# Electrostatics

The study of non-moving electrical charges now forms such a small part of the study of electricity as a whole that it is hard sometimes to remember that, for many centuries, it was the *only* form of electricity that could be studied. It was, however, a necessary step to understanding electrical phenomena as a whole and, as we have seen, has critical implications for the shape and function of many organic molecules.

The laws that govern static charges can be summarized very simply:
• Electrical charges will distribute themselves evenly across a surface.

*This is because...*
• Like charges repel, opposite charges attract; therefore, the identical charges will be equally separated by mutual repulsion.

*The size of the attraction or repulsion is governed by...*
• Coulomb's Law, which, as we have already discussed, states that the force between two charges is directly proportional to the size of the charges and inversely proportional to the square of the distance between them. Put mathematically:

$$F \propto Q_1 Q_2 / d^2$$

here $Q_1$ and $Q_2$ are the size of the respective charges and $d$ is their separation.

## CLINICAL FOCUS

Today, we take for granted electricity in every aspect of our daily – and clinical – lives: light at the flick of a switch, computerized patient records, electromagnetic treatment modalities, diagnostic imaging, electrically powered treatment benches, digital thermometers, ophthalmoscopes, dictaphones, air-conditioned and heated offices – the list could continue for pages; electricity is so much a part of our lives that we only appreciate it when a power cut robs us of access.

One hundred-and-fifty years ago, physicians had no such luxuries. I have, in the corner of my consulting room, a reminder that for our predecessors even something as simple as getting sufficient illumination to make an adequate

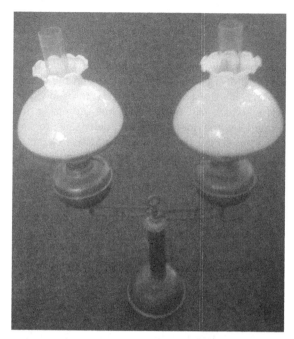

**Figure 7.1** • A doctor's oil lamp, circa 1860, with two double-wicked burners mounted on pivoting arms.

examination could be a major challenge. The doctor's double oil lamp (Fig. 7.1), came with two lamps, each with a double burner, mounted on pivoted arms so the full force of the light could, when required, be brought to bear on the patient. I have tried the lamp – it produced, I would estimate, the equivalent of a 5 watt bulb and had the added disadvantage of setting off the (electric) fire alarms.

At the time it was made, around 1860, neither chiropractic nor osteopathy existed and the term 'physiotherapy' had yet to be coined. Physicians still used leeches and surgical anaesthesia was in its infancy; manual therapy was in the hands of bonesetters.

Interestingly, the founder of chiropractic, Daniel Palmer, originally plied his trade as a 'magnetic healer' in the American mid-west of the 1890s. Over a century later, what has been sneered at as evidence of the 'quack' origins of the profession he began is now under serious investigation as a noninvasive therapy for a range of musculoskeletal and vascular conditions with proven physiological effects on the numerous polar molecules within the human body.

# Electric potential

You will (hopefully) recall from Chapter 2 that potential energy is energy that has been stored. A system with potential energy has the capacity to do work when the stored energy is released. A convenient source of this potential energy is the battery or **electric cell** (Fig. 7.2).

One way of thinking about a battery is that it contains lots of electrons that have been packed close together. Because 'like' charges repel, these negatively charged electrons have potential energy because they do work as soon as they fly apart. If these electrons are put at one end of an electric cable, this repulsive force will cause some of the electrons to move along the wire and work can be done. The more the electrons are packed together, the greater the repulsive force and the greater the electric potential, commonly called the **voltage, V**, because volts are the unit used to measure electric potential. The volt (V) is the potential energy per unit charge (in this case, the electron) and is equivalent to the number of *joules* per *coulomb*. The electric potential can be measured using a **voltmeter**.

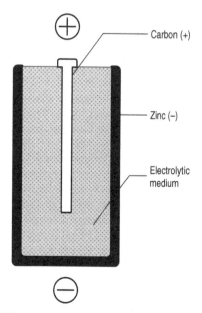

**Figure 7.2** • 'Dry-cell' battery, so-called to differentiate it from the early voltaic piles that employed plates of zinc and either silver or, for economic reasons, copper interspersed with wet paper to provide a medium conducive to electrolysis.

# Conductors and insulators

Although it is tempting to think of the material world as being divided into two – those substances that do conduct electricity and those (**insulators**) that do not – the true picture is more complex by far. We have talked about connecting an electric potential to an electric cable in order to obtain a current but the results we get will be very different, depending on the material from which the cable is made.

## Superconductors

There are actually not two but four classes of conductive substance. The first group comprises **superconductors**. Early in the 20th century, physicists discovered that when certain metals are cooled below their **transition temperatures** (typically less than 20 K), they lose all resistance to electron flow. This means that a current can flow indefinitely without any electrical potential to drive it – it was, and remains, the closest thing to perpetual motion; imagine having a car that, once started, would continue without ever decelerating (the catch, of course, is the amount of energy required to cool to and maintain a temperature of 20 K).

In the 1980s, a breakthrough occurred when it was found that certain ceramic compound materials which, at normal temperatures are extremely poor conductors of electricity, when cooled sufficiently would also act as superconductors. Unfortunately, nobody knows why, which makes the search for high-temperature superconductors a matter of trial and error with increasingly complicated 'designer' molecules.

By 1986, a molecule comprising yttrium, barium, copper and oxygen was exhibiting superconductivity at temperatures of 92 K, above the liquification point of nitrogen. The current record of 138 K is held by a thallium-doped, mercuric-cuprate consisting of the elements mercury, thallium, barium, calcium, copper and oxygen, although recent claims have been made for a lead-doped composite of tin, indium and thulium, which has been reportedly observed superconducting at 181 K, only −92°C. By comparison, the lowest climatic temperature ever recorded is −89.2°C at Vostok in Antarctica in July 1983.

The discovery of a 'room temperature' superconductor would not only have huge implications for power generation and storage but could also revolutionize diagnostic imagine in medicine.

# Conductors

Conventional electrical conductors are those materials that allow the easy transmission of an electrical current. Most conductors are metals and the charge carriers are the outer electrons of the individual atoms, which can move about the atomic lattice formed by the metal without 'belonging' to any one atom. These free-moving, conductive electrons are sometimes referred to as the 'electron gas'. Ionized gases and electrolytic solutions can also act as conductors; here, the charge carriers are ions.

Typically, electric cables are made from copper or aluminium; however, unlike superconductors, these metals do not conduct perfectly – there is **resistance ($R$)** to the electron flow. Using the previous analogy to our perpetually moving car, in the real world the car is slowed by the resistance of the air molecules through which it must move.

Electrical resistance is measured in **ohms ($\Omega$)**. Typically, copper wire offers a resistance of 0.15 $\Omega$ per metre length, although this will depend, amongst other things, on the thickness of the wire. Because of these variable factors, a material will be referred to in terms of its **resistivity ($\rho$)**, calculated by taking the resistance of the wire, multiplied by its cross-sectional area and divided by its length. Conversely, **conductance, $G$,** is measured in **siemens ($S$)** or, occasionally, the 'mho' ('Ohm' spelt backwards).

## Ohm's law

The man after whom the unit of resistance is named, Georg Simon Ohm, was the first to experimentally observe the relationship between voltage, current and resistance. This law states that, for a conductor, the amount of current flowing in a material is directly proportional to the potential difference across the material. The constant of proportionality is the resistance. Thus:

$$V = IR \text{ or } I = {}^{V}\!/_{R} \text{ or } R = {}^{V}\!/_{I}$$

Graphically, this can be demonstrated by plotting current against voltage (Fig. 7.3).

# Insulators

Materials that do not readily conduct electricity are termed **insulators**. In reality, they may be regarded

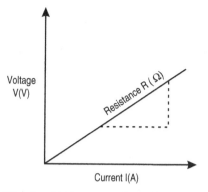

**Figure 7.3** • Graphical representation of Ohm's law demonstrating Georg Ohm's original observations. By altering the potential difference and measuring the current, he demonstrated that the two were directly proportional. The gradient of the resultant curve was the resistance of the material.

as being at the opposite end of a spectrum that starts with superconductors: insulators are in fact merely conductors with extremely high resistivity. Typical examples of such materials are glass, rubber and the plastics that coat electrical cables so that they may be handled without the inadvertent transfer of electricity to the electrician – the classic electric shock! With insulators, the outer electrons are tightly bound to the atoms and are therefore not available to carry charge: the higher the binding energy, the better the insulator.

## Semiconductors

Halfway down our spectrum of conductivity lie materials that have both conductive and insulating capabilities. Therein lies the field of solid state physics, a subject whose scope and complexity lie well beyond the limitations of this text; however, this branch of physics underpins the working of nearly every electronic device: computers, mobile phones, televisions, radios, MP3 players and, increasingly, domestic appliances. Anything with a 'chip' or transistor is reliant upon the atomic and molecular properties of semiconductors and it is therefore worth understanding the basic principles behind semi-conductors.

In **intrinsic semiconductors**, such as germanium and silicon, the outer electrons, which are loosely bound, form covalent bonds with neighbouring atoms. They can, therefore, be released quite

easily if energy is imparted to the system by increasing its temperature. A free electron will leave behind it a 'hole', which may then be filled by another free electron. This 'hole' will therefore move from electron to electron, in effect becoming a positive charge carrier. This arrangement is known as a **hole–electron pair**.

In an **extrinsic semiconductor**, small traces of impurities are deliberately added in a process known as 'doping'. If the impurity is from Group III of the periodic table, such as indium or gallium, when it joins with the semiconductor material there will only be three electrons free to fill four valence bonds (silicon and gallium are both from Group IV). An electron is therefore 'borrowed' from a neighbouring Group IV atom, creating a 'hole' in the same way that a non-doped sample works, albeit more efficiently. This type of extrinsic semiconductor is known as a **p-type semiconductor**.

By contrast, an **n-type semiconductor** is obtained when Group V impurities, such as antimony or arsenic, are added. Once the four valence bonds required by silicon or germanium are satisfied, there is an electron left over, which can then act as a charge carrier. In n-type semiconductors, conduction is therefore mainly due to free electrons, although intrinsic 'holes' will also still carry positive charge in the opposite direction.

Unlike conventional conductors, the resistance of a semiconductor will drop as its temperature rises as the increase in energy creates more charge carriers.

By sandwiching together layers of p-type and n-type semiconductor material, the transistor was invented to replace the large, cumbersome and unreliable valve components of electronic circuits prior to the 1960s. No longer did radios – which could suddenly fit in your pocket – take half a minute to 'warm up'. Finally, it was possible to build a computer that didn't require a room the size of a house to contain it and wouldn't require a component replacement every few hours.

Within a generation, the transistor was replaced by the integrated circuit, which itself became miniaturized, with p-n-p or n-p-n junctions of atomic widths now appearing in the microchips that allow our radios to store thousands of MP3s whilst fitting in our credit card holders, and our computers to fit into hand luggage. A single, modern chip can contain millions of components packed in to a few square millimetres.

# Electrodynamics

The study of moving charges is known as electrodynamics. For our purposes, this will comprise a study of the way in which electricity and electrical components work. This will enable us to understand the operation of such devices as we encounter and rely on in our clinical practice. Clinical tools such as the ophthalmoscope; diagnostic imaging of all types, be it ultrasound, magnetic resonance imaging, conventional x-rays or cutting edge proton emission tomography; and therapeutic interventions such as interferential or TENS machines all rely upon one common factor, the flow of electricity.

## Circuit diagrams

This flow of electricity through a conductive device or apparatus can be best described using a circuit diagram. This is the electrical equivalent of a map and, like a map, it utilizes symbols to describe the topography through which the electricity flows. The most common symbols – and certainly all those you are likely to encounter in the course of your studies and subsequent clinical career – are detailed in Figure 7.4.

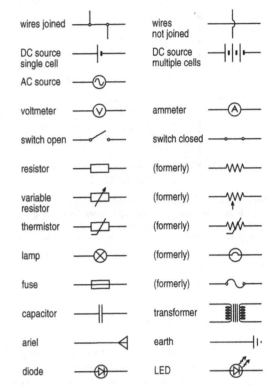

**Figure 7.4** • Circuit diagram symbols.

## Current

This flow of electrons is called a **current, I**, and is measured in amperes (amps; A), one of the seven basic SI units that, as you may recall from Table 1.1, is defined as:

*The current that, if maintained in two wires placed one metre apart in a vacuum, would produce a force of $2 \times 10^{-7}$ newtons per metre of length.*

It is undoubtedly much easier to visualize an amp as being the number of electrons flowing past a point each second; a device that measures this is called an **ammeter**.

The direction in which electric current flows is important; unfortunately, early physicists assumed that positive charges were moving when electricity flowed and so, on a circuit diagram, the current moves from positive to negative. This is known as **conventional current** but takes place in the opposite direction to actual **electron flow**; electrons are of course attracted towards the positive terminal and repelled by the negative. Conventional current is used by electricians and electron flow by physicists. The circuit diagrams you encounter in this book, and most others that you (as clinicians) are likely to read, will be based on conventional current.

In order for a current to flow, there must be a continuous **circuit** running out from and back to the source of the electric potential: electrons will then flow down the potential gradient (Fig. 7.5). If there is a break in the circuit then no current will flow (this is how a switch works). Current flow can also be disrupted by a short circuit (where two wires within the circuit touch in such a way that the continuous flow of electrons is broken).

The type of current provided by a battery gives a continuous flow of electrons (Fig. 7.6A), at least until the battery becomes 'flat' when its charge is exhausted. Unfortunately, this **direct current** is limited in its ability to be generated and transmitted over long distances, which is why domestic electricity comes in a different form, known as **alternating current** (Fig. 7.6B).

The waveform for alternating current is sinusoidal, i.e. it follows the same pattern that you would

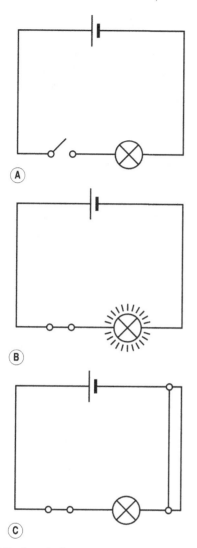

**Figure 7.5** ● In order for a current to flow, there must be a continuous circuit between the two terminals of a battery (B). If there is a break in the circuit (such as that provided by an open switch), no current can flow (A). The same effect is achieved if there is a 'short' in the circuit (C).

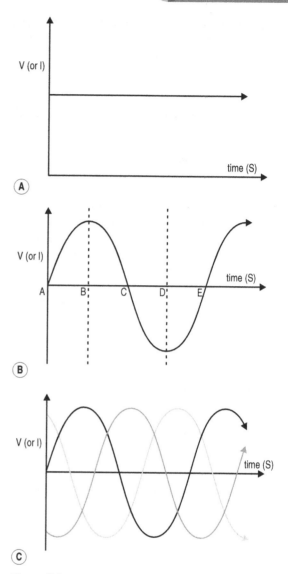

**Figure 7.6** ● With direct current, there is a steady, unbroken flow of electrons (A). With alternating current (B), the current first flows in one direction AB reaching a maximum at B, then diminishing until it reaches zero at C, at which point it reverses direction and repeats the same pattern, CD, until it again reaches zero at E, completing one cycle. With three-phase electricity (C), three loads are transmitted, each 120° out of phase with the other. This form of current is particularly useful in industrial applications for running electric motors; it is also the standard supply for x-ray machines.

get from plotting a graph of angle against its sine value. Electrons start by flowing in one direction, then slow down, stop and flow in the other. This cycle repeats many times per second. Unlike direct current, alternating current has the advantage that it can be **transformed** easily, that is the voltage can be increased and decreased so there is no difficulty in using sufficient voltage, 40 000 V or more, to transmit it via power cables over long distances before reducing it to levels suitable for domestic use.

Alternating current has two obvious drawbacks; the current is not always flowing in the same direction and, at two points in each cycle, the current will be zero. This is not a problem for certain types of electrical device: light bulbs, for example, will glow regardless of the direction of electron flow and will remain incandescent during the brief break in flow. Other types of device, computers for example, will not work if the current supplying them is interrupted.

This problem can, however, be (quite literally) rectified. A **rectifier** is a device than converts AC current into an approximation of DC (Fig. 7.7); however, as can be seen, the approximation by no means gives the linear flow provided by a battery, and a computer screen powered by the mains will still flicker, albeit many times faster than the human eye can detect. This effect can be lessened by incorporating a filter to smooth the waveform (Fig. 7.8). Such a device uses a component called a **capacitor** to store, then gradually release charge, of which more later on.

# Electrical power

At the other end of the scale, alternating current also provides problems for industrial applications. **Electrical power** is given by the product of voltage and current:

$$P = IV$$

As we already know, $V = IR$, therefore the above equation can also be written:

$$P = I(IR) = I^2R$$

However, the **effective power** – measured in watts – is not the same thing as the peak voltage; rather, it is dependent on the magnitude of the peak voltage and the frequency of the positive/negative phase. For our purposes, the effective voltage, also known

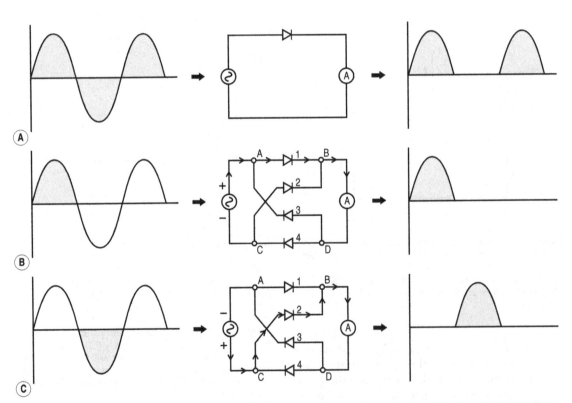

**Figure 7.7** • Alternating current can be simply rectified by using a device called a diode, which allows current to flow in one direction only; however, an alternating current rectified by a single diode will only be 'on' for half the time (A). This is known as 'half-wave' rectification. To allow 'full-wave' rectification, a circuit employing four diodes must be used. When the current is positive (B), it flows to A; the path to D is blocked (by diode 3), so it then flows to the ammeter via diode 1 and B. When the current enters its negative phase (C), it flows to C but the path to D is prohibited by diode 4 so, instead, it flows via diode 2 to B and thence again to the ammeter *in the same orientation as it did during the positive phase*.

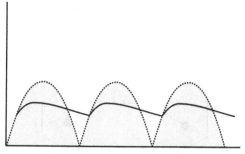

**Figure 7.8** • A full-wave rectifier with a smoothing filter produces a better approximation of direct current.

as the root mean square voltage, is approximately 70% of the peak voltage. It is this value that is quoted when referring to the electrical supply available at the plug socket; therefore, the peak value of the domestic supply is actually 143% ($^1/_{0.7}$) of the quoted value.

Far more power can be obtained from a system that does not drop to zero twice every cycle, and a system whose peak voltage is much higher than its effective value is also more dangerous – if you were unfortunate enough to receive an electric shock, the damage is done by the peak voltage. It is for this reason that industrial supply is 'three-phase'; that is there are three wires, each carrying an alternating current that is one-third of a cycle behind one of its neighbours and one-third of a cycle ahead of the other (Fig.7.6C). Sometimes, there can be four wires – the additional wire is neutral and is used when the load is 'unbalanced', that is the current in the three live wires is not of equal magnitude and/or frequency.

This substantially increases the available power and eliminates the problems caused by the oscillation from positive through zero to negative.

Power surges, caused by fluctuations in the external supply or an unintentional short circuit inside a device, can be dangerous, causing potential damage to the device and its operator. To prevent this, most circuits contain **fuses,** which consist of two terminals connected by a thin strip of wire, traditionally made of tin.

If the current exceeds a certain level (in the domestic setting, usually 3A, 5A or 13A), the resultant heating effect (and remember, power is proportional to the *square* of the current) causes the wire to melt and break the circuit.

# Electronics

This branch of electricity is concerned for the most part with devices that allow a small signal to control

a much larger one. There are a number of everyday components with which we need to be familiar if we are to understand the principles behind the workings of a wide range of electrical devices.

## Resistors

We already know a little bit about resistors from Ohm's law; however, this rule has implications that are not immediately obvious. This is because there is more than one way in which to connect resistors in a circuit; they can be connected in **series** (Fig. 7.9) or in **parallel** (Fig. 7.10).

In the former case, it is easy to see that the total resistance of a series circuit is equal to the sum of the individual resistors:

$$R_{total} = R_1 + R_2 + R_3 + R_4 + \ldots = \Sigma R$$

However, for resistors in a parallel circuit, the splitting of current into several tributaries means that the *inverse* of the total resistance will be equal to the sum of the *inverse* of the resistance in each arm:

$$\frac{1}{R_{tot}} = \frac{1}{R_1} + \frac{1}{R_2} + \frac{1}{R_3} + \frac{1}{R_4} + \ldots = \Sigma^1/_R$$

### Variable resistors

A device that allows you to vary the resistance is called a **rheostat** and this can be used as a **voltage divider** to reduce the potential across the circuit (Fig. 7.11). When rheostats are used in this manner – as they are in dimmer switches and volume controls – they are known as **potentiometers**. As we shall see in Chapter 10, potentiometers have an important role in x-ray machines.

## Thermistors

As discussed earlier, when a semiconductor is heated, its conductance increases owing to the increase in charge carriers. Therefore, when a circuit is switched on, the resistance of a thermistor will be initially high then decrease as it responds to the warming effect of the current.

This device is used to protect sensitive devices such as projector lamp filaments and x-ray tubes from current surges as they are switched on, allowing a gradual increase in current to operating levels and increasing the life of the element.

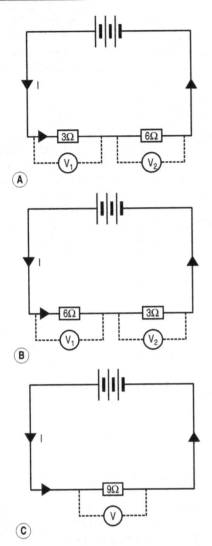

**(A)**

**(B)**

**(C)**

**Figure 7.9** • When resistors are connected in series, all of the current flows through them (it has to, there is nowhere else for it to go). This means the total resistance in the circuits shown below is the same. It does not matter in which order the resistors are placed (**A & B**) or if the 3Ω and 6Ω resistors and replaced with a single 9Ω resistor (3Ω + 6Ω = 9Ω) (**C**). If the potential difference across the circuit is 3 V, then, the current will be $I = V/R = 3/9 = 0.33$ A. In (**A**), the potential across the 3Ω resistor is $V_1 = IR_1 = 0.33 \times 3 = 1$ V and the potential across the 6Ω resistor is $V_2 = IR_2 = 0.33 \times 6 = 2$ V. Therefore, for resistors in series, the total potential difference is the sum of the potentials across the individual resistors $V = V_1 + V_2 + V_3 + \ldots$

## Capacitors

As mentioned earlier, a capacitor is a device designed for short-term storage of electrical charge. Typically, a capacitor consists of two metal plates

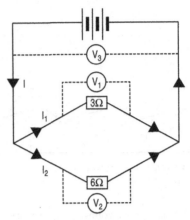

**Figure 7.10** • Resistors in parallel. Resistors behave differently when they are connected in parallel. Here, the potential across each resistor is the same, identical to that of the circuit as a whole. If you study the diagram carefully, you will see that, in effect, there is no difference in the way that $V_1$ or $V_2$ are connected when compared to $V_3$. Both are actually measuring the potential across the terminal of the dry cells, in this case the same as in Figure 7.9, 3 V. When the current reaches the split in the wires, it splits and it does so it proportion to the resistance it faces; the more the resistance, the less current flows so $I = I_1 + I_2 + I_3 \ldots$ As $I = V/R$, the current flowing in through the 3Ω resistor will be 1A and the current through the 6Ω resistor will be 0.5A. The resistance of the circuit is found by adding the inverses of the individual resistors and taking the inverse of the whole; so, $1/R = 1/3 + 1/6 = 2/6 + 1/6 = 1/2$ therefore $R = 2Ω$, which brings us full circle: $V = IR = (I_1 + I_2)R = (1 + 0.5) \times 2 = 3$ V.

separated by an insulator. When this is connected into an electric circuit, one plate will gain electrons and the other lose them, thus storing charge. When the potential difference is removed the stored charge will flow down its potential gradient, creating a temporary current until the charge on the plates is again equal (Fig. 7.12).

As the current is dependent on the potential difference across the plates, it will lessen gradually as the charge decreases in much the same way that a torch bulb will gradually dim over time as a battery runs flat, only with a capacitor the discharge time is measured in fractions of seconds rather than hours. In a capacitor, the manner in which this drop-off occurs is exponential (Fig. 7.13).

A useful analogy for capacitance is a tank full of compressed air. There will be a fixed ratio between the 'charge' of compressed air that is pumped into the tank and the resultant pressure inside it and this ratio will be proportional to the size of the tank – a tank with a large capacity will require a large

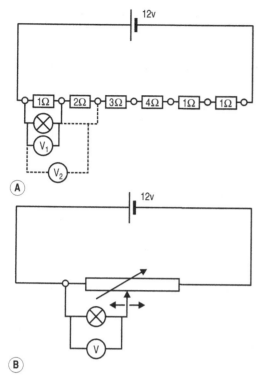

**Figure 7.11** • Voltage diodes. Because the voltage across individual resistors connected in series will be only a fraction of the potential across the circuit as a whole; by choosing to connect across one or more resistors, we can select the voltage we want: in the case of (**A**), using a standard 12 V battery, we can therefore select values of 1 V, 3 V, 6 V, 10 V, 11 V and 12 V.By using a rheostat, which allows us to vary the resistance of the circuit to any value we choose (**B**), we can transition smoothly from any value between 0 V and 12 V. This is how a potential divider works and is commonly found in dimmer switches to control lighting and volume controls on audio devices from phonographs to MP3 players.

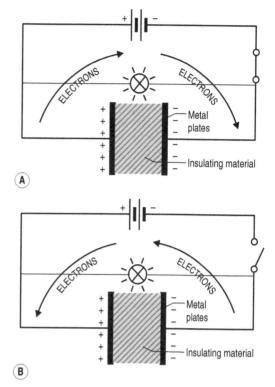

**Figure 7.12** • Capacitance. When a potential difference is placed across a capacitor, the plate connected to the negative terminal of the battery will store electrons whereas the other plate will become electron deficient (**A**). When the potential is removed (here by means of opening a switch), charge is redistributed causing electrons to flow and thus generating a current, which lasts until the stored charge is exhausted (**B**). A capacitor can be thought of as a very short-life battery.

amount of air and one with a small capacity a correspondingly small amount of air to produce the same internal pressure. However, the larger tank will be subsequently capable of doing more work and it is storing more energy. When this energy is released, the 'current' of air leaving the tanks will lessen gradually as the head of pressure drops.

The **capacitance, C,** of any given device is the ratio of the charge on the conductor and its resultant potential (or, in the case of Fig. 7.12, the potential across a capacitor and its resultant stored charge). This can be written mathematically as:

$$C = \frac{Q}{V}$$

and is measured in farads (F)

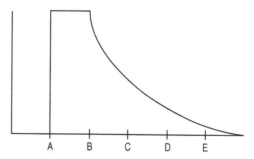

**Figure 7.13** • Capacitor discharge. Although charging of a capacitor takes place almost instantly (**A**), when the charge is 'released' and a current starts to flow from the device (**B**), the charge decays exponentially; this is, after a time (**C**), half the charge will have gone, after a further, equal period of time (**D**), half the remaining charge will have gone and so on.

Although the definition of a farad sounds reasonable enough: *the capacitance of a conductor such that one coulomb of charge would raise its potential by one volt*, it is in reality a derived unit that is hopelessly unwieldy and, in practice, the microfarad, µF, and picofarad, pF are used instead.

The rules for connecting multiple capacitors are opposite to those for resistors. If capacitors are connected in parallel, the potential difference across each capacitor must be the same and so the charge on each capacitor must be the same. As charge and capacitance are directly proportional to each other,

$$C_{TOT} = C_1 + C_2 + C_3 + \ldots = \Sigma C$$

By contrast, the charge across capacitors connected in series will be the same (if it were not, the charge would redistribute itself until it were). Therefore the potential across each capacitor will be different but must total the potential across the circuit as a whole:

$$V_{TOT} = V_1 + V_2 + V_3 + \ldots$$

However, $V = {}^Q/_C$; Q is the same across each capacitor, therefore:

$$V_1 = {}^Q/_{C_1}, V_2 = {}^Q/_{C_2} \text{ etc.}$$

Therefore:

$${}^Q/_C = {}^Q/_{C_1} + {}^Q/_{C_2} + {}^Q/_{C_3} + \ldots$$

So (by cancelling out Q):

$$\frac{1}{C_{tot}} = \frac{1}{C_1} + \frac{1}{C_2} + \frac{1}{C_3} + \frac{1}{C_4} + \ldots = \Sigma {}^1/_C$$

 CLINICAL FOCUS

The functioning of the body's nervous system has often been compared to the functioning of electrical systems. Neurons rely on voltage potentials and charge carriers to operate and anyone who has ever studied a schematic of the brachial plexus cannot help but compare it to a particularly fiendish circuit diagram.

However, one feature of neurons that is usually overlooked in physiology textbooks is that their cell walls actually act like the insulating material found between the charged plates of a capacitor and that much of their electrical behaviour is due to this effect.

Neurons work by generating and transmitting electrical impulses using the **action potential**. Like all cells, nerve cells maintain different concentrations of ions internally in comparison to the environment outside. In particular, they pump out sodium ions ($Na^+$) and pump in potassium ions ($K^+$). In both cases, the ions are transported by means of specialist channels that allow passage of that ion only; however, the potassium channel is slightly leakier than the sodium channel. As a result, there are more positive ions outside the membrane than inside. The membrane is insulated with myelin (the channels exist in small, regularly spaced gaps called *nodes of Ranvier*) and therefore, the inside of the membrane is negative with respect to the outside. The potential difference between the two is, when resting, approximately 70 mV and the cell is said to be **polarized**.

When the axon is stimulated it generates an **action potential**, a wave of negative electrical charge that travels rapidly down the axon in a direction parallel to the way in which electrons travel down an electric wire; however, the mechanism is different and in fact more closely resembles the processes that take place in a semiconductor.

When a stimulus occurs, it causes sodium channels to open briefly, resulting in an influx of sodium ions and lowering the potential difference across the 'membrane capacitor'. If the stimulus is weak, then only a few channels are opened, little charge flows and the temporary change in potential difference is rapidly reversed by the sodium pump. However, when the stimulus reaches a critical point, usually enough to reduce the potential by 20 mV or more, it triggers a major depolarizing reaction. This point is termed the **threshold**. When it is breached, it triggers a massive opening of sodium channels, discharging the 'membrane capacitor' and the inside of the cell in fact becomes temporarily positive with respect to the outside.

Within milliseconds, the sodium channels close and the potassium channels open and potassium floods out, rapidly making the inside of the cell even more negative than it was at rest. After several more milliseconds, the potassium channels close and the pumping mechanism returns the cells to its normal potential; however, until it does, the axon remains hyperpolarized and any further stimuli are unable to create an action potential. This is known as the **refractory period**.

Because the initial opening of sodium channels will trigger the adjacent channels to open, a wave of negative electrical charge jumps from one node of Ranvier to the next and travels rapidly down the axon (because of the refractory period, the sodium channels proximal to the 'wave front' remain closed, so the 'wave' is propagated in one direction only).

The importance of the myelin sheathing is demonstrated by the devastating effects of demyelinating diseases such as multiple sclerosis, which rob nerves of their ability to conduct signals from the central to the peripheral nervous system with catastrophic effect on coordination, balance and muscle control.

## Diodes

As we saw when discussing rectification, a diode is an electrical device that allows the passage of a current in one direction only. It finds a common application in devices such as radios, computers and much medical equipment, where components would be damaged if the power supply were connected the wrong way round, as happens many times a second when the power supply is alternating current. They can also be used to create a back-up system if the main source of power fails (Fig. 7.14).

A special type of diode, called a **light-emitting diode**, gives out light when a current passes through it. They are perhaps better known by their TLA (three-letter acronym); most of us will be familiar

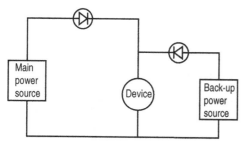

**Figure 7.14** • Diode back-up. In this circuit, the higher voltage main power source will ordinarily power the circuit; however, should this fail, the back-up circuit will take over. This principle is used in dynamo bicycle lamps, which stop generating when the bicycle becomes stationary at junctions and rely on the backup of batteries. It is also the system in operation in laptop computers, which switch seamlessly to battery operation when they are unplugged, and the principle behind large-scale systems such as auxiliary power in hospitals, major internet providers and other places where an uninterrupted power supply is essential.

with LEDs even though some of their uses in seven-segment displays of number in cash-registers, clocks and calculators have been superseded by liquid crystal displays. Their long life and small power requirements also make them ideal for use as indicator lights.

## Systems

The LED is one example of a **transducer**, a device that converts energy from one form to another. Most electronic systems will consist of three parts: an input transducer, a processor and an output transducer. For example, in a CD player, the input transducer is the disc reader; the processor, the amplifier; and the output transducer, the loudspeaker.

There are innumerable input transducers (microphones, thermistors, pickups, switches) and output transducers (lamps, bells, LEDs, meters, electric motors); however, there are only three types of processor with which we need to be concerned.

A **transistor** is a solid state device consisting of three layers of semiconducting material, most commonly n-p-n in configuration. These three layers are known as the *collector* (c), the *base* (b) and the *emitter* (e). There are many types of transistor; however, basically it is a device for magnifying small electric currents and its most common use is in an **amplifier**.

An amplifier is a device in which an input signal is enlarged in terms of voltage, current or power before appearing at the output terminals. A **linear amplifier** has an output signal that replicates the output signal; a **non-linear amplifier** has an output signal that is not a replica of the input signal (Fig. 7.15).

One of the most common types of amplifier is known as the **operational amplifier**, deriving its name from its original use as a device for performing mathematical operations such as addition, multiplication or calculus. It is more commonly referred to as an **OP-AMP.**

An OP-AMP is a high-gain, direct current amplifier. The **gain** of an amplifier is the amount by which the signal is multiplied. The voltage gain of an OP-AMP is typically of the order of tens of thousands. The other feature of an OP-AMP is the fact that it has two inputs, one positive and one negative (with respect to the output terminal).

The OM-AMP has two main uses. It can be used as an **inverter**, whereby the amplified output is opposite in phase to the input. Feedback is used to

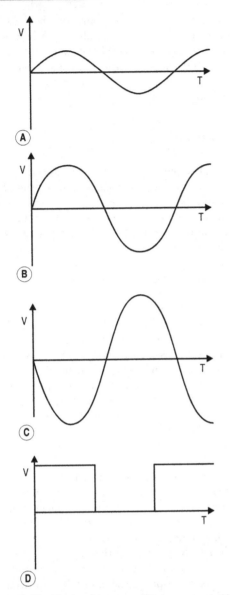

(A)

**Figure 7.15** • The input to an amplifier is represented in (A). In (B), the signal has been amplified but not changed in any other way; this is an example of a linear amplifier. If the signal is changed, as it has been in (C) by means of an inverter, then it is a non-linear signal. Both (B) and (C) are analogue signals whereas (D) has been converted to a digital signal, whereby the voltage is either maximal or depending on the phase of the input.

reduce the gain but to lessen the distortion so that the input is processed more accurately.

If the feedback is removed, an OP-AMP can also be used as a **comparator** to compare two voltages: if the voltage across the negative terminal is greater

than the positive, the output is low; if it is less, then the voltage is high.

The previous output signals discussed have been **analogue signals**, in which the voltage can vary smoothly and have any value between the lowest and highest. A comparator produces a signal that is, to all intents and purposes, **digital**. In a digital system, the output signal can only have certain definite values, usually just *on* or *off* (Fig. 7.15).

A digital signal is also produced by the final type of processor that we shall consider, a **logic circuit**.

The components of a logic circuit generally consist of two digital inputs that generate a single digital output, dependent on the combination of 'ons' and 'offs' at the input, usually referred to as '1' and '0' respectively.

If two switches are connected in series (Fig. 7.16), then current will flow and light the bulb *only* when switch A *and* switch B are closed. This can be analyzed by drawing a table to consider all the possible permutations of the circuit. Such a table is known as a **truth table** (Table 7.1) and this type of logic circuit is called an **AND gate**.

If the two switches are connected in parallel, a different picture arises (Fig. 7.17). Now, the bulb will be lit if *either* switch A *or* switch B is closed.

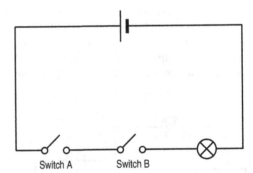

**Figure 7.16** • In this circuit, the bulb will light if and only if both switches are closed. If either one is open, the circuit is incomplete and no current can flow.

**Table 7.1** Truth table for an AND gate

| Switch A | Switch B | Lamp |
|----------|----------|------|
| 1 | 1 | 1 |
| 0 | 1 | 0 |
| 1 | 0 | 0 |
| 0 | 0 | 0 |

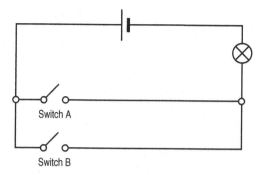

**Figure 7.17** ● In this circuit, the bulb will light if either or both switches are closed as closing a switch will complete one of the two possible circuits.

The truth table for this **OR gate** is detailed in Table 7.2.

The third basic form of gate is different in that it only has one input and one output. If the input is on, the output is off and vice versa. Such a device is known as a **NOT gate** and its (extremely basic) truth table is detailed in Table 7.3.

These three gates can be used to build any logic circuit; however, for the sake of convenience, two other types are used involving combinations of the devices we have already considered. If the output of an AND gate is connected to a NOT gate, the combination is referred to as a NAND gate and its truth table (Table 7.4) is the opposite to an AND gate, the output is only off when both switches are *closed*.

In a similar fashion, a NOR gate is formed when the output from an OR gate is connected to the input of a NOT gate; again, it forms the inverse truth table to that of the OR gate – now the bulb is only on when both switches are *open* (Table 7.5).

Each one of these gates has its own component symbol (Fig. 7.18). Used in combination, they can rapidly develop the circuits that can perform the tasks that we take for granted in our chip-laden civilization, performing complex mathematical functions and, by means of feedback loops, develop memory.

**Table 7.4** Truth table for a NAND gate

| Switch A | Switch B | Lamp |
|---|---|---|
| 1 | 1 | 0 |
| 0 | 1 | 1 |
| 1 | 0 | 1 |
| 0 | 0 | 1 |

**Table 7.5** Truth table for a NOR gate

| Switch A | Switch B | Lamp |
|---|---|---|
| 1 | 1 | 0 |
| 0 | 1 | 0 |
| 1 | 0 | 0 |
| 0 | 0 | 1 |

**Table 7.2** Truth table for an OR gate

| Switch A | Switch B | Lamp |
|---|---|---|
| 1 | 1 | 1 |
| 0 | 1 | 1 |
| 1 | 0 | 1 |
| 0 | 0 | 0 |

**Table 7.3** Truth table for a NOT gate

| Input | Lamp |
|---|---|
| 1 | 0 |
| 0 | 1 |

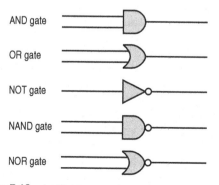

**Figure 7.18** ● Logic components.

**A** SELF-ASSESSMENT

To check your understanding of logic circuits, try developing a truth table for the circuit shown in Figure 7.19. Only one combination of switches will sound the buzzer, which is it? (Answer at end of chapter.)

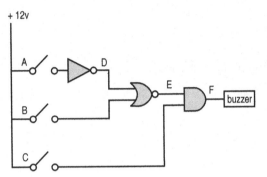

**Figure 7.19** • An arrangement of logic gates that produce a combination lock, can you find the correct combination?

# Magnetism

The form of magnetism with which we are most familiar is that of the Earth. We are brought up to believe that this field is constant, unchanging and allows us to find north at any time by using a compass. In fact, none of these suppositions is correct. The north magnetic pole is currently 11.5° out of alignment with the geographic north pole and wanders about by as much as 150 km per year.

The value of the Earth's magnetic field varies over the surface of the Earth from 0.6 Gauss to as little as 0.3 Gauss and has apparently weakened by as much as 10% since Gauss first measured its value in 1845, and perhaps by as much as a half since 2000 years ago. This weakening may or may not be associated with a forthcoming reversal of the field, which has flipped backward and forwards from north pole to south pole at least 150 times since the dinosaurs died out 65 million years ago, including at least once during the 70 000 year history of modern man. Some biologists think that these events, which may last up to 1000 years, have a major influence on evolution. The sun's cosmic radiation, usually deflected by the Earth's magnetic field, causes genetic damage and increases the rate of mutation (and, incidentally, cancers); it also may be associated with extinction

events – many birds and animals rely on the magnetic field for navigational purposes. In fact, far from the certainties with which we were presented at school, the Earth's magnetism is a force (poorly understood) generated by a mechanism (unknown) that may be about to change (for reasons that remain a mystery).

Although we don't really know how the Earth generates a magnetic field (indeed, according to our understanding of magnetism, the temperature at the Earth's core should be far too hot to allow this to happen), we can create our own magnetic fields quite easily. If we take a **ferromagnetic** substance and stroke it with the north pole of a magnet, then the substance will also become magnetized, causing all of the unpaired electron spins to line up with each other. This process is known as **magnetic induction**.

**AB©** **DICTIONARY DEFINITION**

**FERROMAGNETISM**

Iron, nickel, cobalt, and the rare earth elements gadolinium and dysprosium exhibit a unique magnetic behavior termed *ferromagnetism* after the Latin for iron (*ferrum*), the most common example of such a material. Samarium and neodymium in alloys with cobalt have been used to fabricate very strong rare-earth magnets.

Such an arrangement appears to be a highly stable one as, unless hammered or heated, the material will remain magnetized, often for many years, despite its exposure to the Earth's own magnetic field.

The two magnets will then demonstrate physical properties that have a direct parallel with static electricity. Their field strength obeys the inverse square law and opposite poles will attract each other whilst like poles repel.

There is a second way in which a substance can be magnetized and it is one that is of much more significance to clinicians.

# Electromagnetic induction

We learnt at the start of the chapter that a moving electric charge (i.e., a current) produces a magnetic field, and this fact can be used to create a magnet – indeed it is a simple enough procedure that it can be easily tried at home.

Connect a wire to the positive terminal of a battery. Wrap the wire around a ferromagnetic rod (for convenience, try a six-inch nail) half a dozen times then connect the other end of the wire to the negative terminal. When you disconnect the circuit, you will find that the rod has become a magnet.

The corollary also holds true and is a principle used to generate electricity from the humblest bicycle dynamo to the largest power station. If a loop of wire is rotated between two magnets, it will generate a current; the wire is moving with respect to the magnetic field. This is summarized in the **first law of electromagnetic induction**, which states:

> *A change of magnetic flux through a circuit causes an electromotive force (i.e., a force that causes electrons to move) to be induced in the circuit, which will be proportional to the rate of change of magnetic flux and to the area of the circuit. (Practically, the loop(s) of wire are often made stationary and the magnets rotated around them – the motion is relative: the electrons can't spot the difference!)*

The direction of the current is dependent on two factors: the direction of the magnetic field and the direction of the motion; this is demonstrated by **Fleming's Right-hand Rule** (Fig.7.20).

The implications of this rule are very interesting; if we see what happens at different points during a single revolution of the loop (Fig. 7.21), we can see that the current initially flows in one direction then, as the loop is moving increasingly parallel to the lines of flux, less and less current will be produced. When it passes this point, the current generated will again increase although it will flow in the opposite direction. This process is then repeated for the second half of each revolution. If we plot the current against time, we see a familiar pattern, a sinusoidal waveform: the coil has generated an alternating current.

Whether the coil is spun by a bicycle wheel or a steam turbine, the result is the same, although the frequency of the alternating current will be determined by the number of rotations per second. There are several ways in which the output can be increased, these are detailed in Table 7.6; indeed, the typical output of a power station is measured in gigawatts and the potential difference along a high-tension power cable can be as high as 150 kV. Although this is quite convenient for moving large amounts of electricity across the countryside, it is not a practical voltage for use in domestic and clinical situations; fortunately, induction comes to the rescue once again.

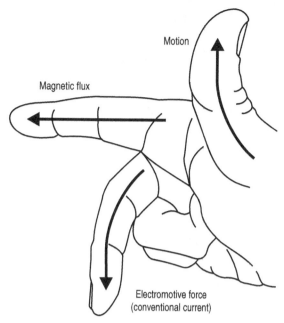

**Figure 7.20** • Fleming's right hand rule for a moving conductor. If you align your right index finger with the direction of the magnetic field (i.e. from north pole to south pole) and your thumb with the direction of movement of the wire, then your middle finger (3rd digit) will indicate the direction of the electromotive force and thus the (conventional) current ... assuming that you haven't dislocated your wrist in the process!

## The transformer

Voltage can be increased or decreased ('stepped-up' or 'stepped-down') easily and efficiently using a device called a **transformer**, which again makes use of the principles of electromagnetic induction (Fig. 7.22). If we have a circuit, part of which is wrapped around one side of a ring of iron, when an alternating current flows though the circuit, it will generate a magnetic field in the iron. Because the current is not just changing (the requirement for magnetic induction) but actually alternating from positive to negative, the magnetic field will vary from north–south, to zero, to south–north, to zero and back to north–south each cycle.

We therefore have changing lines of magnetic flux moving through the iron bar, which has become an alternating electromagnet. If a second loop of wire is passed around the other side of the ring, this changing magnetic field will induce a current inside the wires (remember, even though the wire is static, it is still in motion with respect to the magnetic field ... electrons can't tell the difference).

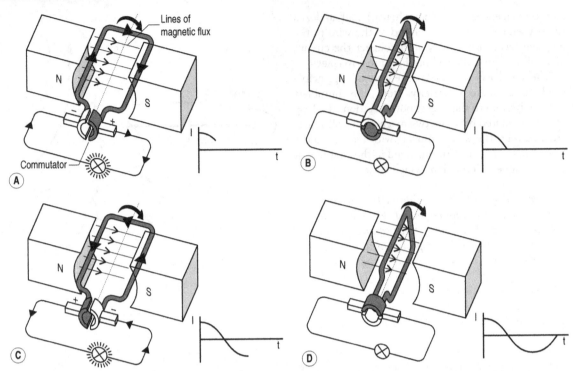

**Figure 7.21** • (A) shows the start of a single revolution of a single coil. At this point, the wire is moving perpendicular to the lines of flux and the maximum possible current is being generated. You can check the direction of flow using Fleming's right-hand rule: in the left half of the loop, which is moving upwards, the current will flow away from the bulb; in the right half of the loop, which is moving downwards, the current is flowing towards the bulb, which will be lit. When the coil has moved through 90° (B), it will be moving parallel to the lines of flux and therefore, during this quarter turn, the current will have diminished to zero and the bulb will have dimmed and gone out. During the next 90° (C), the current will again increase to its maximum, although this time the current will be flowing in the opposite direction (actually it continues to be induced in the same direction but the position of the two pieces of wire have been reversed whilst the remainder of the circuit has stayed the same). Again, you can check this using Fleming's right-hand rule. At (D), the situation will be the same as (B), the current dropping to zero before again reversing to its original direction of flow, reaching a maximum as it returns to its starting point at (A). Note that, although we talk about the bulb going on and off, if the coil is moving at a speed fast enough to induce a current large enough light a bulb, it would have to rotate at many times a second and the residual incandescence of the bulb would ensure that it remained lit.

**Table 7.6** Means for increasing the output of a dynamo, based on the first law of electromagnetic induction

| Action | Effect |
|---|---|
| Increase the speed of rotation | This increases the rate at which the lines of magnetic flux are passed through, thus generating a higher electromotive force |
| Increase the magnetic field | Use stronger (electro)magnets creating a larger magnetic flux<br>Wind the coil on a ferromagnetic core. Again, this will increase the effective magnetic flux |
| Increasing the number of turns in the coil | This increases the area of the circuit |

If we recall the first law of induction, the size of the electromotive force is dependent on the area of wire reacting with the magnetic flux: if there are a lot of coils, the electromotive force will be higher than if there are only a few coils. This means we can choose how much electromotive force we induce in the outgoing circuit; in fact, it is governed by a very simple formula:

$$V_s/V_p = N_s/N_p$$

where $V_p$ and $V_s$ are the voltages in the primary and secondary coil respectively and $N_p$ and $N_s$ are the number of turns in the two coils.

Therefore, if there are fewer coils in the secondary circuit compared to the primary, the device will act as a **step-down transformer**. Such devices can be

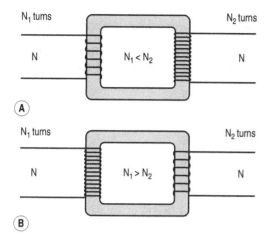

Figure 7.22 • By varying the ratio of turns between the primary ($N_1$) and secondary ($N_2$) coils, a transformer can be used to increase (step-up) (A) or decrease (step-down) (B) voltage. The alternating primary voltage induces an alternating magnetic field in the iron ring. This, in turn, induces an alternating current in the secondary coil; the size of this current is proportional to the cross-sectional area (number of turns).

found in electricity sub-stations to reduce the high-tension transmission voltage to levels more appropriate for domestic and industrial use.

Similarly, if there are more secondary coils than primary, the device will act as a **step-up transformer** of the sort found in power stations to increase the voltage from the level generated to the higher levels required for long distance transport.

 CLINICAL FOCUS

It appears that power transmission may come at a cost to human health. For many years, power companies and governments denied that electricity could be in any way hazardous (other than by direct application – over 400 US citizens die from accidental electrocution every year; in the UK, the figure varies from 25–65). However, there is now a clear epidemiological link between childhood leukaemia and residential proximity to high-tension power cables.

Since these 'clusters' of paediatric cases were first noted, the search for other possible effects of continual exposure to magnetic fields of the order of 0.1–0.4 μT (recall that tesla is the SI unit of magnetic flux density), such as those found within 400 m of pylons. Although there seems to be no link with adult leukaemia, there is now evidence suggesting a link with increased incidence of breast and lung

cancer; depression and suicide; and illnesses associated with air pollution, such as asthma and bronchitis.

Indeed the magnetic fields associated with our electricity supply are, in the UK, now hypothesized to cause 250–500 deaths per year, 10 times the number that are caused by the electricity itself.

# Electricity in the home and clinic

The frequency and voltage of mains supply electricity varies from country to country as do the shape, size and configuration of plugs and plug sockets. This often means appliances purchased overseas simply cannot be connected to the wall outlets at home without changing the plug or using an adaptor. Even then, if the voltage disparity is too great (as would be the case when attempting to use 120 V American appliances in 230 V British sockets), the device not only will fail to operate, but is likely to become a major fire hazard.

Basically, North America and Japan use a low voltage (100–137 V) high frequency (60 Hz) system whereas Europe and most other countries around the world use a high voltage (220–240 V) low frequency (50 Hz) one. The operating parameters for a selection of major countries are given in Table 7.7.

In fact, both systems – which evolved rather than being designed – have faults. Not only is a 50 Hz system 20% less effective in generation that its 60 Hz counterpart, it is also 10–15% less efficient in transmission and requires up to 30% larger windings and magnetic core materials in transformer construction. Electric motors are much less efficient at the lower frequency and must be made more robust to handle the electrical losses and the extra heat generated.

Originally, Europe operated a 120 V supply but, unlike Japan and the US, realized the necessity of a higher voltage to reduce power loss and meet the power demands of modern equipment. Americans opted out of the change; unlike their European counterparts at the time (the mid to late 1950s), many US homes had a fridge, deep-freezer, washing machine and television and the cost – and political unpopularity – of replacing so much domestic equipment was deemed too high.

**Table 7.7** Operating voltage and frequency of domestic and three-phase (industrial) electricity supply in selected countries

| Country | Domestic voltage supply (V) | Domestic frequency (Hz) | Three-phase voltage (V) | Three-phase frequency (Hz) |
|---|---|---|---|---|
| Australia | 240 | 50 | 415 | 50 |
| Austria | 230 | 50 | 400 | 50 |
| Bahamas | 120 | 60 | 206 | 60 |
| Belgium | 230 | 50 | 400 | 50 |
| Bermuda | 120 | 60 | 208 | 60 |
| Brazil | 127/220* | 60 | 220/380/440* | 60 |
| Canada | 120 | 60 | 208/240/600 | 60 |
| Chile | 220 | 50 | 380 | 50 |
| China | 220 | 50 | 380 | 50 |
| Cyprus | 230 | 50 | 400 | 50 |
| Czech Republic | 230 | 50 | 400 | 50 |
| Denmark | 230 | 50 | 400 | 50 |
| Estonia | 230 | 50 | 400 | 50 |
| Fiji | 240 | 50 | 415 | 50 |
| Finland | 230 | 50 | 400 | 50 |
| France | 230 | 50 | 400 | 50 |
| Georgia | 220 | 50 | 380 | 50 |
| Germany | 230 | 50 | 400 | 50 |
| Greece | 230 | 50 | 400 | 50 |
| Hungary | 230 | 50 | 400 | 50 |
| Iceland | 230 | 50 | 400 | 50 |
| India | 230 | 50 | 400 | 50 |
| Indonesia | 230 | 50 | 400 | 50 |
| Iran | 230 | 50 | 400 | 50 |
| Iraq | 230 | 50 | 400 | 50 |
| Ireland (Eire) | 230 | 50 | 400 | 50 |
| Israel | 230 | 50 | 400 | 50 |
| Italy | 230 | 50 | 400 | 50 |
| Jamaica | 110 | 50 | 190 | 50 |
| Japan | 100 | 50/60 ** | 200 | 50/60 ** |

**Table 7.7** Operating voltage and frequency of domestic and three-phase (industrial) electricity supply in selected countries—Cont'd

| Country | Domestic voltage supply (V) | Domestic frequency (Hz) | Three-phase voltage (V) | Three-phase frequency (Hz) |
|---|---|---|---|---|
| Latvia | 230 | 50 | 400 | 50 |
| Mexico | 127 | 60 | 220/480 | 60 |
| Netherlands | 230 | 50 | 400 | 50 |
| New Zealand | 240 | 50 | 415 | 50 |
| Nigeria | 230 | 50 | 400 | 50 |
| Norway | 230 | 50 | 400 | 50 |
| Pakistan | 230 | 50 | 400 | 50 |
| Poland | 230 | 50 | 400 | 50 |
| Portugal | 230 | 50 | 400 | 50 |
| Puerto Rico | 120 | 60 | 208 | 60 |
| Russian Federation | 230 | 50 | 400 | 50 |
| South Africa | 230 | 50 | 400 | 50 |
| Spain | 230 | 50 | 400 | 50 |
| Sweden | 230 | 50 | 400 | 50 |
| Switzerland | 230 | 50 | 400 | 50 |
| Taiwan | 110 | 60 | 190 | 60 |
| Trinidad & Tobago | 115 | 60 | 200 | 60 |
| Turkey | 230 | 50 | 400 | 50 |
| United Kingdom | 240 | 50 | 400 | 50 |
| United States of America | 120 | 60 | 120/208/277/480 | 60 |

*In Brazil, there is no standard voltage. Most states use 127 V for domestic supply and 220 V for three-phase; however a few, mainly north-eastern, states employ a 220 V system for domestic use and 380 V for industrial applications.

**Although the mains voltage in Japan is the same everywhere, the frequency differs from region to region. Eastern Japan uses predominantly 50 (Tokyo, Kawasaki, Sapporo, Yokohoma, Sendai), whereas Western Japan prefers 60 (Osaka, Kyoto, Nagoya, Hiroshima).

The end result is that the US has to cope with the problems of voltage drop-off: light bulbs that burn out rather quickly when they are close to the transformer (127 V) and homes at the end of the line that do not have enough voltage to properly power some of their appliances (105 V).

As a result, all new American buildings now in fact have an effective 240 V system, which is divided between 120 V neutral and hot wires. Major appliances, such as tumble-dryers, kettles, washing machines and ovens, are now connected to 240 V, although the nature of the supply is two-phase, thus further increasing the compatibility problems.

When Nicholas Tesla first designed the three-phase power generation and distribution system, he carefully calculated that the most efficient and practical parameters would be 240 V and 60 Hz. Today, only a handful of countries (Antigua, Guyana, Peru, the Philippines, South Korea and the Leeward Islands) actually follow this system.

In addition to the variation in supply, there are also some 13 different types of plug (and socket) in use in different countries around the world, with either two or three pins, which can be flat, round or square and be of equal or different lengths. In summary, North America and Japan use two flat pins; most of Europe uses two round pins; the UK now uses three square pins. Although many plugs have a wide geographical distribution, some countries, among them Switzerland, Denmark and Israel, have their own unique plugs.

Regardless of the configuration of the power supply and its means of connection, the wiring supply to a domestic residence (or clinic) remains essentially the same. The supply, which is taken directly from the mains cables running below ground or via overhead cables, enters the residence via a **meter**. This records the energy consumed in kilowatt-hours (energy consumed = power (kW) × time (h)).

The wires from the meter supply the **ring main**, also known as the **radial circuit**, from which all the supply is then taken. There are, basically, three circuits inside a typical residence:

• The ring main itself into which heavy-duty machinery such as the electric cooker, shower and boiler (and any x-ray equipment) is directly wired. This is usually protected by a 30A fuse, although the rating can occasionally be higher in countries using a low-voltage supply (32A, 45A or 50A, depending on the power requirement)

• The socket main, providing for the plug sockets, which is protected by a 13A fuse (15A or 20A in low-voltage circuits).

• A lighting circuit, which is protected by a 5A fuse.

In countries employing a three-pin plug system, in addition to the *live* and *neutral* wires, there is an additional *earth* wire, connected to the third pin. This ensures that, in the event of a short circuit to earth, the fuse in the plug will blow, thus disconnecting the supply.

The size of this fuse depends on the power requirement of the appliance attached to the plug – an electric clock uses only $1/1000$ of the power of an electric kettle. A range of typical values for common domestic appliances is shown in Table 7.8.

**Table 7.8** Power requirements for common electrical domestic and office appliances

| Appliance | Power (W) | Current at 120 V(A) | Current at 240 V(A) |
|---|---|---|---|
| Clock | 3 | 0.03 | 0.01 |
| Lamp: energy-saving bulb | 11 | 0.09 | 0.05 |
| TV: 12" black & white | 15 | 0.13 | 0.06 |
| Mobile phone charger | 20 | 0.17 | 0.08 |
| Telephone | 25 | 0.2 | 0.10 |
| DVD Player | 28 | 0.2 | 0.11 |
| Printer: ink jet | 35 | 0.3 | 0.15 |
| Hi-fi | 55–500 | 0.4–4.0 | 0.2–2.0 |
| Lamp: standard bulb | 100 | 0.8 | 0.4 |
| TV: 26" colour | 170 | 1.4 | 0.7 |
| TV: Plasma screen | 300 | 2.4 | 1.2 |
| Refrigerator | 400 | 2.5 | 1.3 |
| Computer & monitor | 460 | 3.8 | 1.9 |
| Vacuum cleaner | 500 | 4.2 | 2.1 |

**Table 7.8** Power requirements for common electrical domestic and office appliances—Cont'd

| Appliance | Power (W) | Current at 120 V(A) | Current at 240 V(A) |
|---|---|---|---|
| Freezer | 1200 | 10.0 | 5.0 |
| Printer: laser | 1200 | 10.0 | 5.0 |
| Hairdryer | 1500 | 12.5 | 6.3 |
| Microwave | 2000 | 16.4 | 8.3 |
| Toaster | 2000 | 16.4 | 8.3 |
| Two-bar electric fire | 2000 | 16.4 | 8.3 |
| Iron | 2500 | 20.8 | 10.4 |
| Tumble drier | 2500 | 20.8 | 10.4 |
| Washing machine | 2800 | 23.3 | 11.7 |
| Kettle | 3000 | 25.0 | 12.5 |
| Cooker | 7000 | 58.3 | 29.2 |

## Learning Outcomes

On completion of this chapter, the reader should fully understand:
- The relationship between electricity and magnetism
- The interaction between statically charged bodies
- The concepts of electric potential and transmission of charge
- Electrical conductivity and resistance and its governance by Ohm's law
- The different classes of electrical conductors and resistors
- Electrodynamic behaviour in relationship to direct current and alternating current in both single and multiple phase transmission
- The function and application of common electronic components
- The function and application of electronic systems and logic circuits
- Electromagnetic induction and voltage transformation.

## CHECK YOUR EXISTING KNOWLEDGE: ANSWERS

Mark your answers using the guide below to give yourself a score:
1 Two equal positive charges are separated by a distance, $d$
   a They will repel each other  [1]
   b It quadruples  [2]
   c It remains the same  [2]
2 What is the total resistance in the circuits shown
   a 10 Ω  [1]
   b 4.8 Ω  [2]
   c 2 Ω  [2]
3 An electric kettle has a power rating of 3 kW
   a $I = 25$ A  [2]
   b $R = 4.8$ Ω  [2]
   c A 30 A fuse  [1]

4 What is:

  a  A thermistor: a semiconductor device whose resistance increases as its operating temperature increases  [2]

  b  A diode: a device that allows current flow in one direction only  [2]

  c  A transducer: a device that converts energy from one form to another  [2]

  d  A linear amplifier: an electrical device whose output waveform is greater in magnitude but the same form as its input  [2]

5 What is the total capacitance in the circuits shown:

  a  0.66 µF  [2]

  b  2 µF  [3]

6 What is the output in the circuit:

  a  Off  [2]

  b  On  [2]

  c  Off  [2]

  d  On  [2]

7 A transformer as a primary voltage of 100 V and 100 turns. What is the output voltage:

  a  10 V  [4]

  b  500 V  [4]

8 Three ways of increasing the output from a dynamo:

  a  Increase the speed of rotation  [2]

  b  Increase the magnetic field  [2]

  c  Increase the number of turns on the coil  [2]

## How to interpret the results:

46–50: You have a firm grasp of the principles and facts contained in this chapter and can move on to the next chapter.

35–45: Although you have understood most of the basic principles involved, you need to add some of the finer details that you will require as a manual therapist.

0–34:  You need to study this chapter in some detail in order to acquire the grounding needed for future chapters.

## A  SELF-ASSESSMENT ANSWERS

| A | B | C | D | E | F |
|---|---|---|---|---|---|
| 1 | 0 | 0 | 0 | 1 | 0 |
| 1 | 1 | 0 | 0 | 0 | 0 |
| 1 | 0 | 1 | 0 | 1 | 1 |
| 1 | 1 | 1 | 0 | 0 | 0 |
| 0 | 0 | 0 | 1 | 0 | 0 |
| 0 | 1 | 0 | 1 | 0 | 0 |
| 0 | 0 | 1 | 1 | 0 | 0 |
| 0 | 0 | 0 | 1 | 0 | 0 |

Successful combination: A = 1, B = 0, C = 1

# Bibliography

Allen, R., Schwarz, C. (Eds.), 1998. The Chambers dictionary, Chambers Harrap, Edinburgh.

Ammari, M., Jeljeli, M., Maaroufi, K., et al., 2008. Static magnetic field exposure affects behavior and learning in rats. Electromagn. Biol. Med. 27 (2), 185–196.

Colbert, A.P., Markov, M.S., Souder, J.S., 2008. Static magnetic field therapy: dosimetry considerations. J. Altern. Complement Med. 14 (5), 577–582.

Eccles, N.K., 2005. A critical review of randomized controlled trials of static magnets for pain relief. J. Altern. Complement Med. 11 (3), 495–509.

Encyclopædia Britannica. Copper processing, Encyclopædia Britannica 2008. Accessed: Encyclopædia Britannica 2006 Ultimate Reference Suite, DVD 13 Feb.

Halliday, D., Resnick, R., Walker, J., 2005. Electric charge. In: Fundamentals of physics, seventh ed. John Wiley, Hoboken, NJ, pp. 561–579.

Halliday, D., Resnick, R., Walker, J., 2005. Currents and resistance. In: Fundamentals of physics, seventh ed. John Wiley, Hoboken, NJ, pp. 682–704.

Hand, J.W., 2008. Modelling the interaction of electromagnetic fields (10 MHz–10 GHz) with the human body: methods and applications. Phys. Med. Biol. 21, 53 (16), R243–R286. Epub 2008 Jul 24.

Harden, R.N., Remble, T.A., Houle, T.T., et al., 2007. Prospective, randomized, single-blind, sham treatment-controlled study of the safety and efficacy of an electromagnetic field device for the treatment of chronic low back pain: a pilot study. Pain Practice 7 (3), 248–255.

Harrington, J.M., Nichols, L., Sorahan, T., et al., 2001. Leukaemia mortality in relation to magnetic field exposure: findings from a study of United Kingdom electricity generation and transmission workers, 1973–97. Occup. Environ. Med. 58, 307–314.

Hay, G.A., Hughes, D.H., 1983. Electricity and magnetism. In: First Year Physics for Radiographers, third ed. Ballière Tindall, Eastbourne, pp. 69–86.

Henshaw, D.L., 2002. Does our electricity distribution system pose a serious risk to public health? Med. Hypotheses 59, 39–51.

Hyland, G.J., 2008. Physical basis of adverse and therapeutic effects of low intensity microwave radiation. Indian J. Exp. Biol. 46 (5), 403–419.

Johnson, K., 1986. Circuits. In: GCSE physics for you. Hutchinson Education, London, pp. 284–303.

Liboff, A.R., 2007. Local and holistic electromagnetic therapies. Electromagn. Biol. Med. 26 (4), 315–325.

Markov, M.S., 2007. Expanding use of pulsed electromagnetic field therapies. Electromagn. Biol. Med. 26 (3), 257–274.

Maslanyj, M.P., Mee, T.J., Renew, D.C., et al., 2007. Investigation of the sources of residential power frequency magnetic field exposure in the UK Childhood Cancer Study. J. Radiol. Prot. 27, 41–58.

Morinaga, H., 1999. Earth's magnetic field, cosmic ray and evolution. Viva Origino 27, 141–147.

Nave, C.R., 2008. Magnetic field of the earth, Hyperphysics, Department of Physics, Georgia State University. Online. Available: hyperphysics. phy-astr.gsu.edu/Hbase/magnetic/ MagEarth.html 4 September 2008, 13:48 BST.

Nave, C.R., Ferromagnetism, Hyperphysics, Department of Physics, Georgia State University. Online. Available: hyperphysics. phy-astr.gsu.edu/Hbase/Solids/ferro. html 4 September 2008 14:22 BST.

Nicolin, V., Ponti, C., Baldini, G., et al., 2007. In vitro exposure of human chondrocytes to pulsed electromagnetic fields. Eur J Histochem 51 (3), 203–212.

Pascoe, R.D., 1976. Semiconductor theory. In: Fundamentals of solid-state electronics. John Wiley, New York, pp. 2–11.

Pascoe, R.D., 1976. The transistor and circuit configurations. In: Fundamentals of solid-state electronics. John Wiley, New York, pp. 41–51.

Pascoe, R.D., 1976. Circuit models. In: Fundamentals of solid-state electronics. John Wiley, New York, pp. 130–154.

Pascoe, R.D., 1976. Symbols for solid state devices. In: Fundamentals of solid-state electronics. John Wiley, New York, pp. 474–476.

Patten, J., 1983. Electrocution statistics: written answer, House of Commons debate 29 July 1983, HM Government Publications, Hansard, London 46:661–2W.

Roach, J., 2004. Earth's magnetic field is fading, National Geographic. Online. Available: news.nationalgeographic. com/news/2004/09/ 0909_040909_earthmagfield.html 4 September 2008, 13:45 BST.

Schauf, C., Moffett, D., Moffett, S., 1990. Excitable membranes. In: Human physiology: foundations and frontiers. Times Mirror/Mosby College, St Louis, pp. 138–163.

Sorahan, T., Nichols, L., 2004. Mortality from cardiovascular disease in relation to magnetic field exposure: findings from a study of UK electricity generation and transmission workers, 1973–1997. Am. J. Ind. Med. 45, 93–102.

Superconductors.org. Superconductive information for beginners, Online. Available: www.supercoductors.org 13 February 2008: 15:35 GMT.

Superconductors.org. Superconductivity over 180K in a Pb-doped Sn-In-Tm Intergrowth, Online. Available: www.supercoductors.org/181K_pat. htm 13 February 2008: 15:45 GMT.

Thorne, J.O., Collocott, T.C. (Eds.), 1984. In: Chambers biographical dictionary. Chambers, Edinburgh.

US Consumer Product Safety. Statistics about electrocution. Online. Available: www.wrongdiagnosis.com/ e/electrocution/stats.htm 6 September 2008, 08:50 BST.

Walker, N.A., Denegar, C.R., Preische, J., 2007. Low-intensity pulsed ultrasound and pulsed electromagnetic field in the treatment of tibial fractures: a systematic review. J. Athl. Train. 42 (4), 530–535.

Wiltshire Fire and Rescue Service. Approximate wattage/amps requirements for common household

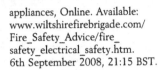

appliances, Online. Available: www.wiltshirefirebrigade.com/ Fire_Safety_Advice/fire_ safety_electrical_safety.htm. 6th September 2008, 21:15 BST.

Wood, A.W., 2006. How dangerous are mobile phones, transmission masts, and electricity pylons? Arch. Dis. Child. 91, 361–366.

World Meteorological Organization. World weather climate extremes archive, Online. Available: wmo.asu. edu/world-lowest-temperature 27th August 2008: 15:00 GMT.

# Chapter Eight

8

# Electromagnetic radiation and radioactivity

## CHAPTER CONTENTS

Check your existing knowledge . . . . . . . . 179
Introduction . . . . . . . . . . . . . . . . . . . 180
The electromagnetic spectrum . . . . . . . . 182
  Radio waves . . . . . . . . . . . . . . . . . . . 182
  Microwaves . . . . . . . . . . . . . . . . . . . . 183
  Infrared radiation . . . . . . . . . . . . . . . . 184
  Visible light . . . . . . . . . . . . . . . . . . . 184
  Ultraviolet . . . . . . . . . . . . . . . . . . . . 184
  X-rays . . . . . . . . . . . . . . . . . . . . . . . 185
  Gamma ($\gamma$) rays . . . . . . . . . . . . . . . . . 186
Radioactivity . . . . . . . . . . . . . . . . . . . 187
  Radioactive half-life . . . . . . . . . . . . . . 187

Sources of radioactivity . . . . . . . . . . . . 187
Types of radiation . . . . . . . . . . . . . . . . 190
Visible light . . . . . . . . . . . . . . . . . . . . 192
  Reflection . . . . . . . . . . . . . . . . . . . . 192
  Refraction . . . . . . . . . . . . . . . . . . . . 193
X-rays . . . . . . . . . . . . . . . . . . . . . . . 194
  X-ray production . . . . . . . . . . . . . . . . 194
  X-ray interaction with matter . . . . . . . . 196
Learning outcomes . . . . . . . . . . . . . . . 199
Check your existing knowledge:
answers . . . . . . . . . . . . . . . . . . . . . . 199
Bibliography . . . . . . . . . . . . . . . . . . . 199

## CHECK YOUR EXISTING KNOWLEDGE

1  What particle is associated with electromagnetic radiation?
2  At what speed does this particle travel in a vacuum?
3  If a beam of light is travelling due north and its associated magnetic field is downward, in what direction will its associated electrical field lie?
4  State the wave equation for electromagnetic radiation
5  Which has higher energy: gamma-rays or microwaves?
6  Which has higher frequency: infrared or ultraviolet?
7  Which has longer wavelength: green light or blue light?
8  Which travels faster: long-wave radio waves or medium wave?
9  How can people sense infrared radiation?
10  If a radioisotope has a half-life of 16 years, how much of it will remain after 64 years?
11  (89)Actinium-227 can undergo radioactive decay in one of two ways. What is its daughter radioisotope if:
  a  It decays by $\alpha$-particle emission?
  b  It decays by $\beta$-particle emission?

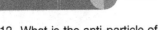

12 What is the anti-particle of:
   a An electron?
   b A proton?
13 If an incident ray of light striking a plane mirror does so at an angle of 40° to the normal, at what angle will the ray reflect?
14 Protanomaly and dichromacy are both forms of which condition?
15 What happens to a beam of light passing from air into glass?
16 Name two means of x-ray production
17 Name four of the five ways in which x-rays can interact with matter
18 What is Bremsstrahlung radiation?
19 What energy will a characteristic photon have?
20 What is attenuation?

# Introduction

We have already touched briefly on the subject of electromagnetic radiation in the previous two chapters; now it is time to examine this phenomenon in detail. As you will see from Table 8.1, as clinicians, we encounter almost the full range of the electromagnetic spectrum both in everyday and medical life. From tuning our car radio to a long-wave station on the way into work, to treating patients undergoing radiotherapy using gamma rays, we use electromagnetic radiation to see, treat and diagnose patients.

A full understanding of this phenomenon is therefore essential to multiple aspects of our clinical performance. Whether evaluating a patient's musculoskeletal status or checking their second cranial nerve, we will be using different parts of the electromagnetic spectrum, and without a comprehensive knowledge of the way in which photons of different energies interact with matter – particularly biological tissue – we cannot hope to maintain and improve a patient's health; or our own!

All electromagnetic radiation is made up of particles called photons, which have neither mass nor charge, and move at a constant speed of $2.997 \times 10^8 \, \text{ms}^{-1}$. By now, you will hopefully have mastered the 'double-think' of wave-particle duality and the unsettling concept of probability waves and have no difficulty in accepting that electromagnetic radiation consists of waves that, unlike the waves we encountered in Chapter 6, which required a medium for their propagation, can travel readily through a vacuum. The waveform consists of oscillating, perpendicular electrical and magnetic fields: the magnetic field produces an electrical field and the electrical field produces a magnetic field, making the system self-sustaining. The direction of propagation is at right angles to the two fields (Fig. 8.1).

You can determine the direction of the fields and its associated photons in a similar way to that for electromagnetic induction: the second finger shows the electromagnetic field direction (rather than the electromotive force), the index finger again indicates the lines of magnetic flux, whilst the thumb determines the direction of propagation (movement). The only difference is that this time you have to use your *left* hand. The reason for this is that electromotive force is associated with *conventional* current (rather than electron movement) and is therefore 'back to front', whilst electric field strength is the 'right way round'. Fortunately, as the left hand is the mirror image of the right, we have a handy self-correcting mechanism. There are plenty of mnemonics to help one stop confusing the two: most *induction* ceremonies involve the *convention* of a handshake (with the *right* hand) whilst when *fielding* in baseball you wear the glove on the *left* hand.

As with all waves, there is a relationship between the distance between each 'peak' (or each 'trough'), known as the **wavelength** ($\lambda$), and the number of times the wave goes up and down each second, known as the **frequency** ($v$ or $f$). We shall be continuing to use $f$ in order to avoid confusion with $v$, our symbol for velocity; note though that the alternative symbol for frequency is not in fact a 'v' but the Greek character 'nu' ($v$).

This relationship is one of inverse proportionality; as can be seen from Figure 8.1: if you double the wavelength, you half the frequency and vice

**Table 8.1** The electromagnetic system

| | E (eV) | f (Hz) | λ (m) | Classification | Common usage | Sources |
|---|---|---|---|---|---|---|
| | $10^{10}$ | $10^{24}$ | $10^{-16}$ | | | |
| | $10^{9}$ | $10^{23}$ | $10^{-15}$ | | | Cyclotrons |
| | $10^{8}$ | $10^{22}$ | $10^{-14}$ | γ–rays | | |
| | $10^{7}$ | $10^{21}$ | $10^{-13}$ | | Megavoltage therapy | |
| Proton emission tomography | $10^{6}$ (1 Mev) | $10^{20}$ | $10^{-12}$ | | Supervoltage therapy | Uranium |
| X-ray | $10^{5}$ | $10^{19}$ | $10^{-11}$ | | Diagnostic x-ray Nuclear medicine | |
| Imaging | $10^{4}$ | $10^{18}$ | $10^{-10}$ | X-rays | Contact therapy | X-ray tubes |
| | $10^{3}$ (1 keV) | $10^{17}$ | $10^{-9}$ (1 nm) | | Grenz rays | |
| | $10^{2}$ | $10^{16}$ | $10^{-8}$ | Ultraviolet | Sunbeds | Very hot bodies |
| Visual imaging | $10^{1}$ | $10^{15}$ | Violet Indigo Blue $10^{-7}$ Green Yellow Orange Red | Visible Light | Sight | Hot bodies Fluorescence |
| | $10^{0}$ (1 eV) | $10^{14}$ | $10^{-6}$ (1 μm) | | Laser therapy | LASERs |
| | $10^{-1}$ | $10^{13}$ | $10^{-5}$ | Infrared | Heat therapy | Warm bodies |
| | $10^{-2}$ | $10^{12}$ | $10^{-4}$ | | | |
| | $10^{-3}$ | $10^{11}$ | $10^{-3}$ (1 mm) | | | Microwave oven |
| | $10^{-4}$ | $10^{10}$ | $10^{-2}$ (1 cm) | Microwaves | Cooking | Radar |
| | $10^{-5}$ | $10^{9}$ (1 GHz) | $10^{-1}$ | | | Cell phone masts |
| | $10^{-6}$ | $10^{8}$ | $10^{0}$ (1 m) | | | TV |
| Magnetic resonance imaging | $10^{-7}$ | $10^{7}$ | $10^{1}$ | | | VHF radio |
| | $10^{-8}$ | $10^{6}$ (1 MHz) | $10^{2}$ | Radiowaves | Communication | MW radio |
| | $10^{-9}$ | $10^{5}$ | $10^{3}$ (1 km) | | | LW radio |
| | $10^{-10}$ | $10^{4}$ | $10^{4}$ | | | |
| | $10^{-11}$ | $10^{3}$ (1 kHz) | $10^{5}$ | | | |
| | $10^{-12}$ | $10^{2}$ | $10^{6}$ | | | |

versa. High frequency equals low wavelength; low frequency equals high wavelength.

The equation that defines this relationship mathematically is called the **wave equation**:

$$\lambda = v/f$$

where $\lambda$ and $f$ have already been defined and $v =$ the speed of the wave.

However, in the special case of electromagnetic radiation, we know that the speed is constant, approximately $3 \times 10^8 \, \text{ms}^{-1}$. So important is this constant that it is given its own symbol, $c$.

Therefore, the wave equation for electromagnetic radiation can be written:

$$\lambda = c/f \ \text{ or } \ f = c/\lambda \ \text{ or } \ c = f\lambda$$

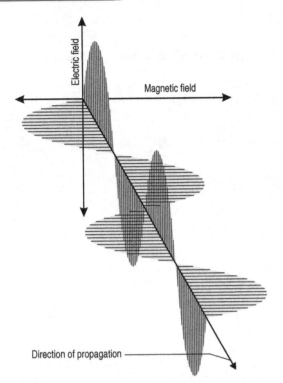

**Figure 8.1 •** Propagation. The waveform for electromagnetic radiation consists of oscillating, perpendicular electrical and magnetic fields: the magnetic field produces an electrical field and the electrical field produces a magnetic field, making the system self-sustaining. The direction of propagation is at right angles to the two fields.

# The electromagnetic spectrum

## Radio waves

At the bottom end of the energy range of electromagnetic radiation are those used for everyday media and communication. It is just as well that these photons have such minuscule amounts of energy; our bodies are penetrated by them every millisecond of every day but with typical energies of $10^{-12}$ to $10^{-6}$ eV they have insufficient energy to cause any damage to the atoms from which we are composed (remember, even at the top end of their energy range, $10^{-6}$ eV is equal to $1.6 \times 10^{-25}$ J !).

Radio (and television) signals are generated by high-frequency alternating currents flowing through the aerial of a *radio transmitter*. If the *receiving aerial*, which can be a simple piece of wire, is placed in the path of the radiation, an electromotive force is induced, causing a current to flow. This current, the *input transducer* that was discussed in Chapter 7, is then amplified in the radio circuitry and the *output transducer* converts the signal to sound waves.

There have traditionally been two means of encoding a radio signal. It is possible to vary the height or *amplitude* of successive waves, known as **amplitude modulation (AM)**, or the *frequency* of the waves, **frequency modulation (FM)**. It is also technically perfectly possible to modulate the *polarity* of individual pulses, that is the angle at which the electric and magnetic fields are oriented; however, this system was never considered commercially even though **ultra-wideband radio** has considerable advantages over conventional radio.

More recently, *digital* signals have started to replace the traditional *analogue* systems. In these, the information is compressed in to 'packets'; these have the advantage that a host of additional information can be encoded – including a request to retransmit the packet if information is lost – thus improving the quality of the output. They have the disadvantage that the software needed to decode the signal is complex and expensive, which is why digital radios and televisions are often many times the price of their analogue counterparts.

Although very long wavelength radio waves are used by the military to communicate with submarines (extremely low frequencies can penetrate seawater, removing the need for submarines to have to surface in order to communicate), the practical maximum wavelength for commercial radio waves is approximately 1 mile (1500 m).

It is the convention that radio stations which utilize AM signals are identified by their wavelength, which can be long wave (> 1000 m) or medium wave (100–999 m). Below this, short wave radio has traditionally been used by the amateur 'ham' radio enthusiast (5–99 m).

By contrast, FM stations are identified by the frequency at which they broadcast (sometimes quoted as the range over which the frequency is modulated). Typically, these will be in the range of tens to hundreds of kHz. The majority of mainstream radio stations eventually moved to FM owing to the superior signal quality.

Television, which needs to encode information relating to pictures as well as sound, is broadcast in the range 10–100 MHz, allowing for broader frequency bands.

# Microwaves

Although some sources define microwaves as part of the radio wave spectrum, their uses are specific and different. Measured in centimetres and millimetres, microwaves were originally a neglected part of the electromagnetic spectrum. This changed during the Second World War, when British physicists and engineers secretly developed RADAR (RA(dio) D(etection) A(nd) R(anging)), enabling them to detect and intercept the waves of German bombers that had been devastating the country's military, industrial and social infrastructure.

## Fact File

### RADAR

RADAR works by transmitting pulses of electromagnetic waves in the microwave spectrum. These are reflected off distant objects, particularly those made of metal, back to the source, thus indicating the presence or absence of the target. By cross-triangulating with other transmitters, the distance and speed of aircraft, ships, and other objects, can be determined.

This was followed in the 1960s by the microwave cooker and, in the last 10 years, by the mobile phone network that now embraces the globe.

## Fact File

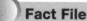

### MICROWAVE OVENS

The question often arises as to why microwave ovens not only cook (and defrost) quicker – because they are more powerful than infrared radiation that is found in conventional cookers – but why they appear to cook from the inside out. Because microwaves are more energetic, they are able to penetrate to the centre of objects more easily, whilst infrared radiation is dependent on conduction to reach the centre of cooking objects. In the same way that the outer layers of, say, a roasting chicken, shield the centre from infrared rays; they insulate the centre of the chicken being cooked by microwaves. Meanwhile, the outer layers of both chickens will radiate energy back into the oven. In the case of the microwaved chicken, which is penetrated more evenly, this means that the insulated inside cooks more quickly than the 'leaky' outside ... good news if you like sponge pudding; not so good if you like your roast beef medium rare.

## CLINICAL FOCUS

As with high-tension cables, mobile phone technology has also been involved in controversy with regard to public health concerns. The difficulty with these is that the symptoms can take a long time to manifest, and therefore even longer to investigate – by which time the technology has almost invariably changed.

A good example of this is so-called first-generation mobile phones. These caused far higher levels of radiation than current phones, and this radiation was held directly over one of the least protected areas of the brain, the ear-hole. By the time the association with brain tumours had been established, the phones were obsolete and many of the victims were dead; whether there are longer-term health issues remains to be seen.

Current concerns focus less on individual handsets and more on radio masts, which are often located on top of residential flats and have an as yet undetermined, largely anecdotal association with clusters of diseases, particularly neoplasms, which, as with high-tension wires, are more prevalent in children.

Mechanisms have been proposed to explain this and the results confirmed in animal experiments, but the masts continued to be mounted close to or on top of family homes. Not only is the research that could answer such questions hard to perform, it is even harder to fund.

As researchers into physical therapies can testify, raising the finance into research that threatens the profits of major international corporations, be they the multi-billion dollar pharmaceutical concerns or the even richer telecommunication giants, is uphill work. Getting money to show that drugs or mobile phones are harmless or even beneficial is far easier – and to controllers of the purse strings have the ability to ensure that negative results never see the light of day.

The truth is, we simply do not know enough about the effects of medium energy electromagnetic radiation to be sure they are safe or not – but it is worth remembering that a generation ago, continual exposure to the ultraviolet radiation of the sun was considered beneficial whilst the generation before were advocating x-rays for curing skin conditions.

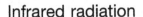 

# Infrared radiation

Produced by moderately hot objects, infrared 'heat rays' are generated by moderately energetic atoms, in much the same way that visible light is produced, albeit with lower energies and longer wavelengths. Classic examples are the conventional ovens discussed above or fires, be they coal, wood or electric; they all radiate infrared, which can be sensed by heat detecting nerve endings in our skin, giving a sensation of warmth. Although mammals cannot see infrared, some fish and most snakes and scorpions have eyes capable of sensing the infrared portion of the spectrum; this means that they can effectively find their prey by the heat that their body radiates, which is particularly useful for hunting in the dark.

Most lay people are perhaps most familiar with infrared through this ability to detect things in the dark by sensing warm objects, such as mammalian bodies. This technology, used in passive infrared (PIR) burglar alarm sensors, has also been widely used by wildlife documentary makers, particularly in the days before photon-multiplying night-imaging technology became easily available.

For the clinician, infrared therapy is a familiar, if largely unproven, technology that is commonly used to treat chronic non-healing wounds and musculoskeletal pain as well as a diverse number of other conditions from haemorrhoids to leukaemia. The technology behind this and the evidence base for infrared therapies is discussed in more depth in Chapter 10.

# Visible light

Although visible light forms only 1% of the electromagnetic spectrum as a whole, it is very important both to us and to a large percentage of the Earth's fauna and flora that rely upon it for vision and as a source of energy.

Visible light falls in the range of wavelengths between 700 nm and 400 nm. Because of its importance, we shall consider this part of the spectrum in its own section later in the chapter.

# Ultraviolet

To a large part of the animal kingdom, ultraviolet radiation forms part of the visible spectrum. Many fish, reptiles, insects, arachnids and all birds can 'see' ultraviolet – it is seemingly only mammals that have problems with this part of the spectrum; indeed, if our eyes are over-exposed to ultraviolet radiation, we develop cataracts that can eventually blind.

Our skin is also sensitive to ultraviolet radiation. Although this has an important function – we cannot make vitamin D without it – it can also cause genetic damage to skin cells and cause neoplastic growths such as basal cell and squamous cell carcinomas and malignant melanomas.

## Fact File

### VITAMIN D

Vitamin D is produced in the body's largest organ, the skin, as a result of exposure to ultraviolet radiation. Without it, we cannot transport dietary calcium across the gut wall adequately and bone mineralization fail causing rickets in children and osteomalacia in adults.

Fortunately, we have a built-in defence mechanism; when ultraviolet radiation strikes the skin, it triggers an endocrine reaction causing cells within the dermis called melanocytes to secrete a pigment that protects against longer-term ultraviolet damage – this is why the hue of a person's skin is related to the latitude of their ethnic origins and also why we tan.

Ultraviolet exposure also has a role to play in the clinician's armoury. Many cases of psoriasis respond well to exposure to ultraviolet – patients will often comment that their skin plaques diminish in the summer and this effect can be maintained by a daily artificial dose in the winter months.

Seasonal affective disorder (SAD) can also be combated by ultraviolet radiation. Everyone shows some physiological response to the diminished light levels of the winter season, and the effect is magnified in populations nearer to the arctic circles. The lack of light entering the eye decreases the stimulation of the pineal gland and reduces production of the neurotransmitter serotonin. Although this is a useful evolutionary device causing torpor, reduced metabolism or even hibernation in the winter months when food sources are low and energy needs to be preserved, it can in some individuals trigger clinical depression. Wintering in tropical or sub-tropical climes or ski resorts (snow reflects ultraviolet better than longer wavelengths, which is why skiers get tanned, or sunburned, so easily) used to be the treatment of choice for the 'December blues'. However, the advent of ultraviolet lamps and, more recently, 'daylight' electric bulbs have helped reduce the dependency on antidepressant medication for the less affluent sections of society.

## CLINICAL FOCUS

The Earth receives considerable protection from ultraviolet radiation through the ozone layer, part of the Earth's stratosphere that lies between 10 and 50 km above the surface of the Earth. Over 90% of the Earth's ozone can be found in this narrow band. Ozone is an irritating, corrosive, colourless gas with a smell something like burning electrical wiring. In fact, ozone is easily produced by any high-voltage electrical arc such as spark plugs, Van der Graaf generators, and arc welders. It is also, in much lower concentrations, what gives that 'seaside smell' near to large bodies of water.

Each molecule of ozone has three oxygen atoms and is produced when normal oxygen molecules ($O_2$) are broken up by energetic electrons or high-energy radiation. The ozone layer absorbs almost 99% of all the sun's ultraviolet radiation; without it, the planet would be sterilized on a daily basis.

Unfortunately, ozone is broken down by the action of freons, chemicals that for many years were used as propellants in aerosols and coolants in refrigerators. This caused significant depletion of atmospheric ozone layers, particularly in the extreme southern hemisphere, where the protection afforded dropped by more than 10%. Although a rapid ban of the use of chemicals has allowed the gas to replenish, the long-term effects on the current generation remain unknown. In the past 10 years, rates of skin cancer in many countries have doubled; in Australia, the most affected country, some authorities estimate that the incidence may peak over the coming decades to 12 times the previous levels.

Public education and better health awareness play a vital role in combating this, and physical therapists – who get to see the skin of their disrobed patients far more often than most other physicians – have an important role to play in this, which is why dermatology forms an important part of most undergraduate syllabuses.

## X-rays

In 1895, a professor of physics at Würzburg University called Wilhelm Röntgen was experimenting with the flow of 'cathode rays' and noted they caused certain materials, such as a piece of barium platinocyanide lying on his work bench, to fluoresce. He also noted that photographic plates, kept wrapped in paper in his desk drawer underneath the tube, were being fogged. He theorized that some unknown radiation was being formed when the tube was in operation, caused by the cathode rays (electrons) striking the glass wall of the tube. Having no idea what the rays could be, he called them 'X-radiation' and, despite an attempt to call them Röntgen radiation in his honour, the name stuck.

 **DICTIONARY DEFINITION**

**CATHODE RAYS**

In 1895, J. J. Thomson hadn't yet got round to discovering electrons; the apparent flow of current through a vacuum, which we now know to be a beam of electrons and successfully used to make television screens work, was then attributed to 'cathode rays' because the 'rays' were given off by the cathode (negatively charged terminal). This is how cathode ray tubes (oscilloscopes) got their name.

Within a month, he had determined most of the ray's properties and taken the first-ever clinical radiograph, an image of his wife's left hand, clearly showing the phalanges and her wedding ring (Fig. 8.2).

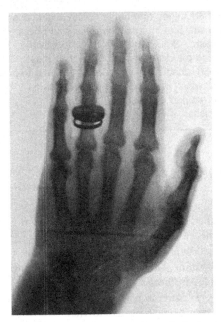

**Figure 8.2** • The world's first ever radiograph, the hand of William Röntgen's wife, clearly showing the differential absorption of air, bone and the metal of Frau Röntgen's wedding ring.

Over 100 years later, and despite the advent of magnetic resonance and advanced ultrasound imaging, the x-ray still represents the most common and important form of diagnostic imaging, of particular use to the manual physician wishing to evaluate skeletal structures.

Because of this, x-rays are dealt with in a separate section later in the chapter.

## Gamma (γ) rays

Unlike the arbitrary differentiation between radio waves and microwaves, the difference between x-rays and gamma rays is not a functional one but rather is based on their method of production. In fact, high-energy x-rays are more energetic than low-energy γ-rays; however, whilst x-rays are produced by the actions of electrons, gamma rays arise from the nuclei of certain radioactive isotopes when they undergo decay. This process is best understood as part of the subject of radioactive decay as a whole.

### Fact File

**X-RAY DIFFRACTION**

Röntgen was unable to make x-rays demonstrate diffraction, and therefore erroneously concluded that they were not in the same class of phenomenon as light. In fact, x-rays do diffract but, because of their short wavelength, no ordinary diffraction grating will cause them to do so. Instead, the gaps in atomic structures such as metallic lattices and crystals will cause x-ray diffraction to occur and they later became a vital research tool in the understanding of the properties of matter. Although x-ray crystallography has been used to determine the atomic and molecular structures of thousands of materials, perhaps the most famous instance was Rosalind Franklin, who used the technique to image DNA. Unfortunately for her, Crick and Watson beat her to the interpretations of her findings. In 1901, Röntgen, was awarded the first-ever Nobel Prize for physics for his discovery. In 1962, Crick and Watson, together with their colleague Maurice Wilkins, won the Nobel Prize for physiology and medicine. Rosalind Franklin never received the honour; Nobel Prizes cannot be awarded posthumously and, in 1958, she had died at the tragically young age of 37 from cancer most probably brought on by exposure to the x-rays with which she worked.

### CLINICAL FOCUS

The primary use of γ-rays is in nuclear medicine. This usage can be divided into two: diagnostic imaging and radiotherapy treatment of cancers.

Standard diagnostic imaging – plain film x-rays, computed tomography and magnetic resonance imaging – can be enhanced, and one way in which this can be done is to use a radioactive isotope, which is taken up by the body. Once the atoms are selectively absorbed by the target structure, their radioactive emissions are detected by the imaging sensors, traditionally photographic plates, in order to produce an enhanced image.

Examples of such tracers include calcium (absorbed by bone), chromium and iron (blood), iodine (thyroid) and Xenon (lung) (Table 8.2).

Radiotherapy uses both x-rays and γ-rays of varying energies depending on the nature of the tumour and its site organ. The primary aim is to target the neoplastic growth whilst limiting damage to surrounding tissue. Commonly used γ-ray sources are given in Table 8.3.

**Table 8.2** Radioactive isotopes used in diagnostic imaging

| Radionucleotide | Half-life (days) | γ-ray photon E (MeV) | Studies |
|---|---|---|---|
| $^{47}$Ca | 4.7 | 0.50, 0.81, 1.31 | Bone |
| $^{51}$Cr | 27.8 | 0.32 | Blood |
| $^{59}$Fe | 45 | 1.10, 1.29 | Blood |
| $^{131}$I | 8.0 | 0.36, 0.64 | Thyroid |
| $^{133}$Xe | 5.3 | 0.08 | Lung |

**Table 8.3** Radioactive isotopes used in nuclear medicine

| Radionucleotide | Half-life (days) | γ-ray photon E (MeV) | Target |
|---|---|---|---|
| $^{60}$Co | 1924 | 1.17, 1.33 | General |
| $^{99}$Te | 0.25 | 0.14 | Acoustic neuroma |
| $^{123}$I | 0.55 | 0.32 | Thyroid |
| $^{198}$Au | 2.7 | 0.41 | Prostate Gynaecology Mouth |
| $^{201}$Tl | 3.0 | 0.07 | Brain Pharynx Larynx |

# Radioactivity

As we saw in Chapter 6, certain isotopes have a ratio of neutrons to protons that is unstable and the **parent nucleide** will undergo spontaneous transformation or disintegration into a **daughter isotope**, often of another element. In doing so, they emit either a particle or a γ-ray. This process of transformation and emission is known as **radioactivity**.

Radioactivity is a property of the atomic nucleus only, so it is unaffected if the isotopes enter into chemical combination (becoming molecules) or undergo physical changes, such as an increase in temperature. Radioactive isotopes are termed **radionuclides** or **radioisotopes**.

# Radioactive half-life

As alluded to in Chapter 6, **radioactive half-life** is a measure of the time that it takes for exactly half of the particles in a sample of a radioisotope to decay or, from the standpoint of measurement, the time taken for the number of disintegrations per second of a radioactive material to decrease by one-half.

For example, a radioactive isotope commonly used for radiotherapy is cobalt-60, which has a half-life of 5.26 years. A 16 g sample of cobalt-60 originally would, after this time, contain only 8 g of cobalt-60 and would emit only half as much radiation. After a further 5.26 years, the sample would contain only 4 g of cobalt-60; after a total of 15.78 years, only 2 g would remain. However, neither the volume nor the mass of the sample visibly decreases because the unstable cobalt-60 decays into nickel-60, which is stable and remains with the still undecayed cobalt.

Half lives vary from as little as $10^{-14}$ seconds, almost too fast to measure, to billions of years, almost too slow to notice.

# Sources of radioactivity

Radioactivity was discovered the year after x-rays, in 1896. Early studies concentrated on pitchblende, a naturally occurring, amorphous, black, tarry form of uraninite, the crystalline form of uranium oxide from which the German chemist Martin Klaproth had isolated uranium as early as 1789. By 1898, the husband and wife team of Pierre and Marie Curie had also identified two further radioactive contents, polonium and radium.

The reason that polonium and radium were present in a sample of a uranium compound is that they form part of a chain or **radionuclide series** of decay.

There are three naturally occurring series in which one unstable radioisotope decays into another until a stable, non-radioactive isotope is obtained (Tables 8.4–8.6). There are varying degrees of stability and instability; for example, in the series being unknowingly investigated by the Curies, there are isotopes of radium and polonium that have half-lives of 1600 years and 139 days respectively (as compared to some radionuclides in the series that have half-lives of as little as $10^{-4}$ seconds). As a result, there will be comparatively more

**Table 8.4** The naturally occurring uranium-238 series

| Parent radioisotope | Particle emitted | Daughter radioisotope | Half-life |
|---|---|---|---|
| (92) Uranium-238 | α | (90) Thorium-234 | $4.5 \times 10^9$ years |
| (90) Thorium-234 | β | (91) Protactinium-234 | 24.1 days |
| (91) Protactinium-234 | $\beta^-$ | (92) Uranium-234 | 1.2 min |
| (92) Uranium-234 | α | (90) Thorium-230 | $2.5 \times 10^5$ years |
| (90) Thorium-230 | α | (88) Radium-226 | $7.5 \times 10^4$ years |
| (88) Radium-226 | α | (86) Radon-222 | $1.6 \times 10^3$ years |
| (86) Radon-222 | α | (84) Polonium-218 | 3.8 days |
| (84) Polonium-218 | α | (82) Lead-214 | 3.1 min |
| (82) Lead-214 | $\beta^-$ | (83) Bismuth-214 | 27.0 min |
| (83) Bismuth-214 | $\beta^-$ | (84) Polonium-214 | 19.9 min |
| (84) Polonium-214 | α | (82) Lead-210 | 22.3 years |
| (82) Lead-210 | $\beta^-$ | (83) Bismuth-210 | 22.3 years |
| (83) Bismuth-210 | $\beta^-$ | (84) Polonium-210 | 138.4 days |
| (84) Polonium-210 | α | (82) Lead-206 | Stable |

**Table 8.5** The naturally occurring uranium-235 series

| Parent radioisotope | Particle emitted | Daughter radioisotope | Half-life |
|---|---|---|---|
| (92) Uranium-235 | α | (90) Thorium-231 | $7.0 \times 10^8$ years |
| (90) Thorium-231 | $\beta^-$ | (91) Protactinium-231 | 1.1 days |
| (91) Protactinium-231 | α | (89) Actinium-227 | $3.3 \times 10^4$ years |
| (89) Actinium-227 | $\beta^-$ | (90) Thorium-227 | 21.8 years |
| (90) Thorium-227 | α | (88) Radium-223 | 18.7 days |
| (88) Radium-223 | α | (86) Radon-219 | 11.4 days |
| (86) Radon-219 | α | (84) Polonium-215 | 4.0 seconds |
| (84) Polonium-215 | α | (82) Lead-211 | $1.8 \times 10^{-3}$ seconds |
| (82) Lead-211 | $\beta^-$ | (83) Bismuth-211 | 36.1 minutes |
| (83) Bismuth-211 | α | (81) Thallium-207 | 2.1 minutes |
| (81) Thallium-207 | $\beta^-$ | (82) Lead-207 | Stable |

**Table 8.6** The naturally occurring thorium-232 series

| Parent radioisotope | Particle emitted | Daughter radioisotope | Half-life |
|---|---|---|---|
| (90) Thorium-232 | α | (88) Radium-228 | $1.4 \times 10^6$ years |
| (88) Radium-228 | β⁻ | (89) Actinium-228 | 5.8 years |
| (89) Actinium-228 | β⁻ | (90) Thorium-228 | 6.1 hours |
| (90) Thorium-228 | α | (88) Radium-224 | 1.9 years |
| (88) Radium-224 | α | (86) Radon-220 | 3.7 days |
| (86) Radon-220 | α | (84) Polonium-216 | 58.0 seconds |
| (84) Polonium-216 | α | (82) Lead-212 | 0.15 seconds |
| (82) Lead-212 | β⁻ | (83) Bismuth-212 | 11.0 hours |
| (83) Bismuth-212 | β⁻ | (84) Polonium-212 | $3.1 \times 10^{-7}$ seconds |
| (84) Polonium-212 | α | (82) Lead-208 | Stable |

radium and polonium (and uranium, which has a half-life of many millions of years) than the other radionuclides in the chain, making them easier to isolate.

In addition to these naturally occurring series, radionuclides are also produced in the upper atmosphere by cosmic ray bombardment (Table 8.7).

Meteorites have also been discovered that contain small amounts of radioactivity. Most meteorites have spent millions of years orbiting the sun with no atmospheric or magnetic protection and can contain radionuclides not found naturally on Earth, such as the short-lived argon-37, which has a half-life of just 35 days.

**Table 8.7** Radioisotopes produced by cosmic ray interaction

| Radionuclide | Half-life (years) |
|---|---|
| $^3$H (tritium) | 12.3 |
| $^7$Be | 0.15 |
| $^{10}$Be | 2 700 000 |
| $^{14}$C | 5720 |

The final source of radioactivity is artificially generated. Obviously, since 1945, nuclear fission – both from the explosion of military devices and from power stations – has contributed to background levels of radioactivity. However, in 1940, before the first mushroom cloud was ever seen, scientists were adding to the periodic table, which, at that stage, finished with uranium, the largest naturally occurring nucleus with 92 protons.

These new 'artificial' elements, which had atomic numbers greater than 92, were called **transuranic elements**. Neptunium ($Z = 93$) and plutonium ($Z = 94$) were the first to be produced and isolated, followed by americium ($Z = 95$). These three elements are radioactive in all of their isotopic forms and, as they are produced artificially, they are said to be *artificially radioactive*.

Finally, it was realized that, in addition to the three naturally accruing radioactive series, a fourth series also exists, called the neptunium series, because neptunium-237 is the most stable radioactive isotope in the series, which starts with polonium-241 and ends with bismuth-209, which is stable.

As with the naturally radioactive series, a quantity of any isotope in the series will eventually decay to become a similar quantity of the stable isotope – in this case bismuth-209.

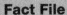

## Types of radiation

The way in which an unstable, and therefore radioactive, nucleus decays and transforms is limited. There are three common types of radiation: gamma ($\gamma$)-rays, which we have already encountered, alpha ($\alpha$)-particles and beta ($\beta$)-particles.

## $\alpha$-particles

The $\alpha$-particle is the nucleus of a helium-4 atom, comprising two protons and two neutrons. It is, in effect, an ion with a charge of +2: $^{4}_{2}\text{He}^{2+}$. When it is ejected from a parent nucleus, it creates a daughter nucleus with an atomic number that is two less than the parent and an atomic mass number that is four less than the parent.

If we take the first step in the uranium-238 series, it can be seen that it is accounted for by alpha particle decay:

$$^{238}_{92}\text{U} \Rightarrow {}^{234}_{90}\text{Th} + {}^{4}_{2}\text{He}$$

The $\alpha$-particle associated with this change, which has a half-life of $4.5 \times 10^{9}$ years, has a typical energy of 4.2 MeV. Note that the equation is in balance, the charges, or number of protons, shown in subscript, are in balance on both sides of the arrow, as are the atomic masses, shown in superscript.

Because $\alpha$-particles are slow moving (approximately $^{1}/_{200}\,c$), double charged and relatively massive, they readily interact with surrounding particles and this means that they have a limited range – typically they will travel only a few centimetres in air and can be absorbed by approximately 100 μm of aluminium.

## $\beta$-particles

$\beta$-particles consist of high-energy electrons, $e^{-}$, but they are not in any way associated with the electrons in the shells orbiting the nucleus. They are best understood if the neutron is regarded as comprising a proton and an electron in combination; this accounts for their neutral charge and the fact that their mass is very slightly heavier than the proton, the tiny difference being equivalent to the mass of the electron. Beta particles are therefore ejected when a neutron breaks up, leaving the nucleus with a new proton.

Beta particle emission happens in the next stage of the uranium-238 series:

$$^{234}_{90}\text{TH} \Rightarrow {}^{234}_{91}\text{Pa} + e^{-}$$

The beta particle is both smaller and less energetic than the $\alpha$-particle. In this transition, which has a half-life of 24 days, the $\beta$-particle has an energy of 0.263 MeV. Note that, whereas the atomic mass has remained the same (the number of nucleons as a whole hasn't changed), the mass number has increased by one as there is now an extra proton.

These particles can also exist in a positive form, $e^+$, called a **positron**. When a positron and a 'negatron' ($\beta^-$ particle) are brought together, they will mutually annihilate each other; the $\beta^+$ particle is the *antiparticle* of the $\beta^-$ particle. If a $\beta^+$ particle is emitted, the atomic number of the daughter radioisotope will be one *lower* than the parent, for example:

$$^{11}_{6}C \Rightarrow {}^{11}_{5}Be + e^+$$

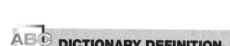 **DICTIONARY DEFINITION**

### ANTIMATTER

Antimatter is the collective term for elementary particles that have the same mass but opposite charge to their more familiar counterparts. In addition to the positron, there is the anti-proton, which has a negative charge, and an anti-neutron, which is made from combining a positron with an anti-proton. Some scientists have predicted that there may be entire galaxies made up from antimatter; however, matter and antimatter cannot coexist at close range for more than a small fraction of a second as they are electrostatically attracted to their anti-particles and annihilate each other with release of gamma radiation. The energy of this radiation is determined by Einstein's famous equation, $E = mc^2$, which was in part verified by the detection of large quantities of electromagnetic radiation of a frequency and wavelength indicating that each $\gamma$-photon carries 511 keV of energy, equivalent to the rest mass of an electron or positron multiplied by $c^2$. In 1995, scientists at the European Laboratory for Particle Physics (CERN) succeeded in creating – very briefly – an anti-atom, comprising anti-protons and anti-neutrons surrounded by shells of positrons.

The lighter, faster-moving (up to 0.65 $c$), less energetic beta particles have only about 10% of the ionization rate of alpha particles and are therefore more penetrating. They can therefore penetrate up to one metre in air and require 1 mm of aluminium to stop them.

## Gamma ($\gamma$) radiation

We already know that $\gamma$-rays are a form of high-energy electromagnetic radiation. The associated particle, the photon, is uncharged and highly penetrative. They easily penetrate aluminium and even

1 cm of lead will only reduce the intensity by 50%. Radioactive $\gamma$ radiation most commonly accompanies $\alpha$ or $\beta$ emission. Although $\alpha$ and $\beta$ decay may proceed directly to the ground (lowest energy) state of the daughter nucleus without $\gamma$ emission, it often results in higher energy (excited) states. In this case, $\gamma$ emission may occur as the excited states then transform to the more stable lower energy states of the same nucleus.

 CLINICAL FOCUS

Radioactive particles – including high-energy photons – interact with biological tissue. The effect of charged particles ($\alpha$- and $\beta$-particles and positrons) and high-energy photons ($\gamma$- and x-rays) on the electron shells of the substances that comprise our bodies is to create ions; the general term for this radiation is thus **ionizing radiation.**

The biomedical effects of ionizing radiation were recognized soon after its discovery. Although the potential medical uses of x-rays were immediately perceived; in 1896, there was no idea that such radiation might have adverse effects.

However, by the end of that year, the first report of an ionizing radiation injury was made; an American electrical engineer, Elihu Thomson, deliberately exposed one of his fingers to x-rays and provided accurate observations on the burns produced. One of Thomas Edison's assistants, Clarence Dally, who was working on the development of a fluorescent x-ray tube, was so badly affected that his hair fell out and his scalp and hands became ulcerated, leading to the eventual amputation of both arms. Eight years later, Dally would be dead from cancer, a fate that befell many early researchers and radiographers.

The need to protect workers from the potential hazards of radioactivity came to a head in the early 1920s. Several thousand women were, at this time, employed in painting watch and clock dials with luminescent paint to enable them to be visible in the dark. Unfortunately, the luminescent agent was radium, which emitted $\alpha$-particles that reacted with zinc compounds causing them to fluoresce. Alpha particles normally only cause surface burns (their high energy and heavy ionization can cause a lot of damage but most are absorbed before they pass through the skin). However, the workers developed a habit of sucking their brushes in order to obtain a fine point on them.

Soon, many became ill with anaemia, lesions of the jawbones and mouth, and gastric disturbances. Many subsequently developed cancers, not just of the mouth and throat but also of the bone and internal organs, as a result of the ingested radium.

This led to the first health and safety legislation dealing with ionizing radiation; because of this and subsequent laws, today, the life expectancy for workers in nuclear power plants, physics laboratories, nuclear medicine and radiography is identical to that of the rest of the population.

Nevertheless, we all receive irradiation all of the time from cosmic rays, the Earth's crust and the atmosphere, which in certain 'hot-spots' can contain significant quantities of the radioactive gas, radon. The dose received can vary quite considerably from one area to another – for example, residents of the high-altitude city of Denver (1600 m) have almost three times the effective exposure to cosmic radiation as someone living at sea level. Atmospheric and airborne radiation can also vary by a factor of four. Areas where the local stone (and, therefore, building material) is granite have higher levels of radioactivity because the rock contains low levels of uranium, which, as we have seen, decays into radon, which can escape from the rock and get trapped in pockets. Although the medical significance of this is debated, there is some evidence that, in the highest concentrated areas, the incidence of lung cancer may be twice as high as in radon-free areas.

# Visible light

As we have already seen in Chapter 6, light behaves as a wave in that it can be diffracted when it passes through narrow slits to produce areas of light and dark showing the interference patterns between its peaks and troughs. Light also exhibits several other wave characteristics, some of which are medically relevant.

# Reflection

We all use domestic mirrors on a daily basis and take them for granted. Medically, mirrors are also used to see or to direct light around corners. We probably understand the laws of reflection instinctively but it is worthwhile being aware of their formal wording.

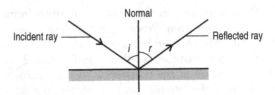

**Figure 8.3** • The laws of reflection. These determine that the angle *i* will be equal to the angle *r* (angle of incidence = angle of reflection) and that incident and reflected rays and the normal all lie in the same plane.

• The angle between the incident (incoming) rays and the normal (90° from the plane of reflection) is the same as the angle between the normal and the reflected (outgoing) ray (Fig. 8.3).
• The normal and the incident and reflected rays all lie on the same plane.

This also has implications for medical tools. As anyone who has used a shaving mirror will know, a mirror with a concave surface will magnify the image, whereas a convex surface will giver a smaller, 'wide angle' view. Oral and laryngopharyngeal examination mirrors often have curved surfaces to obtain these effects.

## CLINICAL FOCUS

The field of fibreoptics, once no more than an interesting optical phenomenon, has exploded over the last two decades. A fibreoptic cable consists of a strand of silica, about the thickness of a human hair, surrounded by a cladding that prevents loss of light by ensuring that when the beam strikes it, it is reflected back into the cable. Light can be transmitted along the fibre over great distances at very high data rates providing an ideal medium for the transport of information and without electromagnetic interference, which is the bane of other methods of signal transmission, such as radio or copper wire linkages. Medically, it has the advantage of being able to transmit light along the length of a flexible tube called a laparoscope. This allows physicians to 'see' around corners, revolutionizing examination techniques. The gastrointestinal tube and bronchi can be seen directly and the vascular system, internal organs and joints can be visualized using only the smallest of incisions. Surgery too has benefited; 'keyhole surgery' is now a standard procedure – the surgeon no longer needs direct access to the target area and the size of operation scars, and resultant trauma and healing time, has significantly decreased.

Our understanding of *how* light was reflected came centuries before our understanding of *why* it was reflected. Visible light reacts in a different manner to radio waves or x-rays when it interacts with matter. When a photon of light strikes an object, it will be absorbed. This can excite the orbital electrons of certain materials, causing a photon to be emitted immediately. If this happens to a high proportion of the incident photons, the surface appears reflective.

Many atoms and molecules will absorb certain wavelengths of light and reflect others, depending on the quantum energy states of their electron shells. Grass appears green because a major constituent, chlorophyll, absorbs most visible light wavelengths whilst reflecting the green wavelengths – this is how we get **colour**. To a physicist, black and white are not colours as they represent either absorption or reflection (respectively) of all visible wavelengths.

If the photons can pass through a material without being absorbed, the material is said to be *transparent*. If all of the photons are absorbed, the material is *opaque*. If the material scatters the photons (thus blurring the transmitted image), or only transmits some of them, the material is said to be *translucent*.

 **CLINICAL FOCUS**

Unlike many other mammals, humans can differentiate between light of different wavelengths – in other words they, or most of them, see in colour. A significant proportion of the population, however, lacks sensitivity to certain wavelengths; they are **colourblind**.

The human eye sees by light stimulating the nerve endings that make up the retina. There are two basic types of nerve ending, *rods* and *cones*. The rods, located in the peripheral retina, give us 'night vision', but cannot distinguish colour. Cones, which are concentrated in the *macula* (the central part of the retina), allow us to perceive colour.

Cones come in three varieties, each containing light-sensitive pigment that is sensitive over a range of wavelengths. Red-sensitive cones are the most common, outnumbering green-sensitive cones by 2:1. Blue-sensitive cones are the least common and form just 10% of the total population.

The coding instructions for these pigments are included in our genes and, if these instructions are wrong, then the wrong pigments will be produced, and the cones will be sensitive to different wavelengths

of light, resulting in a colour deficiency (true colourblindness – seeing in monochrome only – is known as *monochromacy* and is extremely rare).

The incidence of colour deficiency varies between different parts of the world but is far commoner in males (5–8% of the population) than females (0.5%). The commonest forms include:

- **Deuteranomaly (5:100 males):** Weakness of the green cones leads to poor discrimination between the hues in the red, orange, yellow and green region of the spectrum, all of which will be red-shifted. They do not, however, suffer from diminished brightness of the resultant image. Many deuteranomalous individuals are unaware that they have a problem and are able to complete tasks requiring colour vision.

- **Protanomaly (1:100 males):** Weakness of the red cones both in terms of colour and brightness: red, orange and yellow are shifted in hue towards green and appear paler. The red component of violet and lavender is weakened and only the blue component is seen.

- **Dichromacy (2:100 males).** Suffers know they have a colour vision problem, which affects their lives on a daily basis. They see no perceptible difference between red, orange, yellow, and green. All these colours, that seem so different to the normal viewer, appear to be the same colour for this 2% of the population, making tasks such as wiring a plug or negotiating traffic lights potentially hazardous. Dichromacy comes in two forms, of equal incidence:
  - *Protanopia.* The brightness of red, orange, and yellow is much reduced, so much so that reds may be confused with black or dark grey. Violet, lavender, purple and even pink are indistinguishable from various shades of blue – their red components are so dimmed as to be invisible.
  - *Deuteranopia.* The deuteranope suffers the same hue discrimination problems as the protanope, but without the abnormal dimming. Whereas the protanope may be able to use this difference in brightness to differentiate to some extent red from orange, yellow, and green, these names have no meaning to the deuteranope.

# Refraction

When light passes from one medium (for example, air) to another of a different density (glass), some of the light will be reflected and some transmitted.

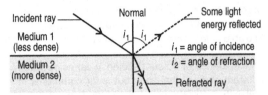

Figure 8.4 • The laws of refraction. When light passes from a less dense into a more dense medium (e.g. air to glass), the beam is refracted so that it is bent towards the normal ($i_1 > i_2$). The reverse is also true, when passing from a denser medium to one that is less dense, the refracted beam will be bent away from the medium ($i_1 < i_2$). This is why curved surfaces can magnify or diminish the appearance of objects; if you construct similar diagrams for convex and concave lenses, you will discover that, no matter what the angle of the incident ray, by the time it has passed from air to glass and back to air the beam will either have converged or diverged.

If the light is not travelling at right angles to the second medium, it will undergo a change of direction. This change of direction, which will be towards the normal in a denser medium and away from the normal in a less dense medium, is called **refraction** (Fig. 8.4). It is a phenomenon that will be familiar to anyone who has been spear fishing and seen the shaft appear to bend at the point where is enters the water.

The amount by which the light is bent also depends on its wavelength: blue light is refracted more than red. This means that when a beam of 'white' light (mixed wavelengths) passes through a refractive substance, such as a glass prism or atmospheric water droplet, it will be split into its constituent wavelengths and form a rainbow.

Refraction is also used in medical optics; concave or convex lenses can be used to correct congenital or acquired faults with the biological lens in the eye.

# X-rays

## X-ray production

X-rays can be produced in one of two ways. When an electron is rapidly decelerated it loses kinetic energy and this energy is dispersed as a photon, which will commonly have an energy lying within the x-ray band of the electromagnetic spectrum. x-rays can also be produced by the movement of electrons between two inner shells, the difference in binding energies being radiated as an x-ray photon.

Both these processes take place within the x-ray tube, wherein high-energy electrons bombard a tungsten target. There are four possible interactions that can then take place (Fig. 8.5).

The first two involve interactions between the incident electron and the outer electron shells:

• **Outer shell excitation.** The incoming electron can interact with an outer-shell electron and give up a small fraction of its energy to excite it to a higher shell. When this electron drops back to its original level it gives off a low-energy x-ray photon, which has the effect of heating the tungsten. The slightly decelerated incident electron continues on its path and is available to take place in further interactions.

• **Outer shell ionization.** If the incident electron imparts sufficient energy to an electron in an outer shell then, rather than merely excite it to a higher shell, it can remove it altogether, creating a (temporary) ion (an electron is readily recaptured from the 'electron gas' within the tungsten lattice) plus a free electron, known as the *secondary electron*. The incoming electron has been slowed, again only slightly. Both primary and secondary electrons may also produce additional ionization or excitation within the tungsten target.

• **Inner shell ionization.** When an incoming electron interacts with an electron from one of the inner shells, we come to the true business of the target, to produce high energy x-rays. In order to remove an electron from an inner shell, it is necessary for the incident electron to have an energy that is equal to or greater than the binding energy of the electron shell (Table 8.8). The difference between this binding energy and the amount of energy transferred from the incident electron is reflected in the kinetic energy of the secondary electron, which can go on to produce additional ionization or excitation. The resultant vacancy in the inner shell is then filled by an electron dropping down from an outer shell. As this happens, a photon is emitted whose energy is equal to the difference in binding energies between the two shells: for example, the transition from the L shell (binding energy 12 keV) to the K shell (69 keV) will result in a photon of $69 - 12 = 57$ keV. This photon is known as a **characteristic photon**, because its energy is directly related to the difference in electron shell binding energies for, in this case, tungsten. This means that only x-rays of 15 different energies can be produced by this means in tungsten, which gives an x-ray spectrum that is unique for each element. That of tungsten is shown in Figure 8.6.

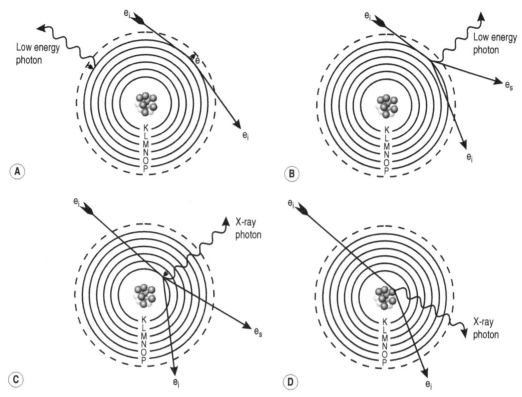

**Figure 8.5** • X-ray production. Possible reactions between high-energy electrons and tungsten atoms. The incident electron ($e_i$) can excite an outer-shell electron, which produces a low-energy photon when it drops back down to its ground state (**A**). It can remove the outer-shell electron, releasing both a low-energy photon and a secondary electron ($e_s$) (**B**). If an inner-shell electron is ionized, a secondary electron again is produced and, as an electron drops down from a higher shell, a photon with characteristic energy (and therefore wavelength) is produced (**C**). If the incident electron reacts with the nucleus and decelerates as a consequence, Bremsstrahlung radiation is produced (**D**).

**Table 8.8** Binding energies and transition values of tungsten electrons (keV).

| Electron transition to shell | Number of electrons | Approximate binding energy* | Electron transition from shell | | | | |
| --- | --- | --- | --- | --- | --- | --- | --- |
| | | | L | M | N | O | P |
| K | 2 | 69 | 57.4 | 66.7 | 68.9 | 69.4 | 69.5 |
| L | 8 | 12 | | 9.3 | 11.5 | 12.0 | 12.1 |
| M | 18 | 3 | | | 2.2 | 2.7 | 2.8 |
| N | 32 | 1 | | | | 0.52 | 0.6 |
| O | 12 | 0.1 | | | | | 0.08 |
| P | 2 | 0.08 | | | | | |

*It is worth recalling that the energies of the *s, p, d* and *f* sub-shells will vary; these figures are therefore averages

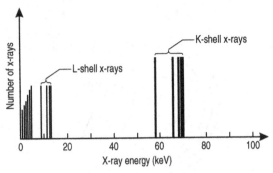

**Figure 8.6** • Characteristic x-ray emission spectrum for tungsten showing the 15 possible photon energies associated with inter-shell transition.

• **Electron–nucleus interaction**. Some of the incident electrons pass through all the electron shells without interaction; they are thereafter strongly attracted by the 74 positively charged protons of the tungsten nucleus, which will slow, deviate or even stop the travelling electron. This change of velocity leads to the production of a photon, whose energy will be identical to the reduction in kinetic energy of the electron. It is easy to see that, in this case, the photon can have any energy between zero (if it passes far enough away to be unaffected) and the maximum value of the electron beam (typically 100 keV). Such radiation is named after the German word for 'braking'. Bremsstrahlung radiation therefore produces a continuous spectrum that is superimposed upon that of the characteristic emission spectrum to create the x-ray profile for a given machine (Fig. 8.7).

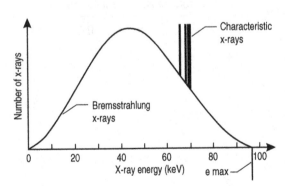

**Figure 8.7** • The x-ray profile for a particular machine is obtained by superimposing the Bremsstrahlung radiation spectrum on top of that for characteristic tungsten x-rays.

# X-ray interaction with matter

In order to fully understand the absorption of x-rays by matter, which forms the basis of radiography, radiotherapy and the associated health and safety of the patient and operator, it is necessary to comprehend the way in which high-energy electromagnetic radiation (x-rays and γ-rays) can interact with matter.

The way in which this happens is, in part, dependent on the energy of the incident photons. It is important to remember that the x-rays from a diagnostic imaging machine produce a heterogeneous beam; that is, one made from a range of values – those shown in Figure 8.7. If the x-rays were all of one energy, we would know exactly how far they can penetrate a given substance before they are absorbed; however, when photons of many energies are mixed together, we can only talk in terms of how much the beam is **attenuated**. The way in which this happens is much like a radioactive half life: if 1 cm of material attenuates 50% of the beam, then 2 cm will attenuate 75% (i.e. half the remaining beam), 3 cm will attenuate 87.5% and so on.

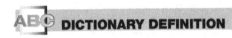 **DICTIONARY DEFINITION**

**ATTENUATION**
Attenuation is defined as the reduction in intensity of a beam as it passes though a medium.
Attenuation is due to *absorption* or *scattering* (or to a combination of the two).

There are five ways in which x-rays can be attenuated:

## Photoelectric effect

When an incident photon has an energy that is equal to or greater than the binding energy of an electron in an atom of the medium with which it is interacting, the photon can ionize the atom by ejecting the electron from its shell; this electron becomes known as a **photoelectron**. In this instance, *all* of the energy from the photon is absorbed by the photoelectron, which has a resultant energy equal to that of the incident photon less the electron's binding energy (Fig. 8.8).

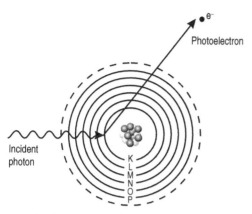

**Figure 8.8** • Photoelectric absorption of an incident x-ray photon leads to the ejection of an inner shell electron.

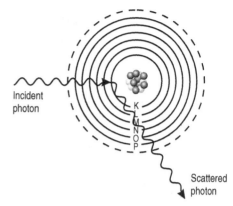

**Figure 8.9** • Classical scattering. Low-energy x-ray photons are absorbed and immediately re-emitted having changed direction but not wavelength.

This transition is accompanied by an outer-shell electron dropping down to fill the vacancy left by the photoelectron and this will be accompanied by the release of a characteristic (for that element) secondary photon whose energy will be equal to the difference between the binding energy of the two shells involved in the transition. This radiation is identical in nature to that which occurs in the tungsten target of an x-ray tube.

The photoelectron is capable of undergoing further interactions as described above; as is the secondary photon, which contributes nothing to the diagnostic value of the x-ray but adds to patient exposure.

The photoelectric effect is comparatively rare; the chances of it occurring decrease with the third power of the photon energy $(1/E)^3$. That means that a photon of 30 keV is *27* times more likely to undergo photoelectric absorption than one of 90 keV.

The chances are also directly proportional to the third power of the atomic number of the interacting material; therefore $_6$C is *216* times more likely to undergo photoelectric absorption than $_1$H.

## Classical (coherent) scattering

When low-energy x-rays (<10 keV) interact with atoms whose electrons have relatively higher binding energies (larger $Z$), they are likely to undergo **classical scattering**, also known as coherent or, occasionally, Thompson (after J.J., who first observed it) scattering.

Because the incident electrons have an energy that is less than the binding energy of the (inner) electron shells, when they interact, the electron does not become excited; rather the incident electron is absorbed and immediately re-emitted. As there has been no transfer of energy, there is no change in the wavelength of the new photon; however, it will be travelling in a different direction – this is what is meant by 'scattering' (Fig. 8.9).

Some degree of this scattering takes place throughout the range of x-rays; however, the only implications for diagnostic imaging are the slight 'fogging' of the film that occurs as a result, causing 'greying' of the photographic plate that detracts from the image contrast.

## Compton (modified) scattering

When the energy of the incident photon is greater than the binding energy of the interacting atoms, **Compton scattering** can occur. If the incident x-ray interacts with an outer-shell electron, it has more than sufficient energy to eject it from the atom, causing the atom to ionize (Fig. 8.10). This secondary electron is called a *Compton electron*.

The photon changes direction (i.e., is scattered) and loses energy. The energy of the Compton scattered x-ray ($E_c$) is equal to the energy of the incident x-ray ($E_i$) less the binding energy of the interacting electron shell ($E_b$) and the kinetic energy of the Compton electron ($E_{ke}$).

The relationship can be expressed mathematically:

$$E_c = E_i - (E_b + E_{ke})$$

Frequently, both the scattered x-ray and the Compton electron have sufficient energy to undergo further interactions before their energies diminish

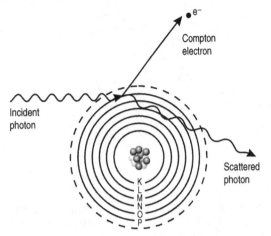

**Figure 8.10** • In Compton scattering, an outer shell electron is ejected gaining momentum at the expense of the incoming x-ray photon, which loses energy and is scattered.

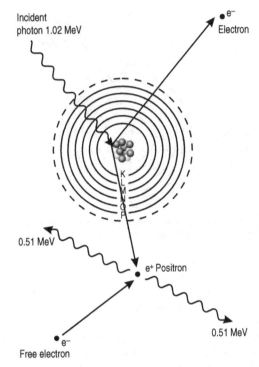

**Figure 8.11** • If the energy of the incident photon is equal to or greater than 1.02 MeV, the x-ray photon can interact with the nucleus to produce a positron and an electron. This is known as pair production.

below any significant threshold; ultimately, the scattered x-ray will undergo photoelectric absorption and the electron will cease to have sufficient energy to ionize or excite other electrons and drop into an electron shell vacated by some other interactive event.

The amount of energy transferred is related to the angle of deflection, which can vary between 0° (no energy transfer) to 180° (whereby a maximum of approximately one-third of the incident energy in transferred). These latter x-rays are referred to as **backscatter radiation** and are responsible for a potential exposure threat to the radiographer.

## Pair production

When an incident x-ray has sufficient energy, it may penetrate close enough to the nucleus to be strongly influenced by the electromagnetic attraction of the nucleus. If the energy of the photon is equal to or greater than 1.02 MeV (the equivalent to the energy of two electrons at rest), the photon will vanish and be spontaneously replaced by an electron and a positron. This process is called **pair production** (Fig. 8.11).

If the x-ray has an energy of less than 1.02 MeV, no pair production can occur; any energy above this level will be equally divided between the two particles and constitute their kinetic energy. If this is

sufficiently high, the electron can interact in the same manner as described above; eventually the electron will be absorbed into a vacancy in an electron shell.

The positron will inevitably meet with its antiparticle, a free electron, and the two will mutually annihilate and the mass of both particles will be converted into energy. Although this process is rare in x-ray production and relatively unimportant in conventional radiography, it is a very important process in the emerging field of positron emission tomography (as we shall see in Chapter 9).

## Photodisintegration

If the energy of the incident x-ray is greater than 10 MeV, it can escape all interactions and be absorbed directly with the nucleus, exciting it to release a nucleon. This process is unimportant for our considerations.

## Learning Outcomes

If you have understood the contents of this chapter, you should now understand:
- The differing parts of the electromagnetic spectrum and their applications
- The concept of radioactive half-life and its implications for a variety of radioisotopes
- The differences in the formation and behaviour of alpha particles, beta particles and gamma radiation
- The behaviour of visible light with regard to reflection and refraction
- The means by which x-rays are produced
- The different ways in which x-rays can react with matter and the physical and medical implications thereof.

## CHECK YOUR EXISTING KNOWLEDGE: ANSWERS

1  The photon   [1]
2  $3 \times 10^8$ ms$^{-1}$   [1]
3  Due west   [3]
4  $\lambda = {}^c/_f$ or $f = {}^c/_\lambda$ or $c = f\lambda$   [2]
5  $\gamma$-rays   [1]
6  Ultraviolet   [1]
7  Green light   [1]
8  They are the same   [1]
9  As heat   [1]
10  6.25%   [3]
11  a) (87)Francium-223 [4]   b) (90)Thorium−227 [4]
12  a) A positron [2]   b) An anti-proton [1]
13  130° (−40° to the normal)   [2]
14  Colour deficiency (colourblindness)   [1]
15  It is refracted towards the normal   [3]
16  a) Slowing of an electron [3]   b) Inner-shell electron transition [3]
17  (Four from) Photoelectric effect, Classical (Coherent) scattering, Compton (Modified) scattering, Pair production, Photodisintegration   [2 each]
18  X-ray radiation produced by electrons being slowed owing to interaction with the positive nucleus   [1]
19  Any energy equal to the transition energies between the electron shells of a given element   [2]
20  The reduction in intensity of a beam of electromagnetic radiation as it passes through a medium (due to absorption and/or scattering)   [1]

### How to interpret the results:

45–50: You have obviously studied this material in some depth before and should be able to apply these principles in the remaining chapters

0–44: These are advanced and interrelated concepts that need to be mastered in order to understand the remaining chapters. Study this chapter in full until you feel comfortable familiarity with the material before moving on

## Bibliography

Absolute Astronomy. Ernest Rutherford. Online. Available: www.absoluteastronomy.com/ quotations/Ernest_Rutherford 14 September 2008, 20:55 BST.

Aetna. Clinical policy bulletin: Infrared therapy. Online. 11 September 2008 15:00 BST.

Allen, R., Schwarz, C. (Eds.), 1998. The Chambers dictionary. Chambers Harrap, Edinburgh, UK.

Allison, W., 2006. Interactions of ionising radiation. In: Fundamental physics for probing and imaging. Oxford University Press, Oxford, pp. 55–84.

Allison, W., 2006. Analysis and damage by radiation. In: Fundamental physics for probing and imaging. Oxford University Press, Oxford, pp. 157–206.

Ammari, M., Brillaud, E., Gamez, C., et al. 2008. Effect of a chronic GSM 900 MHz exposure on glia in the rat brain. Biomed. Pharmacother. 62, 273–281.

Ardell, D., 2008. Rosalind Franklin (1920–1958). The National Heath Museum: Access Excellence Resource Centre. Online. Available: www.accesseXcellence.org/RC/AB/BC/Rosalind_Franklin.php d 12 September 2008 18:35 BST.

Austrian Radiation Protection and Nuclear Safety Agency (ARPANSA) Radiation protection: mobile telephones scientific background. Online. Available: www.arpansa.gov.au/mobilephones/mobiles1cfm 8 September 2008, 20:50 BST.

Belyaev, I.Y., Grigoriev, Y.G., 2007. Problems in assessment of risks from exposures to microwaves of mobile communication. Radiation Biology Radioecology 47, 727–732.

Birch, M.J., Blowes, R.W., 1990. A contact X-ray therapy unit for intracavitary irradiation. Phys. Med. Biol. 35, 275–280.

Bushong, S.C., 2004. Electromagnetism. In: Radiological science for technologists: physics, biology and protection, eighth ed. Mosby, St Louis, pp. 93–107.

Bushong, S.C., 2004. X-ray production. In: Radiological science for technologists: physics, biology and protection, eighth ed. Mosby, St Louis, pp. 147–158.

Bushong, S.C., 2004. Heath physics. In: Radiological science for technologists: physics, biology and protection, eighth ed. Mosby, St Louis, pp. 93–107.

Darling, D., Radioactive species. The Internet Encyclopedia of Science. Online. Available: www.daviddarling.info/encyclopedia/R/radioactive_series.html 13 September 2008, 13:30 BST.

Denman, A.R., Cockerel, T., Phillips, P.S., et al., 2008. Lowering the UK domestic radon Action Level to prevent more lung cancers – is it cost-effective? J. Radiol. Prot. 28, 61–71.

Encyclopædia Britannica. Antimatter. Encyclopædia Britannica 2008. Encyclopædia Britannica 2006 Ultimate Reference Suite, DVD 14 September 2008.

Encyclopædia Britannica. Pitchblende. Encyclopædia Britannica 2008. Encyclopædia Britannica 2006 Ultimate Reference Suite, DVD 13 September 2008.

Encyclopædia Britannica. Röntgen, Wilhelm Conrad. Encyclopædia Britannica 2008. Encyclopædia Britannica 2006 Ultimate Reference Suite, DVD 12 September 2008.

Environmental Illness Resource. Seasonal Affective Disorder. Online. Available: www.ei-resource.org/illness-information/related-conditions/seasonal-affective-disorder-(s.a.d) Accessed 11th September 2008, 16:05 BST.

Garrood, J.R., 1979. Electromagnetic waves and optics. In: Physics. Intercontinental, Maidenhead, pp. 140–176.

Garrood, J.R., 1979. Nuclear and quantum physics. In: Physics. Intercontinental, Maidenhead, pp. 276–314.

Halliday, D., Resnick, R., Walker, J., 2005. Electromagnetic waves. In: Fundamentals of physics, seventh ed. John Wiley, Hoboken, pp. 801–832.

Halliday, D., Resnick, R., Walker, J., 2005. Nuclear physics. In: Fundamentals of physics, seventh ed. John Wiley, Hoboken, pp. 1062–1091.

Hand, J.W., 2008. Modelling the interaction of electromagnetic fields (10 MHz–10 GHz) with the human body: methods and applications. Phys. Med. Biol. 53 (16), R243–R286. Epub 2008 Jul 24.

Harden, R.N., Remble, T.A., Houle, T.T., et al., 2007. Prospective, randomized, single-blind, sham treatment-controlled study of the safety and efficacy of an electromagnetic field device for the treatment of chronic low back pain: a pilot study. Pain Practice 7 (3), 248–255.

Hay, G.A., Hughes, D.H., 1983. Electromagnetic radiation. In: First year physics for radiographers, third ed. Ballière Tindall, Eastbourne, pp. 27–38.

Hay, G.A., Hughes, D.H., 1983. X-rays. In: First year physics for radiographers, third ed. Ballière Tindall, Eastbourne, pp. 139–160.

Hay, G.A., Hughes, D.H., 1983. Interaction of X-rays and gamma rays with matter. In: First year physics for radiographers, third ed.

Ballière Tindall, Eastbourne, pp. 231–259.

Hay, G.A., Hughes, D.H., 1983. X-ray and gamma ray measurement. In: First year physics for radiographers, third ed. Ballière Tindall, Eastbourne, pp. 260–271.

Hay, G.A., Hughes, D.H., 1983. Radioactivity. In: First year physics for radiographers, third ed. Ballière Tindall, Eastbourne, pp. 272–286.

Hunter, J.A., Savin, J.A., Dahl, M.V., 1995. Skin tumours. In: Clinical dermatology, second ed. Oxford, Blackwell Science, pp. 219–245.

Hyland, G.J., 2008. Physical basis of adverse and therapeutic effects of low intensity microwave radiation. Indian J. Exp. Biol. 46 (5), 403–419.

Iwatschenko M. 2005. Calibration of a PET-stack monitor based on coincidence technology. 30th IRMF Meeting, 9 November 2005. National Physics Laboratory, Teddington.

Johnson, K., 1986. Light. In: GCSE physics for you. Hutchinson Education, London, pp. 178–183.

Johnson, K., 1986. Colour. In: GCSE physics for you. Hutchinson Education, London, pp. 222–231.

Johnson, 1986. Physics at work: electromagnetic waves. In: GCSE physics for you. Hutchinson Education, London, pp. 251.

Johnson, K., 1986. Radioactivity. In: GCSE physics for you. Hutchinson Education, London, pp. 372–382.

Kahr, E., 1978. Megavoltage therapy of glioblastoma multiforme. Acta. Neurochir. (Wien) 42, 79–87.

Khan, F.M., 2003. Production of X-rays. In: The physics of radiation therapy: Mechanisms, diagnosis and management, 3rd ed. Lippincott, Williams and Wilkins, Philadelphia, pp. 38–58.

Khan, F.M., 2003. Interactions of ionizing radiation. In: The physics of radiation therapy: Mechanisms, diagnosis and management, third ed. Lippincott, Williams and Wilkins, Philadelphia, pp. 38–58.

Koehler, K.R., Nuclear decay and radioactive series. College Physics for Students of Biology and Chemistry. Online. Available: www.rwc.uc.edu/koehler/biophys/7c.html 13 September 2008, 13:35 BST.

Liboff, A.R., 2007. Local and holistic electromagnetic therapies. Electromagn. Biol. Med. 26 (4), 315–325.

Markov, M.S., 2007. Expanding use of pulsed electromagnetic field therapies. Electromagn. Biol. Med. 26 (3), 257–274.

McCool, R., Introduction to fibreoptics. Jodrell Bank Observatory (University of Manchester). Online. Available: www.jodrellbank.manchester.ac.uk/research/fibre/intro2fibre.htm 15 September 2008, 14:25 BST.

National Aeronautical and Space Administration. The ozone layer. Online. Available: www.nas.nasa.gov/About/Education/Ozone/ozonelayer.html 11 September 2008, 15:45 BST.

National Institutes of Health. Dietary Supplement Fact Sheet: Vitamin D. Office of Dietary Supplements. Online. Available: www.ods.od.nih.gov/factsheets/vitamind.asp. 11 September 2008, 15:20 BST.

Nave, R., Electromagnetic radiation. Department of Physics and Astronomy, Georgia State University. Online. Available: hyperphysics.phy-astr.gsu.edu 8 September 2008 11:25 BST.

Nelson, S., 1998. Lightning-Associated Deaths – United States, 1980–1995. MMWR. Morb. Mortal. Wkly. Rep. 47, 391–434.

Nicolin, V., Ponti, C., Baldini, G., et al., 2007. In vitro exposure of human chondrocytes to pulsed electromagnetic fields. Eur. J. Histochem. 51 (3), 203–212.

McQuillin, B.R., 1982. Geometrical optics. In: Robertson, A.J. (Ed.), Rapid revision notes A-level physics: heat, light and sound. Celtic Revision Aids, London, pp. 47–83.

McQuillin, B.R., 1982. Physical optics. In: Robertson, A.J. (Ed.), Rapid revision notes A-level physics: heat, light and sound. Celtic Revision Aids, London, pp. 93–113.

Rabin, J., Color vision fundamentals. USAF School of Aerospace. Online. Available: www.colorvisiontesting.com 17 September, 12:30 BST.

Siwiak, K., McKeown, D., 2004. Generating and transmitting UWB signals. In: Ultra-wideband Radio. John Wiley, Hoboken, pp. 55–88.

Takebayashi, T., Varsier, N., Kikuchi, Y., et al., 2008. Mobile phone use, exposure to radiofrequency electromagnetic field, and brain tumour: a case-control study. Br. J. Cancer 12, 98, 652–659.

Thorne, J.O., Collocott, T.C. (Eds.), 1984. In: Chambers biographical dictionary. Chambers, Edinburgh.

University of Bristol. Ecology of vision: Exploring the fourth dimension. Department of Biological Sciences. Online. Available: www.bio.bris.ac.uk/research/vision/4d.htm 11September 2008, 15:15 BST.

Yochum, T.R., Rowe, L., 1996. Skeletal radiology: a historical perspective. In: Yochum, T.R., Rowe, L.J. (Eds.), Essentials of skeletal radiology. Williams & Wilkins, Baltimore, xxv–xxix.

Walker, N.A., Denegar, C.R., Preische, J., 2007. Low-intensity pulsed ultrasound and pulsed electromagnetic field in the treatment of tibial fractures: a systematic review. J. Athl. Train. 42 (4), 530–555.

Wood, A.W., 2006. How dangerous are mobile phones, transmission masts, and electricity pylons? Arch. Dis. Child 91, 361–336.

# Chapter Nine

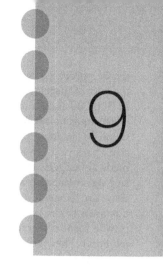

# Diagnostic imaging

## CHAPTER CONTENTS

Introduction . . . . . . . . . . . . . . . . . . 203
The x-ray machine . . . . . . . . . . . . . . 204
   Thermionic emission . . . . . . . . . . 204
   Electron production . . . . . . . . . . . 205
   Electron energy . . . . . . . . . . . . . 206
   Production of x-rays . . . . . . . . . . 207
   Quantity of x-rays . . . . . . . . . . . 209
   Quality of x-ray . . . . . . . . . . . . . 210
   Patient exposure . . . . . . . . . . . . 211
   Radiation dosage . . . . . . . . . . . 214
   The x-ray image . . . . . . . . . . . . 216
Computed tomography . . . . . . . . . . . 218
   Spiral CT . . . . . . . . . . . . . . . . . 220

Magnetic resonance imaging . . . . . . . . 221
   Introduction . . . . . . . . . . . . . . . . 221
   Magnetic resonance . . . . . . . . . . 221
Positron emission tomography (PET) . . . . 226
Diagnostic ultrasonography . . . . . . . . . 227
   Obstetric ultrasonography . . . . . . . . 229
   Musculoskeletal ultrasound . . . . . . . 230
   Doppler ultrasonography . . . . . . . . . 231
Learning outcomes . . . . . . . . . . . . . . 231
Bibliography . . . . . . . . . . . . . . . . . . 231

## CHECK YOUR EXISTING KNOWLEDGE

1 Are you a qualified radiographer?

If you are not, the chances of you having acquired the requisite knowledge included in this chapter are remote; a physics degree will probably enable you to skip the section on x-ray production, otherwise this is a section of the book to be studied from beginning to end.

If you are, then proceed to Chapter 10.

## Introduction

Since Röntgen first took the blurred, indistinct image of his wife's hand at the end of the 19th century, diagnostic imaging has changed beyond all recognition. Patient (and practitioner) exposure has decreased, quite literally, by an order of magnitude; meanwhile, imaging quality has been enhanced to the point where it is now possible, using computed tomography, to produce three-dimensional colour films … where films are used at all; digitization means that most images are now read on computer screens. This means that they can be instantly magnified and exposure parameters modified as required.

Over the past 30 years, it has become possible to image not only bone but soft tissues as well, revolutionizing the diagnosis and management of injury and disease processes. These changes have, inevitably come at a price. Whereas a new x-ray machine can be purchased and installed for under $100 000, the cost of magnetic resonance imagers start at over $1 500 000 and positron emission tomography costs many times more. The recent development of ultrasound as an imaging modality has started to drag costs back and offer some relief to over-stretched medical budgets. However, as patient expectations and the population age profile both increase, clinicians are being forced into cost/benefit decisions unknown to the previous generation (though not to private manual therapists working with self-funding patients). They must also now become familiar with a raft of different imaging modalities based on a much wider array of underlying principles (i.e. physics) and understand how and why their patients would benefit from referral.

In some manual disciplines, practitioners might also be expected to competently interpret and clinically correlate advanced imaging findings – in both instances, without understanding the fundamentals behind how the images are generated, produced and recorded, the task becomes a feat of memory rather than the consequence of understanding.

This chapter begins with traditional, plain film x-ray in which the basic principles have remained largely unchanged since Victorian times. We will then consider the consequences of the arrival of silicon chip technology, which allowed sufficient computing power to assimilate data into multiple, sequential images, both from x-rays and from the behaviour of individual atomic nuclei within the body, which can be detected, recorded and accurately interpreted. The chapter concludes with consideration of a new application for old technology; ultrasound, which is now providing a cheap, portable, non-invasive alternative to evaluate both injury and illness.

## The x-ray machine

We have already considered the basics of x-ray production in the previous chapter – take some electrons; accelerate them so that they have lots of energy; smash them into a piece of tungsten and, hey presto, x-rays!

It is now time to understand how those elements work in practice.

## Thermionic emission

As we have already discovered, many metals have, at room temperature, a 'sea' of disassociated electrons within their lattice structure. These 'free' electrons can move around in response to an applied electromagnetic field; however, under normal conditions the negative charges on all these electrons are cancelled out by the positive charges on the atoms of the metal.

If the metal is heated, however, the electrons gain kinetic energy. Occasionally, one electron will gain so much energy that it is capable of overcoming the attraction of the nuclei and can fly off into the metal's surroundings. When this happens, the electron-deficient metal develops a positive charge resulting in an electrostatic attraction between the (negatively charged) electrons that have leapt out of the metal and the (positively charged) metal they have left.

The result of this is the production of a **space charge**. The hot metal becomes surrounded by a 'cloud' of electrons that have jumped out of the metal before being drawn back by the attraction between the electron and the metal. We see this effect every time we switch on a conventional electric light bulb.

Taken overall, the system remains electrically neutral – sum the charges of electron cloud and metal at any moment, and the result will still be zero. This process of 'boiling off' electrons is known as **thermionic emission**.

In an x-ray machine, the thermionic filament is traditionally made from tungsten. This element is particularly useful in this context, not only because it is relatively inexpensive and easily available but because of its work function profile (Fig. 9.1) and

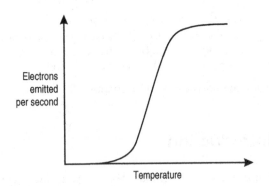

**Figure 9.1** • The thermionic emission profile for tungsten. Until the threshold temperature is reached, no electrons are produced; thereafter, a relatively small increase in temperature (current) produces a large increase in electron emission. When the field charge effect reaches saturation, mutual repulsion between the electron cloud and newly emergent electrons means that further increases in temperature do not liberate additional electrons.

its high melting point (3683K). When the x-ray machine is switched on, the filament is heated only slightly by a current that is low enough that it is below the threshold for thermionic emission. It is further protected from too rapid heating by a *thermistor*, described in Chapter 8 as a device whose conductance increases with temperature.

Once the filament current is high enough for thermionic emission to occur, we can see from Figure 9.1 that it takes only a very small increase in temperature (produced by the heating effect of the current) to effect a very large increase in the number of electrons produced. There is an upper limit to electron production. This is determined by the mutual repulsion between the electron cloud and the electrons within the filament that are trying to escape, the **space charge effect**. Beyond this point, very few further electrons are produced, regardless of how much additional current is introduced. The risk of vaporizing the tungsten also increases, thus limiting the effective filament current to below this level.

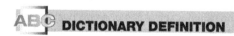

## DICTIONARY DEFINITION

**WORK FUNCTION**

You have, of course, already encountered this concept in Chapter 6 when discussing the photoelectric effect. Work function is defined as the minimum amount of energy required per electron to remove it from the surface of a solid. It is given a symbol, the Greek letter phi ($\Phi$).

In order to improve the performance of the tungsten, it is coated with graphite to give it a smooth surface. It is also mixed with 2% of radioactive thorium oxide, which has the effect of lowering the work function of the filament by a third from the 4.5 eV of pure tungsten to around 1.5 eV.

The equation that predicts the number of electrons per square metre of available surface ($J$), the *Richardson-Dushman equation*, is complicated and does not need to be memorized or scrutinized in detail. However, it states that:

$$J \propto T^2 e^{-\Phi/T}$$

Where T is absolute temperature and $e$ is the base of the natural logarithm (if you do not already know

what this is, it matters not, just accept that it is a constant = 2.718).

The effect of this can be twofold. If we lower the work function from 4.5 to 1.5, it means that, if our filament is heated to, say 2000K, a typical operating temperature, we can produce more electrons for the same energy. It also means that we could lower the threshold temperature at which thermionic emission begins, thus extending the life of the filament ... or, as happens in reality, do a little bit of both.

## Electron production

Practical considerations mean that most commercial x-ray machines have filament currents that are in the range of 3–6A. The heating effect of this current is used to generate thermionic emission in the tungsten filament. It is important not to confuse the *filament current* with the **tube current**, which is the number of electrons per second travelling from the filament to the target, measured in mA. This is one of three defining factors for an x-ray exposure and is pre-set by the operator, usually in increments of 50 mA. For musculoskeletal radiography, this range will usually cover from 50 mA (for extremities) to 300 mA (for lumbopelvic views of obese patients).

Radiographers invariably refer to the tube current as the 'mA'; however, by itself it does not tell us how many electrons are available for x-ray production, merely how many are being directed at the target per second.

This brings us to the second defining measure of a patient's exposure, the length of time over which electrons are produced, which will mirror the length of time over which x-rays are produced and therefore the amount of exposure. The exposure time is measured in seconds although, in reality, it will usually be fractions of a second. These two factors are usually combined to reflect the number of electrons produced, the **mAs**, which again is referred to in terms of its units ('em-ay-ess').

Thus, an mAs of 100 can be produced by a filament current of 100 mA operating for one second or by a filament current of 200 mA operating for half a second or 250 mA for 0.4 s.

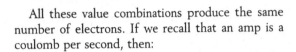

All these value combinations produce the same number of electrons. If we recall that an amp is a coulomb per second, then:

**100 mAs = 100 mCs/s = 100 mC**

There are $1.6 \times 10^{-19}$ C per electron, therefore there are:

**$1/1.6 \times 10^{-19} = 6.25 \times 10^{18}$ electrons per coulomb**

Therefore, 100 mC has $6.25 \times 10^{17}$ electrons.

Usually, the radiographer will be provided with a set of protocols with measurements related to the thickness of individual body parts. These protocols allow them to ascertain the optimum mAs for a patient of any size; they must then determine the best combination of tube current and exposure time; for example, if a cervical spine x-ray is taken at 16 mAs and the radiographer chooses to take it at 200 mA, then the exposure time will be:

$$^{16\ mAs}/_{200\ mA} = 0.08\ s$$

Because the filament is producing negative electrons that are going to be accelerated towards the (positive) target, the filament is termed the *cathode*. It has one further component of which we should be aware, the **focusing cup**. The filament is housed within the focusing cup, which is negatively charged. Although this increases the space charge effect, this disadvantage is offset by the directionality it gives to the electron beam, which otherwise tends to rapidly spread out (owing to mutual repulsion) to the point where many electrons miss the target altogether.

## CLINICAL FOCUS

No two patients are identical and the radiographer must consider a number of factors when determining the patient exposure. If a patient moves during the course of an exposure, the result is the same as it would be in conventional photography: the resulting image is blurred.

Unlike conventional photography, which is merely collecting reflected light, radiography involves significant doses of ionizing radiation passing through the patient before being collected on the film, which is placed behind them. Everything

possible is therefore done to ensure a minimum number of repeated exposures.

As a rule, x-rays are taken at the fastest possible exposure time. This needs to be balanced against using the tube at unnecessarily high mA values, which shortens the tube life (generally, there is little to be gained by taking a 3 mAs radiograph of a foot using an exposure of 0.01 s/300 mA when 0.03 s at 100 mA is fast enough to preclude the possibility of any motion artifact).

There are considerations that may affect this decision. A patient with a parkinsonian tremor or other conditions of involuntary movement, may require a faster than usual exposure time to 'freeze' the joint being imaged.

Although in hospitals most x-rays are taken with the patient lying down, manual physicians want to elicit as much biomechanical information as possible from the resultant films and this often involves x-raying the patient standing up. They then have to overcome the difficulties posed by patients with antalgia, ataxia, balance and respiratory problems, as well as the higher doses often necessitated by upright films. This is particularly true of films of the lower spine (when a spinal film of an overweight patient is taken with the patient lying prone, the fat is pushed to the side by their own weight leaving less soft tissue to penetrate).

## Electron energy

As we saw in the last chapter, when electrons interact with matter, there are a number of events that may occur. As we are only interested in the production of diagnostic quality x-rays, i.e. those capable of penetrating the patient and being detected once they have done so, we should be particularly keen to avoid electron interactions that produce heat and weak Bremsstrahlung radiation.

This involves having electrons with high energies, which means in turn that they must be accelerated to a high speed. This is done by sealing the filament and the tungsten **target** at which the electrons will be fired in a sealed glass cylinder containing a vacuum. This comprises the **x-ray tube**. The absence of air prevents the electrons interacting with the molecules of nitrogen, oxygen, carbon dioxide and trace elements, which would only produce low-energy x-rays (small nuclei, therefore lower electron shell binding energies) and limit the number and energy of those electrons reaching the target.

The electron energy comes from placing a high voltage across the two ends of the x-ray tube. We have already termed the filament the cathode; the other end of the potential gradient is the tungsten target, the *anode*. Electrons are repelled from the cathode and attracted to the anode, the higher the potential difference between the two, the greater the electrons' energy when they strike the target.

In order to do this, a number of obstacles must be overcome. The first of these relates to the voltage supply to the room in which the x-ray is located. We have already seen how the nominal voltage can vary depending how far one is from the nearest substation. It can also vary from hour to hour and from one season to another depending on demand: a frost warning on the weather forecast can cause a sudden dip in power as millions of heaters and boilers are all turned on at once, before power stations can adapt to the increased demand.

Most x-ray machines operate on 220 V but this can easily vary by 5% or more, which does not help the production of consistent, high-quality x-ray beams. The problem is overcome by the insertion of a **line compensator**, which measures and monitors the incoming voltage and will automatically adjust the incoming voltage to be exactly 200 V at all times.

It does this by being wired to the next x-ray component, the **autotransformer**. Although this works on a subtly different principle from the transformers that we considered in Chapter 7, the underlying physics remains the same – a primary voltage induces a magnetic field in a shared ferromagnetic core. This, in turn, induces a secondary voltage. By adjusting the ratio of the number of coils around the core in the primary and secondary circuits, the secondary voltage can be increased or decreased compared to the primary.

In a typical x-ray machine, the transformer steps up the voltage by a factor of 500 to produce voltages of up to 110 kV across the length of the tube. This secondary voltage is referred to in terms of 'kilovolts peak' ($kV_p$) and, once again is referred to in terms of its units ('kay-vee-pee'), the third and last of the factors determining exposure.

Although there are now plenty of available electrons and the means to impart significant amount of energy to them, there remains one further obstacle. The mains supply to the x-ray machine, whether single phase or multi-phase, is in the form of alternating current. This means that 50 or 60 times per second, it fluctuates from positive to zero to negative and back to zero. This means that the electrons are

bounced up and down the x-ray tube and spend at least half their time travelling in the wrong direction.

The solution is, of course, to include a rectifier in the circuit immediately after the transformer (remember, direct current cannot be transformed). As it would be unproductive to have the tube sitting idle for half the time, *full wave rectification* is used, and this ensures that the filament end of the tube is always negative and the target always positive.

High-voltage capacitors are then used to smooth the circuit to deliver a constant, controllable, high voltage across the vacuum between cathode and anode (Fig. 9.2).

---

### Fact File

#### THE THERMIONIC TUBE

The x-ray 'tube' got its name because it works on the same principle as a diode, one of the electrical components that were considered in Chapter 8.

In the days before semiconductors, such elements were provided by an evacuated glass tube – in the case of the diode, electrons could only flow from the negative end to the positive one, never the other way around, thus creating a 'one-way system'. Although in the UK, they were referred to as 'valves' (hence 'valve radio'), in the US they were called 'tubes'. The most familiar example of such a tube is not a diode but a conventional television set ... hence the expression 'spending an evening in front of the tube'.

---

## Production of x-rays

There are a number of considerations that must be made regarding the x-ray target before electrons are haphazardly smashed into it. The first is the choice of material. Why tungsten? The element scores highly on a number of essential characteristics. In addition to being relatively cheap and easily available, tungsten has a high atomic number. This means a high K-shell binding energy and, therefore, a greater number of high-energy (and, thus, diagnostic) x-rays. It also has a high liquefaction point – almost three times that of copper – which means that it can withstand high tube current without melting, pitting or vaporizing (a common cause of tube failure). Finally, tungsten has good thermal conductivity. It is therefore efficient at dissipating the heat away from the immediate area of electron contact.

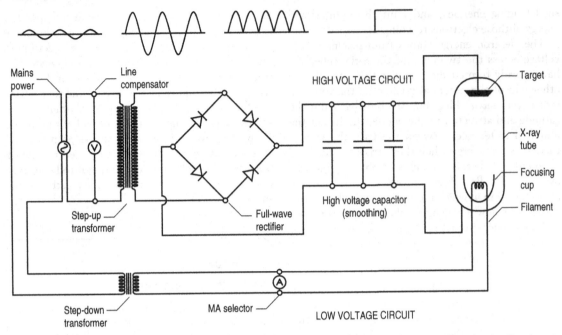

Figure 9.2 • X-ray circuit. Schematic diagram of the modification of mains supply to an x-ray machine showing the stages required for the high-voltage circuit to the tube and the low voltage circuit to the filament and focusing cup.

Although in dental x-ray machines, the low exposures mean that a fixed target can be used, in medical machines, capable of imaging a pelvis, if the electron beam were always centred on a single spot, that area would soon become damaged and degraded and the (expensive) tube, ruined.

One way around this problem is to rotate the target, thus spreading the area of electron bombardment around the whole of the circumference of the circular target. This can increase the potential target area from just 5 mm$^2$ to more than 1500 mm$^2$. Typically, x-ray targets rotate at speeds of 50 revolutions per second.

### Heel effect

The x-ray target must also be carefully shaped (Fig. 9.3A) in order to direct as many of the x-rays as possible towards the target (patient) rather than randomly, in which event they will be absorbed by the protective lead casing of the tube rather than used for their intended purpose. The edge of the rotating anode is bevelled – usually at an angle of about 6° – in order to direct the x-rays towards the *aperture*, the hole through which the radiation is directed at the patient. Metal sliding panels called *collimators* can cover all or part of the aperture to further limit the spread of the beam and to ensure that only the targeted area is exposed.

Unfortunately, for every innovation there is a consequence, and the sloping of the target means that the x-rays that are produced have varying amounts of tungsten to penetrate before emerging from the target and therefore a higher chance of interacting with other tungsten atoms before emerging. This means that the x-ray beam that emerges from the aperture will be more intense on the cathode side than the anode side, the *heel* of the target (Fig. 9.3B). This will have an effect on the x-ray penetration of the patient and the final image, which can be under-exposed on one side and over-exposed on the other.

### CLINICAL FOCUS

The 'heel effect' can be used to work for the radiographer rather than inevitably detracting from the final quality of the images produced. Many regional views include areas that differ in thickness from top to bottom or have varying densities and the heel effect can be employed to compensate for this; however, this requires appropriate orientation of the aperture.

For abdominal films, the upper abdomen is thicker than the pelvis and lower abdomen. The cathode should therefore be superior to balance this and ensure a more even optical density is obtained.

By contrast, when taking chest x-rays, the upper thorax is thinner than the lower. By positioning the cathode inferiorly, this effect can be minimized. This effect applies, to some extent or other, to almost every body part from the foot (the calcaneus is thicker than the metatarsals and phalanges) to the cervical spine (C7 is larger than C1 and surrounded by denser soft tissues).

---

### Fact File

#### X-RAY MACHINE TARGETS

In fact, tungsten is not the only target material used in x-ray machines, although it is almost ubiquitous in the tubes of medical diagnostic apparatus. However, for specialist machines dedicated to mammography, molybdenum and rhodium are often used because of the lower x-ray energies required for soft tissue imaging.

When high-energy x-rays are required – usually for medical purposes – a uranium target may be used. For x-ray crystallography, low-energy x-rays can be produced using targets of copper or cobalt.

## Quantity of x-rays

The intensity of an x-ray beam is most commonly measured in roentgens (R), even though this is not an official SI unit. A typical diagnostic x-ray exposure produces x-ray intensities of 5 mR per mAs giving a variation from 15 mR for a hand x-ray to 1.2 R for a lumbar spine lateral view.

### ABC DICTIONARY DEFINITION

#### ROENTGENS

As an x-ray beam passes through air, it interacts with air molecules in the ways described in Chapter 8 and produces ions by exciting electrons to the point where they become disassociated with their parent atoms.

One roentgen is defined as the amount of radiation needed to liberate positive and negative charges of one electrostatic unit of charge in 1 cm$^3$ of air at standard temperature and pressure. This corresponds to the generation of approximately $2.08 \times 10^9$ ion pairs.

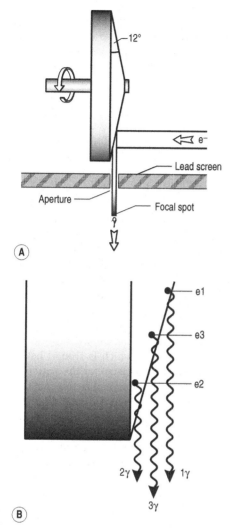

**Figure 9.3** • The heel effect. x-rays interact with the surface of the tungsten target, which is sloped in order to help direct the maximum number of x-ray photons towards the aperture. Those that are emitted in other directions are absorbed by the lead lining of the x-ray tube housing (A). In close up (B), it is easy to see that, because of this slope, not all the x-rays that are produced by the electron interactions with the tungsten will travel the same distance through the tungsten before they emerge. The greater the distance they travel – here, $\gamma_1$ travels less distance than $\gamma_2$ and $\gamma_3$ – the more chance of them interacting with tungsten atoms and being photoelectrically absorbed or Compton scattered and thus failing to reach the aperture. This means that the density of the emergent beam will be higher on the cathode side than on the anode side.

A number of factors can affect the quantity of x-rays reaching the patient. We have already discussed mAs, which is directly proportional to the quantity of x-rays (if the mAs is increased, the number of electrons hitting the target increases as does the number of x-rays produced).

The relationship between x-ray quantity and $kV_p$ is slightly more complicated. If the $kV_p$ is altered, then the ratio of the new x-ray beam intensity to the previous beam is proportional to the square of the *ratio* of the change in $kV_p$. This is best understood by looking at a couple of examples. If the $kV_p$ is increased from 70 to 90, the intensity of the x-ray beam will increase by:

$$\left(\text{Final kVp}\middle/\text{Initial kVp}\right)^2 = \left(\frac{90}{70}\right)^2 = 1.65$$

This is the ratio by which the beam intensity increases; that is, a 29% increase in tube voltage, will give an increase of 65% in the number of x-rays produced. In a similar vein, if the $kV_p$ is reduced from 100 to 92, the x-ray intensity will decrease to:

$$\left(\frac{92}{100}\right)^2 = 0.85$$

Therefore, an 8% decrease in $kV_p$ will create a 15% drop-off in x-ray intensity. The relationship to image is even more complicated because, at higher $kV_p$ values, the x-rays have more energy and so more will penetrate the patient to reach the film and expose it.

The final consideration when determining the number of x-ray photons reaching the patient is that of **source-image distance (SID)**, yet again referred to by its acronym ('ess-eye-dee'). The x-ray beam spreads out as it travels from the point source of the tube aperture and the manner in which it does this is governed by the inverse square law.

Typically, diagnostic x-rays are taken at distances of between 90 cm and 150 cm; the distance is often fixed to remove the necessity of allowing for yet another variable when determining the x-ray factors for a given patient's exposure. However, it is quite easy to appreciate that if the SID is doubled, the mAs must be increased by a factor of four; if tripled, by a factor of nine.

## Quality of x-ray

The quality of an x-ray beam is referred to in terms of its **penetrability,** that is, its ability to permeate

matter: the higher the quality of the x-rays, the higher the penetrability. This can be quantified by using the *attenuation* of the x-ray beam.

You will recall from the last chapter that x-rays are attenuated exponentially; that is, if 50% of x-rays of a given energy are stopped by 1 cm of a given material, then 75% (i.e., half the remaining x-rays) will be stopped by 2 cm, 87.5% by 3 cm and so on. The amount of material required to reduce the beam by 50% is known as the **half-value layer** (HVL) of the material.

Unfortunately, this mathematical relationship breaks down when considering a diagnostic x-ray beam, which is not homogeneous but consists of x-rays of a wide range of energies. The situation is further complicated by the fact that the patient is also non-homogeneous; bone has a different HVL to blood or fat or muscle. The HVL characteristic of an individual x-ray machine is therefore determined by experiment rather than calculation, using (homogeneous) aluminium filters. A diagnostic x-ray beam usually has a HVL of approximately 4 mm for aluminium, which is around half that of the average soft tissue matrix of the patient.

There are, once again, several factors that can affect the quality of x-rays. Before discussing these, it is worth noting that neither mAs nor SID have any effect on the quality of the beam, only the quantity of x-rays produced. $kV_p$ does affect the quality, as might be expected. Increasing the energy of the electrons hitting the target results in the production of more high-energy x-rays, which means the spectrum of x-ray energies is shifted to the right and more high-energy characteristic x-rays will be produced. There is no direct linear relationship between $kV_p$ and HVL; however it is *approximately* proportional (Fig. 9.4).

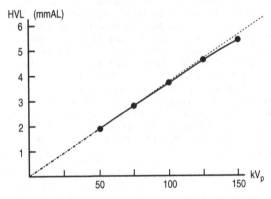

**Figure 9.4** ● The relationship between $kV_p$ and half-value layer (HVL) is approximately linear.

As is implicit from the discussion of HVL, **filtration** can also affect the quality of the beam. If a filter is placed between the x-ray source and the target then a greater proportion of low-energy x-rays will be attenuated than high-energy x-rays. Although this will reduce the quantity of x-rays reaching the patient, it will *increase* their quality. The most commonly selected material for x-ray filters is aluminium; it is cheap and, because of its relatively low atomic number ($Z = 13$), allows through a relatively high proportion of high-energy x-rays but will stop low-energy x-rays through the photoelectric effect.

The thicker the filter, the more photons are stopped and the higher the energy profile of the photons remaining in the emergent beam; however, practical considerations limit the thickness of filters – if the quantity of x-rays is diminished too much, not enough photons reach the patient to obtain a diagnostic image within a realistic timeframe.

There are two types of filter employed in the x-ray room. *Inherent filtration* is included in the x-ray tube as is a combination of the glass screen over the aperture and added aluminium, usually a thin sheet placed between the target and aperture to remove as many low-energy x-rays as possible without significantly affecting the quantity of photons. As this filtration is fixed, its effects can be incorporated in the exposure protocols for a given machine. The effects of this collimation are shown in Figure 9.5.

*Compensating filters* are also employed by the radiographer. These are often wedge-shaped and are used to gradate a beam. For a body part that is, itself, wedge shaped, such as the thoracic spine or foot, the filter (which is placed over the emergent beam) is aligned so that the thickest part of the filter is over the thinnest part of the anatomy.

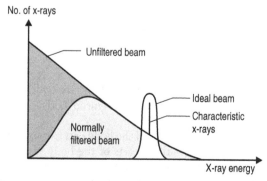

**Figure 9.5** • Filtration can have a considerable effect on reducing the number of low-energy, non-diagnostic x-rays from reaching the patient.

**Table 9.1** Factors that affect the quality and quantity of x-rays

| Factor | Effect upon | |
|---|---|---|
| | X-ray quantity | X-ray quality |
| mAs | Increases in direct proportion | None |
| SID | Decrease according to inverse square ratio | None |
| $kV_p$ | Increases in proportion to the square of the ratio of the increase | Increases approximately proportional |
| Filtration | Decreases exponentially | Increases |

The factors that affect x-ray quality and quantity are summarized in Table 9.1.

## Patient exposure

In Chapter 8, we examined the ways in which x-rays can interact with matter. In diagnostic radiography, only two of these are important: the Compton and photoelectric effects. They are, however, only important in a negative sense – it is the x-rays that pass through the patient *without* undergoing any interaction with matter that form the image of the patient in which we are interested.

It is the photoelectric effect that gives us the image of the patient; if all x-rays were to pass through the patient, the resultant image would be uniformly dark or **radiolucent**. If all the x-rays were to be absorbed, the image would be uniformly white or **radio-opaque**. It is the fact that x-rays are **differentially absorbed** in the photoelectric effect that is important to the clinician.

You will recall that the chance of the photoelectric effect occurring was inversely proportional to the cube of the x-ray's energy and to the cube of the atomic number of a given atom. Differential absorption therefore *increases* as the $kV_p$ is decreased; however, if it is decreased by too much, not enough x-rays will pass through the patient to form a diagnostic image.

The effective atomic number of different soft tissues is dependent on the relative proportion of atoms within their matrix. Bone, for example, is made from hydroxyapatite, which contains calcium ($Z = 20$) and phosphorus ($Z = 15$). It has an

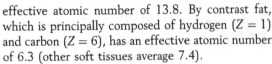

effective atomic number of 13.8. By contrast fat, which is principally composed of hydrogen ($Z = 1$) and carbon ($Z = 6$), has an effective atomic number of 6.3 (other soft tissues average 7.4).

Therefore, photoelectric absorption is:

$$\left(\frac{13.8}{6.8}\right)^3 = 8.36 \text{ times more likely to occur in bone than in fat.}$$

## CLINICAL FOCUS

The increased absorption of x-rays by higher atomic numbered atoms is utilized by the introduction of contrast agents to radiology. Chemicals such as barium ($Z = 56$), which is ingested to image the gut, and iodine ($Z = 53$), which is injected into the blood to allow visualization of a variety of vessels and organs.

The much larger atoms are several hundred times more likely to react photoelectrically with incident x-rays than the soft tissues of the surrounding organ and appear radio-opaque, allowing differentiation of structures that would otherwise transmit a homogeneous beam.

---

The chance of interactions is also related to the **mass density** of the material — bone is denser than fat and therefore there are more atoms with which the x-rays can interact. So, the probability of x-ray interactions (of either type) is directly proportional to the mass density of the material (Table 9.2). This is why interaction is much more likely in lung tissue than in air, despite the fact that their effective

atomic numbers are almost identical. The actual chances of either Compton scattering or the photoelectric effect occurring in lung tissue is:

$$\frac{320}{1.3} = 246 \text{ times more likely than in air.}$$

This also means that the photoelectric effect is *not* 8.3 times more likely to occur in bone that fat because we have not considered the contribution mass density will make to the chances of interaction:

$$\frac{1850}{910} = 2.0 \text{ times more likely.}$$

Therefore, the chances of the photoelectric effect occurring in bone are actually:

$$8.3 \times 2.0 = 16.6 \text{ times more likely.}$$

Therefore, bones are very much more radio-opaque than fat, which is why they appear white on x-ray images and the surrounding soft tissues are darker.

By contrast, Compton scattering – the alteration in direction of an incident photon after an interaction with an outer-shell electron – contributes nothing to the diagnostic quality of the image; rather, it detracts from it. Scattered x-ray photons create **film fogging**, degradation of the diagnostic image by photons that do not relate to the absorption or transmission by body parts. A Compton scattered photon might land anywhere on the receptor (or, indeed, miss it altogether) and detract from the optical contrast.

The Compton effect is independent of atomic number but is directly proportional to the mass density; the Compton effect also *increases* with increasing $kV_p$.

This means that, at lower $kV_p$ values, the photoelectric effect dominates, whilst, at higher values, the Compton effect is more important. Increasing the $kV_p$ also increases the percentage of x-rays that pass through the patient (Table 9.3).

Another consideration with regard to scatter radiation is the size of the beam. As the area of the beam increases, the relative intensity of the scatter radiation also increases. The x-ray beam can be **collimated** in order to limit its width and height and ensure only the required body part is exposed to ionizing radiation.

Finally, the thickness of the body part can contribute to scattering – thick parts of the body result in more scattering than thin parts; the same body part will create less scatter in a thin patient than an obese one. Various techniques exist to compress tissue in overweight subjects to limit this effect.

**Table 9.2** Effective atomic number and mass densities of different body materials

| Tissue type | Effective Z | Mass density (kg m$^{-3}$) |
|---|---|---|
| Bone | 13.8 | 1850 |
| Muscle | 7.4 | 1000 |
| Fat | 6.3 | 910 |
| Lung | 7.4 | 320 |
| Air | 7.6 | 1.3 |

**Table 9.3** Effect of decreasing kV$_p$ on Compton scattering, photoelectric absorption and x-ray transmission

| kV$_p$ | Percent interaction Photoelectric | Percent interaction Compton | Total | Percent transmission |
|---|---|---|---|---|
| 50 | 78.9 | 21 | 99.998 | 0.002 |
| 60 | 69.9 | 30 | 99.9 | 0.1 |
| 70 | 59.8 | 39.8 | 99.6 | 0.4 |
| 80 | 46 | 52 | 98 | 2 |
| 90 | 38 | 59 | 97 | 3 |
| 100 | 31 | 63 | 94 | 6 |
| 110 | 23 | 70 | 93 | 7 |
| 120 | 18 | 73 | 91 | 9 |

 CLINICAL FOCUS

It is the duty of any radiographer to limit the patient dosage to the minimum levels consistent with obtaining a diagnostic series. This process starts with the decision whether or not to x-ray, which has to be assessed on a risk/benefit ratio.

This may vary from one clinical discipline to another. Current medical practice is to refrain from taking high-dose x-rays of the lumbar spine in the absence of 'red flag' signs of pathology; however the manual and, in particular, the manipulative physician will have different criteria behind any such decision. Radiographs that may not affect the decision to prescribe analgesics or NSAIDs may contain information that is important to consider before prescribing exercise regimes or undertaking spinal manipulation. This is the key to the decision making process; although formal guidelines exist (Table 9.4), they can be summarized by a single clinical question: are the x-ray results likely to affect the patient's plan of management?

**Table 9.4** Clinical indicators for x-ray

### General considerations

- Significant trauma
- Failure to respond to treatment
- Unexplained weight loss of 4.5 kg or more over the preceding 6 months
- Unexplained pyrexia of more than 3 days' duration
- Unrelenting pain at rest
- Evolving neurological deficit
- Known history of cancer
- Use of corticosteroids, IV drugs, blood thinners
- Known endocrine diseases
- Pinpoint bony tenderness
- Patient over age 50
- Suspected joint instability

### Spinal x-rays

#### All regions

- Trauma to or potentially involving the spine
- Pain or limitation of motion
- Planned or prior surgery to the spine
- Evaluation of suspected primary and secondary malignancy
- Arthritis
- Suspected congenital anomaly and associated syndromes
- Evaluation of spinal anomaly seen on other imaging
- Follow-up of previous spinal anomaly
- Suspected spinal instability

#### Cervical spine

- Shoulder or arm pain from suspected radiculopathy
- Occipital headache

#### Thoracic spine

- Pain radiating around chest wall
- Osteoporosis with suspicion of compression fracture
- Evaluation of scoliosis and kyphosis

#### Lumbar spine

- Pain radiating into legs
- Osteoporosis with suspicion of compression fracture
- Evaluation of scoliosis and kyphosis
- Paediatric limp, refusal to bear weight or complaint of hip pain

The use of filters, consideration of the heel effect and patient positioning can all help to limit patient exposure but one of the most important considerations is beam collimation. Standard practice involves selecting the appropriate film size(s) for the body part to be imaged and to collimate to the size of the film prior to positioning the patient. However, by further limiting the beam size to include only the area of diagnostic consideration, a further and considerable saving in unnecessary patient exposure can be made. This practice also reduces the amount of scatter, which leads to decreased film fogging and better optical density in the final image.

# Radiation dosage

It is the duty of the radiographer to protect not only their patient from unnecessary exposure but also themselves; their staff and ancillary workers; and any members of the public that might be in the x-ray room (parents, for example, assisting with a paediatric patient).

The principles of radiation protection were originally devised for workers in nuclear energy but find equal application in the healthcare setting (Table 9.5). The first and last of these principles finds particular application in the x-ray room: exposure time is always kept to a minimum, although this is more to limit the chances of any *motion artifact*. Shielding is used extensively in and around the x-ray room (Table 9.6). The source image distance is usually fixed in radiography; however, this principle can be applied to scattered radiation by placing the control console as far away as possible from the patient.

**Table 9.5** The principles of radiation protection

| Principle | Rationale |
|---|---|
| Minimize the exposure time | Total exposure = exposure rate × exposure time |
| Maximize the distance to the source | Exposure reduces according to the inverse square law |
| Use shielding | At 60 kV$_p$ the HVL of lead is 0.11 mm; even a thin layer of lead can offer substantial protection from both primary and scattered radiation |

**Table 9.6** Use of x-ray shielding

| Location | Purpose |
|---|---|
| Lead-based plaster on walls | Protection of patients and staff in adjacent rooms |
| Lead glass/walls around control console | Protection of radiographer |
| Lead aprons | Protection for staff or other persons required to be in x-ray room |
| Body shielding | Protection of radio-sensitive organs (e.g. gonads) |
| Filtration | As discussed previously, filtration is primarily used to improve the optical density when imaging a body part of variable thickness; however, it also has the benefit of reducing patient exposure |

 **DICTIONARY DEFINITION**

**MOTION ARTIFACT**

An *artifact* is something that has been produced artificially; in radiography, it is something that appears on the film that should not be there.

Many x-ray exposures, particularly those involving the spine, are relatively lengthy. A lumbopelvic lateral view may take up to a second to acquire – plenty of time for even the most cooperative patient to inadvertently move. Even a cervical spine exposure may be $^1/_{10}$ to $^1/_{20}$ of a second; contrast that with the $^1/_{60}$ of a second regarded as the minimum necessary in conventional photography to eliminate camera shake or subject movement.

If a radiographic image is blurred, it is as useless as a snapshot with a fuzzy image. The difference is that the latter did not require exposure to ionizing radiation to obtain. For this reason, radiographers always use the shortest exposure time possible to acquire images and minimize the risk of motion artifact that would require retaking of the x-ray.

We have seen already that the intensity of the x-ray beam is measured in roentgens. It is possible to consider patient exposure in terms of the intensity of x-ray photons falling per unit area of skin; however, this is a misleading figure as it tells us nothing about what happens after that point – x-rays that pass through the patient without interacting produce no biological effect; we also have to consider the secondary effects produced by photoelectrons and internally scattered x-rays.

We must therefore start thinking in terms of the **absorbed dose**. This is traditionally measured in *rads*, although its SI unit is the **gray (Gy)**. The difference between the exposure intensity and the absorbed dose is related to the concept of differential absorption that we encountered earlier in the chapter: bone has a higher effective atomic number than soft tissue because it is composed of elements with a higher $Z$ number.

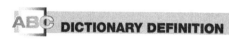 **DICTIONARY DEFINITION**

**ABSORBED DOSE**

The absorbed dose is the energy imparted by radiation per unit mass of the absorbing medium. It is measured in grays (Gy), the definition of which is:

*The absorbed dose of one joule per kilogram of the given medium.*

Traditionally, the unit of the rad has been used; a rad is simply $1/100$ of a gray:

**100 rad = 1 Gy.**

Absorbed dose is also dependent on the $kV_p$ of the incident beam. At lower values, the photoelectric effect will predominate, and this is proportional to the cube of the atomic number of the interacting atom; the absorption by bone is therefore much higher than by soft tissue. At higher $kV_p$ values, Compton interactions predominate and the absorbed doses of bone and soft tissue are similar.

However, the absorbed dose does not take into account the ionizing effect of different types of radiation: an α-particle is much more highly ionizing than an x-ray photon, even if it is much less penetrating. To counter this, different types of radiation are given different **radiation weighting factors ($W_r$)**. The fact that x-rays are assigned a radiation weighting factor = 1 makes the physics (and mathematics) considerably easier as this is the only form of radiation we need to consider as manual physicians.

The absorbed dose also fails to take into consideration the relative sensitivity of different body tissues: thyroid cells are five times more sensitive to ionizing radiation as skin cells; gonadal cells, in turn, are four times more sensitive than thyroid cells (Table 9.7).

This now gives us the information required to calculate the **effective dose (E),** which is used to determine occupational and patient exposure levels. Effective dose is measured in **seiverts (Sv)** or, traditionally, *rem*. It is a sobering thought that the limits for occupational exposure have decreased from a recommended maximum of 10 mSv per day in 1902 to a statutory 50 mSv per *year*! For non-radiation workers, this limit is even lower, just 1 mSv per year.

There is no maximum permitted dose for either diagnostic x-rays or other forms of medical exposure; this is always determined by weighing the risk to the patient against the potential benefit and is, as such, a clinical decision to which no formula can be applied.

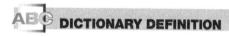 **DICTIONARY DEFINITION**

**EFFECTIVE DOSE**

The effective dose (E) takes into account the radiation weighting factor ($W_r$) of differing types of radiation (= ×1 for x-rays) and the tissue weighting factor ($W_t$), a measure of the relative sensitivity of different organ tissue types:

**E = Absorbed dose × $W_t$ × $W_r$**

It is measured in sieverts (Sv) (or more practically in millisieverts (mSv)); traditionally, the rem (Roentgen Equivalent Man) has been used:

**100 rem = 1 Sv**

**Table 9.7** Weighting factors for different human tissues

| Organ or tissue | Tissue weighting factor ($W_t$) |
|---|---|
| Gonads (testes or ovaries) | 0.2 |
| Red bone marrow | 0.12 |
| Colon | 0.12 |
| Lung | 0.12 |
| Stomach | 0.12 |
| Bladder | 0.05 |
| Breast | 0.05 |
| Liver | 0.05 |
| Oesophagus | 0.05 |
| Thyroid | 0.05 |
| Skin | 0.01 |

 CLINICAL FOCUS

The effects of radiation can be considered in two areas: acute exposure and chronic exposure. The effects of acute exposure on the blood cells, gastrointestinal tract and central nervous system will be inevitably and rapidly fatal at exposures above 50 Gy; however, x-ray beams are not capable of providing these levels of exposure, which are associated with major disasters such as the explosion at the Chernobyl nuclear reactor or the nuclear bombings of Hiroshima and Nagasaki. Even at doses of 10 Gy, death is inevitable, although, after the appearance of initial symptoms of vomiting, nausea and diarrhoea, victims appear to make a recovery (the *latent period*) before succumbing days or weeks later.

Below this value, there is individual variation and clinicians talk in terms of the **LD$_{50}$**, the **L**ethal **D**ose that will kill 50% of any given population (in terms of acute exposure, within 60 days of the exposure taking place; the LD$_{50/60}$). The LD$_{50/60}$ for humans is 3.5 Gy; interestingly, for cockroaches it is 100 Gy, making them the most likely evolutionary starting point for any post-holocaust repopulation.

Of more interest to clinicians are the effects of chronic, low-level radiation exposure, which can damage skin and cause depilation; damage the haemopoietic system, depressing the immune system and predisposing to leukaemia; cataracts;

and genetic damage, which can result in short-term infertility and long-term predisposition to fetal abnormalities at levels as low as 100 mGy.

Of particular concern is the risk of exposing fetal tissue to ionizing radiation. Such exposure, at levels again as low as 100 mGy, can cause spontaneous abortion; congenital abnormalities; mental and physical retardation; and genetic mutation.

Of particular importance is exposure in the first trimester of pregnancy, when exposure to diagnostic levels of radiation can produce an 830% increase in risk of developing childhood leukaemia.

It is for this reason that radiographers apply the **10 day rule**, whereby sexually active females of childbearing capability are only x-rayed within 10 days of the onset of menstruation, when pregnancy is physiologically impossible. Radiographs performed outside of that time scale need be done on a risk/benefit ratio: a suspected spinal fracture in a sexually active female taking the contraceptive pill will carry very different considerations to a routine x-ray on a woman known to be trying to conceive.

# The x-ray image

The manner in which the radiographic image is obtained can have a significant bearing on the amount of exposure the patient has to undergo.

## Grids

The number of scattered x-rays reaching the x-ray detector can be reduced significantly by using a **grid** (Fig. 9.6A). This consists of a grille made from narrow strips of lead approximately 0.1 mm thick, 5 mm high and spaced at 0.5 mm intervals. In order to allow maximum reception of transmitted x-rays whilst minimizing scattered x-rays, the gaps in the grid can be angled to reflect the divergence of the primary beam (Fig. 9.6B). This is known as a **focused grid** and explains why the source–image distance is usually fixed; the angle of the gaps will be dependent on the amount of divergence, and the amount the beam has diverged will depend on the distance it has travelled from its source (the aperture).

In order to prevent the grid from leaving narrow, radio-opaque strips on the final image, the grid is housed in a **Bucky**, which moves the grid across the film and back again during exposure.

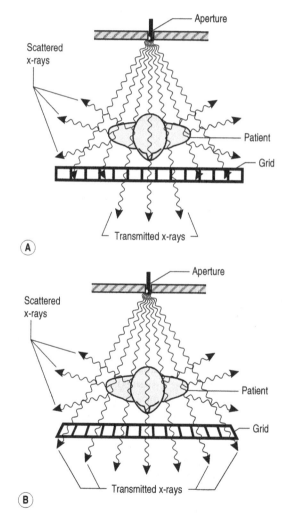

**Figure 9.6** • An x-ray grid, made from strips of lead, prevents many of the scattered x-rays from reaching, and thus fogging, the film (**A**). By angling the grid interspaces to coincide with the angle of divergence of the primary x-rays beam (**B**), the maximum number of transmitted x-rays can reach the film.

## Intensifying screens

Traditionally, x-rays have been taken using photographic film. This film would be placed in a cassette, a rigid, hinged case that has a thin front cover of carbon fibre (to minimize beam attenuation) and a back cover made from heavy metal (to minimize scatter).

The front cover of the cassette also contains an **intensifying screen**, through which the x-ray photons must pass. This screen contains a layer of luminescent material (traditionally phosphor but now using oxysulphides of rare earth elements such as yttrium, lanthanum and gadolinium).

As an x-ray passes through the luminescent layer, it interacts with the outer-shell electrons of thousands of atoms. On each occasion, it gives up a little of its energy to ionize the atom; a free electron then drops back into the 'hole' created and emits a photon as it does so. This photon, whose energy will be associated with the energy level of the electron shell, will have a characteristic wavelength. It is these photons, which have wavelengths of visible light, that are responsible for the majority of the film's exposure. Modern intensifying screens can reduce patient exposure to as little as $1/400$ of that required by an exposure without any screen.

As ever, this comes at a price. The luminescent photons are emitted in random directions; this causes blurring of the image (Fig. 9.7). However, because the layer of luminescent material is thin and the separation from the film small, the benefit in reduced patient exposure easily outweighs the slight reduction in *spatial resolution*, the ability to image small objects that have high subject contrast, such as the interface between bone and soft tissue.

## Image receptor

The device that converts the x-rays leaving the patient into an image capable of being viewed by a radiologist is called an **image receptor**. Traditionally, this has been the combination of the *intensifying screen* and radiographic film, which consists of a thin layer of emulsion mounted on to a flexible base some 50 times thicker than the emulsion.

The emulsion consists of a mixture of gelatin and the active ingredient, silver halide crystals – a lattice of silver ions ($Ag^+$) alternately interspersed with bromine ($Br^-$) and iodine ($I^-$). The physics behind the formation of the **latent image** is still not fully understood but involves the interaction between incident photons (whether x-ray or luminescent) and the atoms of silver, iodine and bromine.

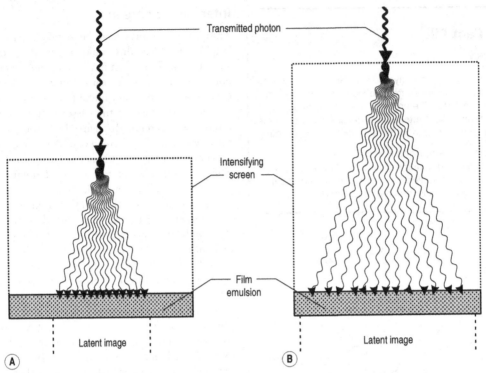

**Figure 9.7** • The intensifying screen allows for interaction between the x-ray photon and outer-shell electron. One high-energy electron can produced many thousands of lower-energy photons in the visible light spectrum. These secondary photons are emitted at random angles; however, if the thickness of the intensifying layer is kept to a minimum, this blurring effect will not detract significantly from the spatial resolution of the final image as can be seen in the difference in latent image size between the thin screen of (**A**) and the thicker screen of (**B**).

If the x-ray is absorbed photoelectrically or undergoes a Compton interaction, then a secondary electron will be produced. These electrons can combine with the silver ions to produce silver atoms, which disrupts the lattice and liberates the silver. The more silver present to react with the developer, the darker the **manifest image** will be when viewed.

Increasingly, digital technology has replaced conventional film. The image receptor consists of a matrix of rows and columns; each cell within this matrix is called a pixel and contains a detector that can count the number of photons incident upon it. This information can be converted into an image in the same way as a digital camera works; it has the advantage that the manifest image requires neither developing nor a view box and is therefore available immediately on the radiologist's computer. The image can also be easily manipulated to compensate for any exposure deficiencies or to instantly magnify and enhance areas of clinical interest. It has one further advantage; no longer are large rooms with endless rows of shelves required to store patients'

images, which can now be stored on hard drives and recalled at the touch of a button.

## Computed tomography

Computed tomography (CT) was developed during the 1970s primarily in answer to the problem of obtaining a radiographic image of the abdominal contents (and other soft tissues). The low contrast offered by the amount of scatter radiation and the superimposition of abdominal structures made this area difficult to image using conventional techniques.

Although the technology behind CT has improved dramatically, the principles remain the same: the patient is placed in a ring of solid-state x-ray detectors and x-rays are taken from multiple angles using a very tightly collimated beam, exposing only a thin slice of the patient. A computer is then used to assemble information from each exposure and produce a digital image of a transverse slice through the body (Fig. 9.8). By moving the beam and detectors a

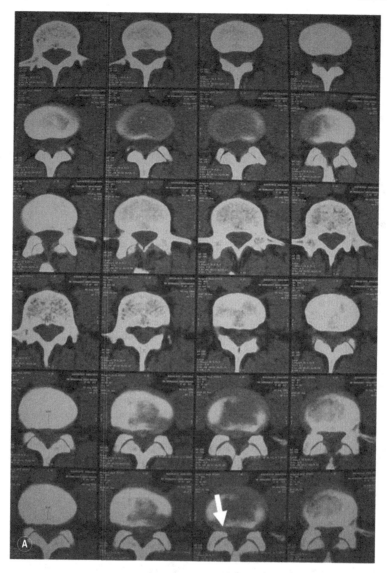

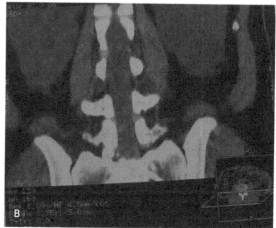

**Figure 9.8** • Computed tomography of the lumbar spine showing a slice by slice progression through the vertebrae (A). These views demonstrate the **soft tissue window**: the osseous structures appear as homogeneously white, whilst the discs, muscles and other soft tissues occupy the grey scale allowing for the radiologist to assess these for abnormalities such as the central and right foraminal disc herniaton seen here (arrow). The images can be reconstructed to any plane. **(B)** demonstrates the lumbar spine in the coronal plane. Once again, this is a soft tissue window; the proximal psoas muscles are particularly well visualized. Courtesy of Michelle Wessely, IFEC, Paris.

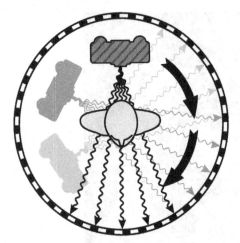

**Figure 9.9 •** A fourth-generation CT scanner involves a stationary array of detectors and a moving x-ray tube. In fifth-generation machines, either can move – as can the patient. The principles however remain the same, multiple films are taken from different angles and the information from each exposure is used to compute a transverse slice through the body.

few millimetres inferiorly or superiorly between each group of exposures, it is possible to build a sequence of films that allow evaluation of both soft tissue and osseous structures, slice by slice (Fig. 9.9).

The physics behind the image acquisition is beyond the scope of this text; however, the principles are easily understood and many of the concepts that apply to conventional x-ray also apply to CT, from x-ray production to dose limitation – but the multiple exposures mean that the patient's effective dose from a CT scan can be higher by an order of magnitude than that from a conventional x-ray.

## Spiral CT

At the end of the 1990s, spiral (or helical) CT was introduced. Instead of the x-ray tube circling the patient whilst stationary and then the patient (or tube) advancing to collect the next 'slice' of the image, the camera circles continuously whilst the patient moves past; this creates a 'spiral' of imaging data.

This has a number of advantages over conventional 'step and shoot' CT. In particular, it reduces motion artifacts, partly because of the increased speed of acquisition and partly because of the way

in which the signal is processed; this is particularly useful when imaging the lung – with conventional CT, a patient, who often had a degree of pulmonary compromise, would have to hold their breath for as much as 45 seconds. Even then, the 'slice by slice' approach left gaps that could lead to neoplastic nodules being poorly imaged or missed altogether. Spiral CT leaves no gaps, although it does not collect enough raw data to allow for an image to be produced in the normal way. Instead, spiral CT uses the increase in computing power to *interpolate* the data, that is 'fill in' the missing information by using the information available from adjacent and overlapping detectors.

By placing two or more cameras side by side, creating a DNA-like double helix, even less information is missed. Because the process is so much quicker, it not only allows for faster imaging of the relevant anatomy, but often means that more anatomy can be imaged in the same time. Most spectacularly of all, spiral CT allows for stunning three-dimensional images of internal structures, allowing the radiologist or clinician to take a virtual tour around the site of pathology (Fig. 9.10).

The system is not without its drawbacks, however. The x-ray tube needs to be larger and more robust; it will regularly be in continuous operation for up to a full minute, and this adds considerably to cost whilst detracting from longevity. Processing time is also increased owing to the amount of data collected and the complexity of the algorithm needed to produce the image.

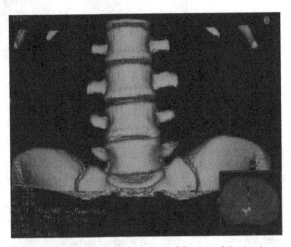

**Figure 9.10 •** A three-dimensional CT scan of the lumbar spine. Note the reduction in L4/5 disc height seen in this anterior view. Courtesy of Michelle Wessely, IFEC, Paris.

# Magnetic resonance imaging

## Introduction

Like CT, magnetic resonance imaging (MRI) is a comparatively new technology, which uses powerful computer algorithms to generate multiplanar slices through the body; however, it provides a greater degree of contrast between the different soft tissues of the body than does CT, which makes it particularly useful in cardiovascular, musculoskeletal, neurological and oncological imaging.

Unlike CT, MRI does not use ionizing radiation, offering a modality that can be used without risk to the patient for both diagnostic imaging and assisting the clinician in management, allowing repeat imaging to monitor the course of a condition or the response to treatment.

Instead of x-rays, MRI uses a powerful magnetic field to align the fields of atoms within the body. Radiofrequency fields are then used to modify the alignment, which causes the atomic nuclei to produce a rotating magnetic field that is detectable by receptors inside the scanner. This signal can then be manipulated to build sufficient information to construct an image of the body.

## Magnetic resonance

As we saw in Chapter 6, subatomic particles such as protons have the property of spin, causing the particle to act as a magnetic dipole, with north and south poles. If two such particles pair up, the laws of magnetic attraction and repulsion mean that they will point in opposite directions and cancel each other out, so that the resultant particle has no overall magnetism. Certain nuclei, such as $^1$H, which consists of a single proton, $^3$He, $^{13}$C, $^{23}$Na or $^{31}$P, have an uneven number of protons and neutrons, and therefore have an unpaired particle, giving the nucleus an overall magnetism, known as the magnetic moment.

This effect is particularly strong in hydrogen, which does not have other particles to 'dilute' the relative strength of its magnetic moment; it is this nucleus therefore that is of primary importance in MRI. Hydrogen has two spin states, sometimes referred to as 'up' and 'down'. When these spins are placed in a strong external magnetic field, such as that found in an MRI scanner, they precess around an axis along the direction of the field (Fig. 9.11). Most protons have low energies and will align with the magnetic field; however, a small number have sufficient energy to have an anti-parallel alignment.

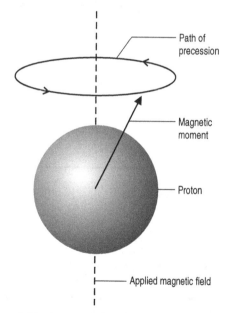

**Figure 9.11** • Precession. The magnetic moment of the proton precesses about the flux lines of the applied magnetic field.

The frequency with which the protons precess ($\omega_0$) is directly proportional to the strength of the magnetic field (B). In a typical scanner field of 1 tesla, hydrogen atoms will precess at precisely 42.6 MHz, which is in the radiowave band of the electromagnetic spectrum (Table 8.1). This value, which varies from nucleus to nucleus as well as with magnetic field strength, is known as the *Larmor frequency*.

## Energy absorption

By applying a radiofrequency pulse of this value at 90° to the magnetic field, it causes the hydrogen nuclei, *and only the hydrogen nuclei*, to resonate; other nuclei – even if they have dipoles – will have their own unique resonant frequency for a given magnetic field. The hydrogen nuclei absorb energy from the pulse, which increases their net energy and, therefore, the number of high-energy anti-parallel protons. If exactly the right amount of energy is applied, this will result in the equal magnetic fields of the combined hydrogen magnetic moments cancelling each other out; effectively the **net magnetization vector** of the hydrogen nuclei lies at 90° to the applied field.

## Phase coherence

The applied radiofrequency pulse also causes the rotating magnetic moments of the hydrogen nuclei to move into phase with each other; this is known as **phase coherence**. It affects all of the nuclei, so the low-energy 'spin up' protons are in phase both with each other and with the high-energy 'spin down' protons. This means that the net magnetization vector now precesses in exactly the same way as the individual protons at the Lamor frequency.

---

**Fact File**

**FLIPPING**

Lay explanations of MRI often refer to the hydrogen nuclei being 'flipped'. It is a key learning point that these protons **do not move**. They are not flipped on to their sides, nor are they turned upside down at any point.

It is *only* their magnetic moments that move, in exactly the same way that the reversal of the Earth's magnetic poles over history (Ch. 6) has never affected the orientation of the planet or the direction of its rotation.

---

## The MR signal

The image detector in MRI is an electromagnetic coil, which acts as a receiver. It is placed at 90° to the applied magnetic field in what is known as the **transverse plane**; the direction of the magnetic field is the **longitudinal plane.**

Whilst the net magnetization vector lies in the transverse plane, its precession means that it passes across the receiver, inducing a voltage in the coil. This is the **MR signal**. Because the motion of precession is circular, it induces an alternating current in exactly the same way that a spinning magnet induces an alternating current in a power-generating coil.

When the radiofrequency pulse is removed, the protons begin to lose energy, and the difference between the numbers of spin up and spin down protons increases again until the net magnetization vector lies in the longitudinal plane. As this happens, the MR signal decays: remember, electromotive force is *only* induced by the component of the magnetic field lying perpendicular to it – the longitudinal component of the vector induces no current in the receptor coil. This decrease in the magnitude of the MR signal is called **free induction decay** ('free' because it happens when the hydrogen nuclei are free of the radiofrequency pulse).

The removal of the radiofrequency pulse also causes the net magnetization vector to stop precessing. This loss of phase coherence is called **transverse (or $T_2$) relaxation** whereas the recovery of longitudinal magnetization is called **longitudinal (or $T_1$) relaxation.**

## Contrast

Molecules, as we know, are constantly in motion; the greater the motion, the greater the inertia.

Most molecules in the body contain hydrogen; amongst the commonest of these are fat and water. Water molecules are small and therefore have low inertia; however, they have a high inherent energy, which makes it more difficult for them to absorb more energy efficiently. By contrast, fat molecules consist of long chains of hydrocarbons – a central chain of interlinked carbon atoms with hydrogen attached to the sides. They therefore have high inertia and also possess a low inherent energy, meaning that they readily absorb additional energy.

These characteristics mean that the different tissues in the body have different relaxation times and this is used to produce contrast: areas of high signal (which appears white), medium signal (grey) and low signal (black) which reflect the strength of the MR signal recovered from different locations within the sample.

In addition to relaxation times, contrast is also affected by a number of other factors, including the relative density of the excited hydrogen and the **extrinsic factors** controlled by the radiographer. The two most important of these are the **repetition time (TR)** and the **echo time (TE)**.

## Repetition time (TR)

This is the time between the *applications* of the radiofrequency pulses and is measured in milliseconds (ms). The TR affects the length of the relaxation period.

## Echo time (TE)

This is the length of time between the start of a radiofrequency pulse and the collection of the MR signal; it is also measured in milliseconds. The TE affects the relaxation times after the *removal* of

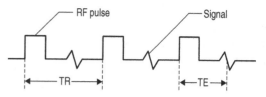

**Figure 9.12** • Pulse sequences. The radiofrequency pulse (RF) is applied at regular intervals. The repetition time (TR) is the time between the applications of the pulse. The echo time (TE) is the time from the application of the pulse to the collection of the magnetic resonance signal.

the radiofrequency pulses and also the peak of the signal induced in the receiver coil.

The differentiation of these factors is shown in Figure 9.12.

The precise design of the imaging pulse sequences allows one contrast mechanism to be emphasized while the others are minimized. This ability to choose different contrast mechanisms is what gives MRI its tremendous flexibility. In the spine (Fig. 9.13), the spinal canal structures have very different appearance

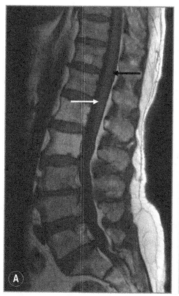
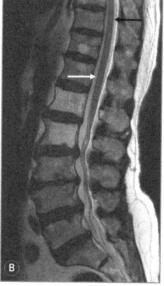

**Figure 9.13** • Two midsagittal MR images of the lumbar spine. (A) $T_1$-weighted image. Note how the neurons of gray matter (black arrows), have a medium intensity (grey) signal whilst the cerebrospinal fluid (white arrows) appears dark. These contrasts are reversed in the $T_2$-weighted image (B). Of incidental note is the higher intensity signal in the body of the T11 vertebra on both $T_1$-weighted and $T_2$-weighted images; this represents a haemangioma. Courtesy of Michelle Wessely, IFEC, Paris.

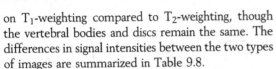

on $T_1$-weighting compared to $T_2$-weighting, though the vertebral bodies and discs remain the same. The differences in signal intensities between the two types of images are summarized in Table 9.8.

There are conditions in which it is not possible to generate enough image contrast to adequately show the anatomy or pathology of clinical interest by adjusting the imaging parameters alone. In such cases, a contrast agent may be administered. This may be as simple as getting the patient to drink a glass of water to assist in imaging the stomach and small bowel; however, most of the contrast agents used in MR are selected for their specific magnetic properties.

The most common paramagnetic contrast agent used is gadolinium. Gadolinium-enhanced tissues and fluids appear extremely bright on $T_1$-weighted images and this provides high sensitivity for detection of vascular tissues such as tumours and permits assessment of brain perfusion in cases of cerebrovascular incidents. The addition of gadolinium adds a considerable degree of invasiveness and potential toxicity to the imaging procedure and is contraindicated in patients with impaired kidney function (nephrogenic fibrosis).

## Proton density weighting

By reducing $T_1$-weighting and $T_2$-weighting effects using a long TR and a short TE respectively, it is possible to create an image that reflects the relative proton density of different tissues. A high signal is produced in areas that have a high proton density and vice versa; this can be used to identify certain pathologies.

**Table 9.8** Signal intensities seen in $T_1$-weighted and $T_2$-weighted images

| Structure | $T_1$-weighting | $T_2$-weighting |
|---|---|---|
| Air | No signal | No signal |
| Avascular necrosis | Low signal | High signal |
| Calcification | No/low signal | No/low signal |
| Cortical bone | No/low signal | No/low signal |
| Cysts | Low signal | High signal |
| Degenerative fatty deposition | High signal | Low signal |
| Fast-flowing blood | No signal | No signal |
| Fat | High signal | Low signal |
| Haemangioma | High signal | High signal |
| Infarction | Low signal | High signal |
| Infection | Low signal | High signal |
| Lipoma | High signal | Low signal |
| Scar tissue | No signal | No signal |
| Sclerosis | Low signal | High signal |
| Slow-flowing blood | High signal | High signal |
| Tendons | No signal | No signal |
| Tumours | Low signal | High signal |

 CLINICAL FOCUS

Although MRI is generally safe and noninvasive, there are circumstances where it is contraindicated.

### MRI contraindications or relative contraindications

- Brain aneurysm clip
- Implanted neural stimulator
- Implanted cardiac pacemaker or defibrillator
- Cochlear implant
- Ocular foreign body (e.g. metal shavings)
- Other implanted medical devices: (e.g. Swan Ganz catheter)
- Insulin pump
- Metal shrapnel or bullet
- First trimester pregnancy
- Patients with unstable angina.

Claustrophobia, which affects up to 10% of patients, used to be regarded as a relative contraindication and patients would often need sedation before being able to enter the scanner. Recent improvement in scanning technology has allowed the advent of the 'open' scanner whereby, instead of entering a narrow tunnel, patients lie between two plates that are open to the sides (Fig. 9.14).

Certain patients are contraindicated for the administration of MRI contrast agents:
- Lactating women
- Patients with haemoglobinopathies
- Renal disease (decreased glomerular filtration rate).

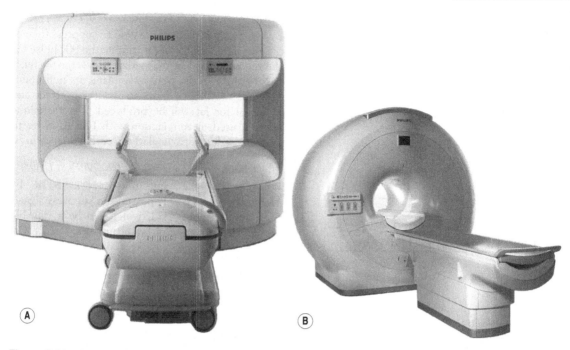

**Figure 9.14** ● Recent improvements in receptor analysis have allowed the development of open-sided MRI scanners (**A**), which ameliorate the effects of claustrophobia – a condition that affects up to 10% of people and can preclude the use of a conventional scanner (**B**). Courtesy of the Cheltenham Imaging Centre.

## Pulse sequences

There are a number of ways in which the operator can further manipulate the image. A pulse sequence is defined as a series of radiofrequency pulses, which may be further modified by the application of **gradients**, a change in magnetic flux density along the length of the scanner, and intervening time periods.

The main purpose of these pulse sequences is to manipulate the TE and TR to produce different types of contrast and to re-phase the spin of the hydrogen nuclei, which tend to gradually un-phase owing to inhomogeneities in the applied magnetic field causing signal decay.

### Spin echo (SE)

**Spin echo (SE)** uses a radiofrequency pulse to re-phase in the manner already described; however, in addition to the initial 90° pulse, a second pulse is added at 180° to rephase any nuclei that have decreased their precessional frequency and reform the net magnetization vector. This regenerates the induced MR signal, which had been decaying, and this regeneration can be measured. The regenerated signal is called an **echo** and, because a radiofrequency pulse has been used to generate it, it is specifically termed *spin echo*. Spin echo is use to produce $T_1$-weighted (short TR, short TE) and $T_2$-weighted (long TR, long TE) images. By adding an additional 180° pulse (these pulses do not effect TR, which is still defined as the gap between the application of 90° pulses), it is possible to produce two images per pulse. Both will have a long TR; however the first will have a short TE and produces a proton density weighted image. The second has long TR and TE and is used to produce a standard $T_2$-weighted image (Fig. 9.15). This is known as a **dual echo** sequence.

The main problem with methods of image acquisition is the length of time taken; this can be reduced by **fast** or **turbo spin echo (FSE/TSE)** whereby a chain of 180° re-phasing pulses are applied in between the 90° pulses. This can reduce the imaging time by factors of as much as 16; however, there is an inevitable trade-off with image quality and artifacts from blood flow, which usually is not imaged but can be 'frozen' if the image acquisition is fast enough. This technique depends on altering the *gradient* between each pulse so that the phase is slightly shifted and can be differentiated by the computer algorithm.

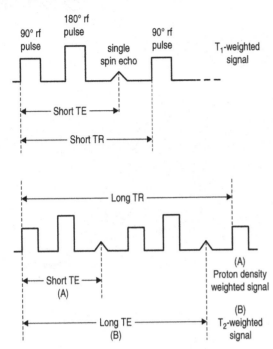

**Figure 9.15** • Pulse sequences used to produce T1-weighted, T2-weighted and proton density weighted signals using spine echo and dual echo sequences.

## Inversion recovery (IR)

If, instead of beginning with a 90° radiofrequency pulse, a spin echo sequence begins with a 180° pulse then the net magnetization vector will be inverted (the TR now becomes the time interval between successive inverting 180° pulses). This pulse is then followed by a second pulse at 90°, which creates a magnetic resonance signal in the induction coils. The time between the two pulses is called the **time from inversion (TI)** and this process is called **inversion recovery**. If this signal is then rephased as before with a rephasing 180° pulse (as distinct from the *inverting* 180° pulse; this pulse does *not* influence TR), then an echo pulse can be produced.

There are three inversion sequences that are in common diagnostic use.

## Fast inversion recovery

This is a mixture between inversion recovery and fast spin echo, which has the advantage of reducing image acquisition time, which can otherwise be lengthy. The gap between the turbo pulses can be made shorter (for $T_1$-weighting) or longer (for $T_2$-weighting).

## Short TI inversion recovery (STIR)

By using a short TI, it is possible to suppress the net magnetization vector of fat, timing the 90° pulse for the moment that net magnetization vector for fat is passing through the transverse plane, its null point. The pulse will then have no induction effect and no signal for fat will be produced. The technique is often used in conjunction with FSE in order to evaluate oedema, particularly in cerebral structures.

## Fluid attenuated inversion recovery (FLAIR)

Using exactly the same principles as STIR, by *lengthening* the TI, it is possible to suppress signals from cerebrospinal fluid, which can be a valuable tool in the evaluation of brain tumours.

# Positron emission tomography (PET)

Used in both nuclear medicine and neurological and physiological research, PET is an imaging technique that produces a three-dimensional image of functional processes in the body. The principle on which it works is the introduction into the body of a positron-emitting radionuclide tracer by means of a biologically active molecule (you will recall from Chapter 8 that a positron is the anti-particle of the electron).

Once the molecule, most commonly a glucose analogue, fluorodeoxyglucose (FDG), is absorbed into the body's systems, the scanner then detects pairs of γ-rays emitted indirectly by the tracer. The relative intensity of the gamma-ray pairs allows images of tracer concentration in three-dimensional space within the body to be reconstructed by computer analysis. In modern scanners, this reconstruction is often accomplished with the aid of a CT x-ray scan performed on the patient during the same session, in the same machine.

PET is used heavily in clinical oncology both to image tumours and to search for metastases and for clinical diagnosis of certain diffuse brain diseases such as those causing various types of dementias. It is also an important research tool to map normal human brain and heart function.

Unlike some imaging scans such as CT and MRI, which isolate organic anatomical changes within the body, PET is capable of detecting areas of molecular biology detail at a stage prior to an actual anatomical change. PET does this by using radiolabelled

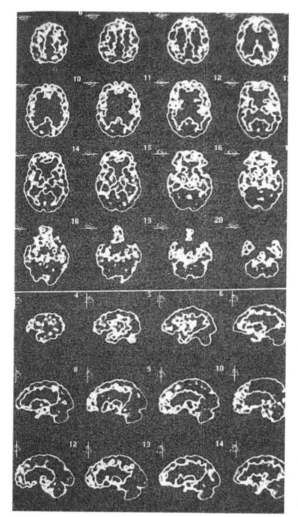

**Figure 9.16** • PET of the cranium showing vascular structures in the axial (upper 16 images) and sagittal (lower 12 images) planes. Reproduced from Youmans Neurological Surgery Online, 5th edition, edited by H. Richard Winn, 2004, Elsevier Churchill Livingstone, with permission.

molecular probes that have different rates of uptake, depending on the type and function of tissue involved. Changes in the regional blood flow in various anatomical structures can be detected, visualized and relatively quantified with a PET scan (Fig. 9.16).

PET is a particularly valuable technique for certain conditions, because it is can target the radiochemicals used for particular bodily functions (Table 9.9). The protocols for PET scanning remain the same: following the introduction of the **short-lived** radioactive tracer isotope, usually into the patient's bloodstream, there is a latent period whilst the marker is absorbed; this varies from minutes to

a few hours (for the most commonly used molecule, FDG, the waiting period is approximately 1 hour). Once the active molecule has become concentrated in the tissues of interest, the research subject or patient is placed in the imaging scanner, which is not dissimilar in appearance to that of a CT scanner.

As the radioisotope undergoes decay, it emits positrons ($\beta^+$). These almost immediately meet with electrons; as we know, the result of their mutual annihilation is a pair of photons in the $\gamma$ radiation spectrum (511 keV), which move in diametrically opposite directions. These are detected by scintillating material in the scanning device, creating a burst of light, which is detected in similar ways to CT or digital x-rays. The technique is dependent upon the simultaneous detection of photon pairs; photons that do not arrive within a few nanoseconds of each other are ignored.

PET scans are increasingly read alongside CT or MRI scans, giving the clinician both anatomical and metabolic information; indeed, modern PET scanners are now available with integrated CT scanners. Because the two scans can be performed in immediate sequence during the same session, with the patient not changing position between the two types of scan, the two sets of images can be perfectly correlated. This is particularly useful in showing detailed views of moving organs or structures with higher amounts of anatomical variation.

In order to limit patient exposure, the radioisotopes used in PET scanning typically have short half-lives: such as $^{11}C$ (20 min), $^{13}N$ (10 min), $^{15}O$ (2 min), and $^{18}F$ (110 min). The main limitation to the widespread use of PET is the high costs of the cyclotrons needed to produce the short-lived radionuclides used in PET scanning, in addition to the costs of the scanners themselves. This limitation restricts clinical PET primarily to the use of tracers labelled with $^{18}F$, which has a sufficiently long half-life (110 min) to be transported a reasonable distance before use. It has the advantage that, with modern processing power, it can produce a unique three-dimensional, real-time insight into metabolic activity of a wide range of cell types.

# Diagnostic ultrasonography

Ultrasound is one of the most widely used diagnostic tools in modern medicine and has been used to image the human body for at least 50 years. The technology has a number of advantages over the other forms of diagnostic imaging that we have encountered in this

**Table 9.9** Medical applications for positron emission tomography (PET)

## Oncology

PET scanning with the tracer fluorine-18 (F-18) fluorodeoxyglucose (FDG), is widely used in clinical oncology. This tracer is taken up by cells that utilize glucose, which are metabolically much more active in rapidly growing malignant tumours. FDG is trapped in any cell which takes it up until it decays; this results in intense radio-labelling of tissues with high glucose uptake, such as the brain, liver and many neoplasms. This allows the technique to be used for diagnosis, staging, and monitoring treatment of cancers. It is of particular use in:
- Lung cancers
- Hodgkin's disease
- Non-Hodgkin's lymphoma
- Metastatic disease

It is also a useful means of assessing the patient's response to cancer therapy: the risk to the patient from lack of knowledge about disease progress is much greater than the risk from the test radiation.

## Neurology

Neuroimaging in PET is based on the assumption that areas of high blood flow in the brain, as detected by an $^{15}O$ or FDG tracer, are associated with brain activity. It is also now possible to use new radio-tracers that allow neuroreceptor pools to be visualized, which may have significant consequences for a wide range of neurological pathologies. At present, the principle use of PET in neurology is the detection of Alzheimer's disease and other conditions of dementure, which can be done at an earlier stage than with MRI.

## Neuropsychology and psychiatry

The same selective neuroreceptor binding tracers that have been developed for neurological use also allow the examination of links between specific psychological processes or disorders and brain activity. Compounds that bind selectively to dopamine, serotonin andopioid receptors have been used successfully to evaluate:
- Schizophrenia
- Substance abuse
- Mood disorders

## Cardiology

The applications of PET in detecting atherosclerosis and vascular disease and determining the risk of cerebrovascular incidents has been determined but its cost-effectiveness remains unclear.

## Pharmacology

In pre-clinical trials, it is possible to radio-label a new drug and inject it into animals. The uptake of the drug, the tissues in which it concentrates, and its eventual elimination, can be monitored far more quickly, humanely and cost effectively than the older technique of killing and dissecting the animals to discover the same information.

chapter (Table 9.10). It does require some care in its application: ultrasonic energy can enhance the inflammatory response and heat soft tissue.

Ultrasonographic scanning in medical diagnosis uses exactly the same principles as sonar. Pulses of high-frequency ultrasound (> 1 MHz), created by a piezoelectric transducer (see Chapter 10) are directed into the body toward the target structure.

In the same way in which we have seen other waves behave, as the sound waves traverse the internal structures of the body, they can be reflected, absorbed or transmitted. It is the reflected waves that are used to form the diagnostic image; the intensity and time delay of the reflections can be analyzed to obtain information regarding the internal organs and surrounding structures. Transmitted waves are useful in the passive sense in that they are free to continue on their journey and to interact with deeper tissues.

The absorption of the sound wave is the limitation of ultrasonography. Although greater resolution can be obtained by using higher frequencies, one of the properties of waves is that higher frequencies tend to be much more strongly absorbed and it is this trade-off that ultimately limits the clarity, contrast and detail that can be obtained with medical ultrasonography.

There are a number of modes in which the ultrasound scanner can operate and these offer different diagnostic information to the clinician:

**Table 9.10** Advantages of ultrasonography over other forms of diagnostic imaging

| Feature | Advantage |
| --- | --- |
| Portable | The scanner can be easily transported to the patient and the scan carried out in situ |
| Cheap | The costs of an ultrasonography machine is just a few percent of that of an x-ray unit and only a few per mil of CT, MRI or PET scanners |
| Training | The training required for an ultrasonographer is much shorter, easier and cheaper than for other forms of diagnostic imaging |
| Non-invasive | Ultrasound uses no ionizing radiation or contrast media and does not require enclosure in a scanner. This has made it the first choice for obstetric scanning for two generations |
| Fast | Because of the lower costs and easier availability, waiting times for ultrasonography in public health care can often be much shorter |
| Data acquisition | The data from an ultrasound scan is displayed in real time on a screen and can be recorded electronically |
| Speed | An ultrasound scan usually takes just a few minutes, comparable with x-ray but significantly faster than CT, PET or MRI |

## A-scan mode

This technique uses a single transducer to scan along a line in the body with the resultant echoes being plotted as a function of time. This technique is primarily used for mensuration to determine the sizes of internal organs.

## B-scan mode

Rather than a single transducer, the B-scan mode utilizes a linear array of transducers to scan a plane in the body; the resultant tomograph is displayed on a television screen as a two-dimensional plot.

## M-scan mode

This mode is used to record the motion of internal organs, for instance, cardiac imaging, where the technique can offer invaluable information in the investigation of heart dysfunction.

# Obstetric ultrasonography

Because it does not use ionizing radiation, ultrasound has become one of the staples of obstetric diagnosis (Fig. 9.17) and is now performed routinely at least once during nearly all pregnancies (normally at 12 weeks post-conception). In some countries, it is now also the practice to carry out a second scan at 20 weeks (Table 9.11).

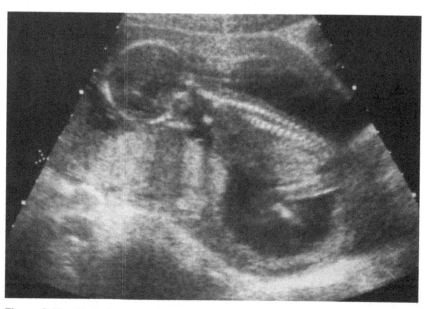

**Figure 9.17** ● Obstetric ultrasound. The fetal spine is particularly clearly seen – note the absence of lordotic or kyphotic curves.

**Table 9.11** Purposes of obstetric ultrasound

- Assess foetal growth and development
- Check for foetal movement
- Confirmation foetal viability
- Determination of gestational age
- Determination of the baby's sex
- Determination of the number of fetuses (multiple pregnancy)
- Location of foetus (intrauterine versus ectopic)
- Location of the placenta in relation to the cervix
- Identify major physical abnormalities
- Identify foetal heartbeat

Ultrasonic imaging is also utilized during the process of drawing off amniotic fluid to test for birth defects. The high-resolution, real-time images are used to guide the needle and minimize the chances of damage to the fetus or surrounding tissue.

## CLINICAL FOCUS

Fetal imaging by ultrasound has become increasingly common since the 1960s and is now a routine part of obstetric management in many Western countries. Although it was originally regarded as entirely without risk to the fetus, some evidence is now emerging that the procedure is not without some side-effects. An epidemiological study in Sweden has shown that men whose mothers underwent scanning during pregnancy were significantly more likely to be left-handed than those who had not had a scan. After 1975, when a second, later scan was introduced as routine practice, there was a 32% increase in the likelihood of left-handedness when compared to a control group.

Animal experiments have also verified changes in fetal cells, including cell death, neuronal migration and gastrointestinal bleeding in animal experiments, although these are often hard to translate into possible human effects.

Recent reviews have concluded that, although there is no direct evidence of harm, obstetric ultrasound should not be used for non-medical purposes (e.g. fetal 'snapshots'). They also acknowledge that carrying out the research on humans to verify the animal findings presented ethical problems that were 'almost certainly insurmountable'.

Most studies conclude that the potential benefits to maternal and fetal well-being outweigh any risks, although they also suggest that it would be prudent to eliminate unnecessary or unwarranted imaging and to apply risk/benefit decision making in the same manner as other diagnostic imaging procedures.

## Musculoskeletal ultrasound

Musculoskeletal ultrasound (MSU) is an excellent technique for evaluating soft tissue and cortical involvement in many conditions, particularly those affecting the extremities. The usefulness of MSU has been increasingly recognized by rheumatologists and orthopaedists over the past decade and the technique is now regularly used to detect and monitor early erosions and joint effusions in rheumatoid arthritis and other inflammatory arthropathies. MSU can also provide valuable information in the location and evaluation of trauma both to soft tissues and osseous structures. Because of the lack of ionizing radiation, there is no impediment to bilateral comparative imaging: the sonographer can compare the injured side to the good side to help identify abnormalities (Fig. 9.18).

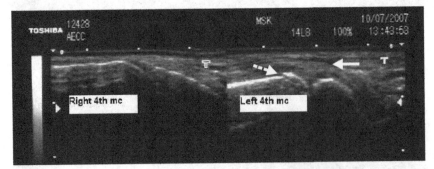

**Figure 9.18** • Musculoskeletal ultrasound of the 4th metacarpal. Comparison with the normal right side allows easy identification of a fracture (dotted arrow) and associated soft tissue swelling (arrow). Figure courtesy of Jane Cook, AECC, Bournemouth UK. © *Clinical Chiropractic* 2008.

# Doppler ultrasonography

Ultrasonic Doppler techniques have become very important in evaluating conditions that involve hae-modynamics (blood flow). If an ultrasound beam is reflected off an oncoming pulse of arterial blood, it undergoes a Doppler shift of a few kilohertz and this can be easily detected or, in some cases, even heard directly by the sonographer physician.

Using this technique, it is possible to detect and monitor the heartbeat of a fetus long before a stethoscope can pick up the sound. Arterial diseases such as arteriosclerosis and vascular conditions such as deep vein thrombosis can also be diagnosed, and the healing of blood vessels can be monitored following surgery.

By combining B-scan and Doppler imaging (known as duplex scanning) blood flow can be measured; this is used extensively to diagnose heart valve defects.

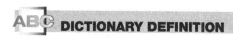 **DICTIONARY DEFINITION**

**THE DOPPLER EFFECT**

When waves leave a source, the speed at which they do so is a combination of the speed of the sound plus (or minus) the speed of the object from which they are emitted. The most everyday aspect of this phenomenon, first described by

Austrian physicist Christian Doppler in 1842, is seen as an emergency vehicle passes. As the vehicle approaches, the pitch of the siren appears to be higher; as it passes and moves away, the pitch lowers.

This is because the speed of the vehicle is initially added to the energy of the waveform; then, as it moves away, it is subtracted from it. However, the speed of many waves is fixed: the speed of light, $c$, is a constant; the speed of sound, whilst dependent on the medium through which the waves are being propagated, is also constant for that medium ($340 \text{ ms}^{-1}$ through the atmosphere at sea level). This change in wave energy is therefore represented by changes to the frequency (and, obviously, wavelength).

The Doppler effect is used in astronomy to measure the speed of other stars and galaxies and to determine whether they are moving away from us and, if so, how fast. This is what is meant by 'red shift': stellar objects moving away from the Earth have their spectra shifted towards the lower frequency (red) end of the visible spectrum.

In Doppler ultrasound, the speed of the arterial pulse adds to the velocity of the reflected waves and increases its frequency. The difference between the emitted ultrasound pulse and the reflected one can be easily detected.

 Learning Outcomes

If you have understood the contents of this chapter, you should now understand:
- How x-ray machines work, their applications and limitations
- The health risks for patients and operators exposed to ionizing radiation
- The evolution and usage of computer tomography
- The means by which nuclear magnetic resonance occurs and how this can be used to obtain diagnostic images of varying types of tissue
- The physics relating to the formation of nuclear positrons and how they can be generated and detected
- The medical uses for ultrasonography.

# Bibliography

Abramowicz, J.S., Barnett, S.B., Duck, F.A., et al., 2008. Fetal thermal effects of diagnostic ultrasound. Journal of Ultrasound Medicine 27, 541–559.

Absolute Astronomy. Thermionic emission. Online. Available from: www.absoluteastronomy.com/topics/Thermionic_emission 28 September 2008, 11:35 BST.

Allen, R., Schwarz, C. (Eds.), 1998. The Chambers dictionary. Chambers Harrap, Edinburgh.

Allison, W., 2006. Interactions of ionising radiation. In: Fundamental physics for probing and imaging. Oxford University Press, Oxford, pp. 55–84.

Allison, W., 2006. Analysis and damage by irradiation. In: Fundamental physics for probing and imaging. Oxford University Press, Oxford, pp. 157–206.

Allison, W., 2006. Imaging with magnetic resonance. In: Fundamental physics for probing and imaging. Oxford University Press, Oxford, pp. 207–226.

Allison, W., 2006. Medical imaging and therapy with ionising radiation. In: Fundamental physics for probing and imaging. Oxford University Press, Oxford, pp. 233–268.

Allison, W., 2006. Ultrasound imaging and therapy. In: Fundamental physics for probing and imaging. Oxford University Press, Oxford, pp. 267–306.

American College of Radiology, 2003. ACR guidelines for the performance of spine radiographs in adults and children. Online. Available from: www.acr.org 4 October 2008, 20:15 BST.

Atlee, Z.J., Gager, R.M., 1972. Method of manufacturing of x-ray tube having thoriated tungsten filament. United States Patent 3846006, 24 December.

Balint, P., Sturrock, R., Musculoskeletal ultrasound imaging: a new diagnostic tool for the rheumatologist? Br. J. Rheumatol. 36, 1141–1142.

Bushong, S.C., 2004. The x-ray imaging system. In: Radiological science for technologists: physics, biology and protection, eighth ed. Mosby, St Louis, pp. 108–127.

Bushong, S.C., 2004. The X–ray tube. In: Radiological science for technologists: physics, biology and protection, eighth ed. Mosby, St Louis, pp. 128–146.

Bushong, S.C., 2004. X-ray production. In: Radiological science for technologists: physics, biology and protection, eighth ed. Mosby, St Louis, pp. 147–158.

Bushong, S.C., 2004. The radiographic image. In: Radiological science for technologists: physics, biology and protection, eighth ed. Mosby, St Louis, pp. 190–314.

Bushong, S.C., 2004. Digital radiography. In: Radiological science for technologists: physics, biology and protection, eighth ed. Mosby, St Louis, pp. 108–127.

Bushong, S.C., 2004. Computed tomography. In: Radiological science for technologists: physics, biology and protection, eighth ed. Mosby, St Louis, pp. 441–457.

Bushong, S.C., 2004. Health Physics. In: Radiological science for technologists: physics, biology and protection, eighth ed. Mosby, St Louis, pp. 93–107.

Cook, J., Wessely, M., 2008. Wrist pain in a chiropractor: case discussion. Clinical Chiropractic 11, 111–114.

DeVries, R.M., Manne, A., 2003. Cervical MRI. Part I: a basic overview. Clinical Chiropractic 6, 137–143.

Deyo, R.A., Diehl, A.K., 1986. Lumbar spine films in primary care: current use and effects of selective ordering criteria. J. Gen. Intern. Med. 1 (1), 20–25.

Encyclopædia Britannica. Gray. Encyclopædia Britannica, 2008. Encyclopædia Britannica 2006 Ultimate Reference Suite. DVD 6 October 2008.

Encyclopædia Britannica. Positron emission tomography. Encyclopædia Britannica, 2008. Encyclopædia Britannica 2006 Ultimate Reference Suite. DVD 6 October 2008.

Encyclopædia Britannica. Sievert. Encyclopædia Britannica, 2008. Encyclopædia Britannica 2006 Ultimate Reference Suite. DVD 6 October 2008.

European Nuclear Society, Tissue weighting factor. Online. Available from: www.euronuclear.org 6 October 2008, 10:30 BST.

aus der Fünten, K., Cook, J., 2008. Correlation between musculoskeletal ultrasound, magnetic resonance imaging, arthroscopic and clinical findings in a 30-year-old male with a medial meniscus ganglion: a case report. Clinical Chiropractic 11, 83–89.

Garrood, J.R., 1979. Electricity and electrostatics. In: Physics. Intercontinental Book Productions, Maidenhead, pp. 171–231.

Garrood, J.R., 1979. Electromagnetism. In: Physics. Intercontinental Book Productions, Maidenhead, pp. 232–275.

Garrood, J.R., 1979. Nuclear and quantum physics. In: Physics. Intercontinental Book Productions, Maidenhead, pp. 276–314.

Halliday, D., Resnick, R., Walker, J., 2005. X-ray diffraction. In: Fundamentals of physics, seventh ed. John Wiley, Hoboken, pp. 909–918.

Halliday, D., Resnick, R., Walker, J., 2005. Magnetic resonance. In: Fundamentals of physics, seventh ed. John Wiley, Hoboken, pp. 1015–1016.

Hay, G.A., Hughes, D.H., 1983. Electromagnetic radiation. In: First year physics for radiographers, third ed. Ballière Tindall, Eastbourne, pp. 127–138.

Hay, G.A., Hughes, D.H., 1983. Thermionic emission and x-ray tubes. In: First year physics for radiographers, third ed. Ballière Tindall, Eastbourne, pp. 161–196.

Hay, G.A., Hughes, D.H., 1983. X-ray control and indicating equipment. In: First year physics for radiographers, third ed. Ballière Tindall, Eastbourne, pp. 219–230.

Hay, G.A., Hughes, D.H., 1983. Interaction of x-rays and gamma rays with matter. In: First year physics for radiographers, third ed. Ballière Tindall, Eastbourne, pp. 231–259.

Hay, G.A., Hughes, D.H., 1983. Radiological protection. In: First year physics for radiographers, third ed. Ballière Tindall, Eastbourne, pp. 287–304.

Hay, G.A., Hughes, D.H., 1983. Ultrasound. In: First year physics for radiographers, third ed. Ballière Tindall, Eastbourne, pp. 320–332.

Health Canada. In: Radiation: Safety Code 34, Radiation Protection and Safety for Industrial X-Ray Equipment, Appendix II - Recommended Dose Limits for Ionizing Radiation. December 2007. Online. Available from: www.hc-sc.gc.ca.

Health Physics Society, Regulatory dose limits. 2 July 2008. Online. Available from: hps.org.

Helms, C.A., 2005. Unnecessary investigations. In: Fundamentals of Skeletal Radiology, third ed. Elsevier, Philadelphia, pp. 1–6.

Hirshfeld, Jr., J.W., Balter, S., Brinker, J.A., et al., 2004. ACCF/AHA/HRS/SCAI clinical competence statement on physician knowledge to optimize patient safety and image quality in fluoroscopically guided invasive cardiovascular procedures. A report of the American College of Cardiology Foundation/American Heart Association/American College of Physicians Task Force on Clinical Competence and Training. J. Am. Coll. Cardiol. 44, 2259–2282.

HM Government (UK), 2000. Statutory Instrument 2000 No. 1059: The Ionising Radiation (Medical Exposure) Regulations 2000. HMSO, London.

Lauterbur, P.C., 1973. Image formation by induced local interactions: examples of employing nuclear magnetic resonance. Nature 242, 190–191.

Klunk, W.E., Engler, H., Nordberg, A., et al., 2004. Imaging brain amyloid in Alzheimer's disease with Pittsburgh Compound-B. Ann. Neurol. 55, 306–319.

Matthews R. 2001. Ultrasound scans linked to brain damage in babies. Epidemiology 12, 618.

Stratmeyer ME, Greenleaf JF, Dalecki D, et al., 2008. Fetal ultrasound: mechanical effects. Journal of Ultrasound Medicine 27:597–605.

The Nobel Foundation, 1964. Felix Bloch: the Nobel Prize in physics 1952 From: Nobel Lectures, Physics 1942–1962. Elsevier, Amsterdam. Online. Available from: nobelprize. org/nobel_prizes/physics/laureates/ 1952/bloch-bio.html 10 October 2008 17:00 BST.

The Nobel Foundation, 1964. E. M. Purcell: the Nobel prize in Physics 1952. From: Nobel Lectures, Physics 1942–1962. Elsevier, Amsterdam. Online. Available from: nobelprize. org/nobel_prizes/physics/laureates/ 1952/purcell-bio.html 10 October 2008 17:05 BST.

Westbrook, C., 2002. Alignment and precession. In: MRI at a glance. Blackwell Science, Oxford, pp. 16–17.

Westbrook, C., 2002. Resonance and signal generation. In: MRI at a glance. Blackwell Science, Oxford, pp. 18–19.

Westbrook, C., 2002. Image contrast. In: MRI at a glance. Blackwell Science, Oxford, pp. 20–27.

Westbrook, C., 2002. Pulse sequences. In: MRI at a glance. Blackwell Science, Oxford, pp. 28–47.

Young, H., Baum, R., Cremerius, U., et al., 1999. Measurement of clinical and subclinical tumour response using [18F]-fluorodeoxyglucose and positron emission tomography: review and 1999 EORTC recommendations. Eur. J. Cancer 35, 1773–1782.

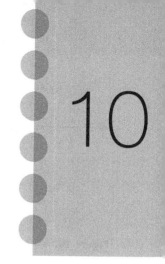

## Chapter Ten

# Making it better

## CHAPTER CONTENTS

Check your existing knowledge . . . . . . . . 235
Introduction . . . . . . . . . . . . . . . . . . . 235
Ultrasound . . . . . . . . . . . . . . . . . . . 235
   Thermal effects . . . . . . . . . . . . . . . . . . 237
   Non-thermal effects . . . . . . . . . . . . . . . 237
Cryotherapy . . . . . . . . . . . . . . . . . . . 238
Electromagnetic field therapies . . . . . . . . 238
   Short-wave diathermy . . . . . . . . . . . . . 238
   Microwave diathermy . . . . . . . . . . . . . 238

Infrared therapy . . . . . . . . . . . . . . . . . . 239
Visible light and ultraviolet therapies . . . 239
Laser therapy . . . . . . . . . . . . . . . . . . . 239
Magnetic field therapy . . . . . . . . . . . . . 239
TENS . . . . . . . . . . . . . . . . . . . . . . . . 240
Interferential . . . . . . . . . . . . . . . . . . . 240
Electrical muscle stimulation . . . . . . . . . 241
Learning outcomes . . . . . . . . . . . . . . . 241
Bibliography . . . . . . . . . . . . . . . . . . . 242

## CHECK YOUR EXISTING KNOWLEDGE

There is no formal assessment of knowledge base for this section: either you do know how modalities function and how they achieve their physiological results or you don't.

Depending on your musculoskeletal specialty, syllabus and personal preference, it may also be appropriate to 'cherry pick' certain modalities and ignore others, although, even if you are not intending to use them yourself, you should be aware of their effects as patients who have already undergone these therapies and part of their previous management may well present to you.

## Introduction

Over the last 50 years, many physical therapists have increasingly adopted the use of modalities into their clinical practice. They are useful in that they provide a range of treatment alternatives; however, whilst training in their indications, contraindications and usage is necessarily thorough, the physics behind their interaction with the patient and the machines themselves is often scanty or lacking altogether.

In this final chapter, we shall be taking a brief overview of the most common physical modalities, explaining the principles of how the machines operate and their physiological effects. We shall also briefly summarize their usage and the evidence for efficacy in different conditions.

## Ultrasound

We have already discussed ultrasonography as a tool for diagnostic imaging; however, it is also the oldest and most widely used of the physical modalities. The term *ultrasound* refers to cyclic sound pressure with any frequency greater than that of the upper

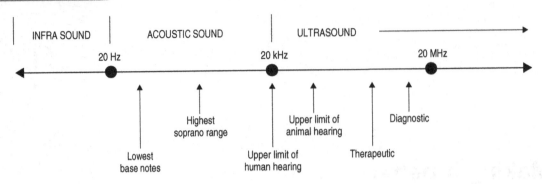

**Figure 10.1** • The range of sound waves.

limit of human hearing. Although this limit varies between individuals and genders and decreases with age, it is approximately 20 kHz (20 000 hertz) in healthy young adults and this figure serves as a useful lower limit in describing ultrasound (Fig. 10.1).

Although therapeutic ultrasound has been used for over 50 years in physical therapy, its application within the clinical environment has changed significantly over the last 20 years. Whereas, in the past, it was employed primarily for thermal effects, this is no longer the case; now it is much more widely used for its physiological effects, especially in relation to tissue repair and wound healing.

Whether used for diagnostic or therapeutic purposes, ultrasonography begins with the production of the sound waves. This takes place in the **transducer**, the component of the ultrasound equipment that is placed in direct contact with the patient's body. It contains piezoelectric material, which converts the electrical impulses received from the **pulse generator** into sound waves. These can be continuous (therapeutic usage) or pulsed (therapeutic and diagnostic usage). In diagnostic imaging, the transducer also contains a second piezoelectric element that, when echo pulses return to the body surface, are converted back into electrical pulses that are then processed by the system and formed into an image.

As with all waves, the ultrasound wave has a wavelength and reciprocally related frequency. It also has amplitude and a velocity that will vary according to the density of the medium through which it is passing (Table 10.1).

The power and intensity of the beam are also considerations: you will recall from earlier chapters that power is the rate of energy transfer and is expressed in units of watts. **Intensity** is the rate at which power passes through a specified area and is expressed in units of watts per square centimetre. Intensity is

**Table 10.1** Velocity of ultrasound waves in selected human tissues

| Material | Velocity ($ms^{-1}$) |
|----------|---------------------|
| Fat | 1450 |
| Water | 1480 |
| Soft tissue | 1540 |
| Bone | 4100 |

the rate at which ultrasound energy is applied to a specific tissue location within the patient's body. It is the quantity that must be considered with respect to producing biological effects and safety. The intensity of most diagnostic ultrasound beams at the transducer surface is on the order of a few milliwatts per square centimetre; this rises to as much as 2 $Wcm^{-2}$ for therapeutic purposes.

In order to be of medical use, it is necessary to provide a medium through which the ultrasound can freely pass in order to reach the patient's tissues. Unless this is done, ultrasound will be reflected at the metal/air interface found at the transducer head. This medium is referred to as a **coupling medium,** and several different types are used in practice including water, various oils, creams and gels. Ideally, the coupling medium should be sufficiently fluid to fill all available spaces, relatively viscous so that it stays in place and should allow the transmission of ultrasound waves with minimal absorption, attenuation or disturbance.

Once the beam enters the body, it can be absorbed, transmitted or reflected by the tissues therein. We have already dealt with this in regard to ultrasonographic imaging in Chapter 9; however, there are additional considerations for therapeutic usage.

In order to have a therapeutic effect, *absorption* of the applied energy is necessary; therefore the effectiveness of the modality will vary according to a tissue's capacity to absorb the applied energy. The rate of absorption is related to protein content; tissues with a higher protein content (e.g. ligaments, tendons and scar tissue) will absorb ultrasound to a greater extent whilst tissues with high water and low protein content (e.g. blood and fat) absorb much less energy.

These absorption characteristics have also to be balanced against the wave reflection at the tissue surface. Although cartilage and bone also have a high-protein-low-water profile, a significant proportion of ultrasound energy striking the surface of structures composed of these tissues is likely to be reflected.

## Thermal effects

When ultrasound is absorbed, it generates heat within the absorbing tissue. The amount of heat will depend on the protein content of the tissue and the frequency of the applied ultrasound; the higher the frequency, the greater the absorption rate. A biologically significant thermal effect can be achieved if the tissue temperature is raised to 40–45°C for at least 5 minutes.

Although controlled heating can produce beneficial effects, including pain relief, decreased joint stiffness and increased local blood flow, ultrasound is relatively inefficient at generating sufficient thermal change to achieve a therapeutic effect at commonly applied clinical doses, and there are tissue heating methods available in clinical practice that are better at achieving the desired thermal changes.

## Non-thermal effects

A number of trials and meta-analyses produced during the 1980s and 1990s increasingly challenged the routine use of therapeutic ultrasound, showing it to be no better or, in some cases worse, than placebo for the treatment of a number of acute musculoskeletal injuries, as well as more chronic problems such as osteoarthritis, most probably owing to its heating effects, which can increase local inflammation.

At the same time, interest started to become focused on the use of ultrasound as a rehabilitative tool to assist tissues that were healing. The production of scar tissue is a complex series of cascaded, chemically mediated events that results in the deposition of collagen at the site of tissue damage.

The effects of ultrasound during the repair process are thought to vary, according to the primary events that are occurring in the tissues. Once tissue bleeding has ceased (ultrasound can increase blood flow, presumably through heat effects, and thus perpetuate this phase of injury response), it is appropriate to start using ultrasound as soon as is feasible. During the inflammatory phase, ultrasound has a stimulating effect on the mast cells, platelets and white blood cells, which mediate the inflammatory response; however, this intervention is not intended to increase the inflammatory response as such (though if applied with too greater intensity at this stage, this can be a complication) but rather to 'optimize' the inflammatory response, which is essential for the effective repair of tissue and inhibition of which can inhibit the repair phases that follow.

Dosage, intensity, pulsation, timing and the preferential absorption of the damaged tissue are all factors that must be considered carefully to make the initial earliest repair phase as efficient as possible, and thus have a promotional effect on the healing process as a whole. Despite the tendency for osseous structures to reflect rather than absorb ultrasound waves, it appears that the modality can also be of use in reducing fracture healing time.

During the proliferative phase, in which scar tissue is produced, ultrasound can also have a stimulative effect; the targets now are the fibroblasts, endothelial cells and myofibroblasts, the cells that activate collagen production in wound healing. Pulsed ultrasound appears to be more effective in encouraging fibroplasia and collagen synthesis than a continuous dose application.

Ultrasound may also have a beneficial role during the remodelling phase of repair, which can last for up to a year after the original injury. The proliferative stage produces a 'generic' scar, which is then refined so that it adopts some of the functional characteristics of the tissue that it is repairing. Although a scar in tendon will not become tendon itself, it will behave more like tendinous tissue. This is achieved mainly by the orientation of the collagen fibres in the developing scar and also to the change in collagen type, from predominantly type III to type I collagen, which has greater mobility and higher tensile strength.

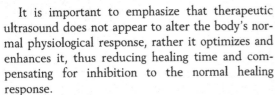

It is important to emphasize that therapeutic ultrasound does not appear to alter the body's normal physiological response, rather it optimizes and enhances it, thus reducing healing time and compensating for inhibition to the normal healing response.

Most recently, it has been discovered that ultrasound has a role in aiding and targeting drug uptake by enhancing membrane transport and increasing vascular and soft tissue transportation.

## Cryotherapy

By contrast to ultrasound, the application of cooling agents to an area of injury aims to limit the inflammatory response and its vascular, mechanical and biochemical nociceptive consequences. Cryotherapy is usually applied by means of a gel pack, containing material that remains pliant at the temperatures generated by domestic freezers ($-20°$ to $-26°C$) or by the application of cooling gel, a substance with a high latent heat of vaporization, which achieves a similar effect by carrying heat away from the injured area as it evaporates.

There is good evidence that this approach, when used in the acute phase of injury, can reduce pain and ischaemia and increase mobility and return to normal activity; this may be at the expense of slightly longer secondary healing phases. Dosage and application need to be carefully monitored, particularly when the procedure is being performed by the patient in an unsupervised manner: 5 minutes for superficial and 15 minutes for deep structures appears to represent the maximum beneficial period for application and a latent period of 30–90 minutes for the local physiology to normalize also appears optimal.

The most common complication of cryotherapy is soft tissue damage from over-cooling. This can produce epidermal damage ('cold burns') and local ischaemic effects – it is therefore important for the clinician to monitor the duration and frequency of application as well as ensuring that ice packs are not applied directly to the unprotected skin.

## Electromagnetic field therapies

There are a number of techniques in physical therapy that involve the application of an electromagnetic field of varying strengths to a variety of tissues. Generally, these fields are induced by high-frequency alternating currents and the application is either via pads placed on the skin over the area to be treated or, in less portable machines, by a transducer head that can be positioned on or directly above the skin.

## Short-wave diathermy

Diathermy is simply the process of producing heat in the body by the application of external energy, most usually using electromagnetic fields, although, technically, ultrasound is also a form of diathermy.

However, with short-wave diathermy, the energy levels are substantially higher than with ultrasound; typically up to 100 times more energy is applied and the technique is therefore used to apply 'deep heat' to areas where the thermal effects of ultrasound are considered ineffective either because of the size of the area involved or the depth of the tissue.

Most typically, two pads are applied to the area and a high frequency current generated to produce electromagnetic radiation in the 25–50 MHz range, that of shortwave radio (hence the name). This produces a heating effect; however, given the comments above regarding heating effect and the detrimental action it can have when used inappropriately, it is not perhaps surprising that use of diathermy as a therapeutic modality has declined in recent years.

It does, however, still have a place in the physical therapist's repertoire: there is some evidence that it can ease the pain associated with chronic degenerative conditions.

There are, however, a significant number of contraindications, most particularly metal implants, and overheating to the point of tissue damage is the most frequent complication.

## Microwave diathermy

By increasing the energy of the radiation in to the microwave spectrum, still greater heating effects can be achieved. Even greater care needs to be taken when applying this modality and the list of contraindications is even longer: microwave diathermy is also used in surgery for ablation!

## Infrared therapy

Usually applied using light-emitting diodes (LEDs), this modality again uses heating effect; however, as the photons begin to become more energetic, they also become less penetrating. Infrared therapy therefore produces more surface heating and relies on conduction for any deep heating effect.

Although the same comments apply as to other heat-based therapies; infrared is also used in treatment of dermatological conditions and in plastic surgery.

## Visible light and ultraviolet therapies

Although these modalities are used within medicine, they are mainly for dermatological conditions and, in the latter case, seasonal affective disorder (SAD). They are of limited use in the field of manual therapy.

## Laser therapy

As well as lamps and LEDs, phototherapy in the infrared to ultraviolet part of the spectrum may also be generated by lasers. This modality has the advantage of being able to produce very specific wavelengths of electromagnetic radiation in a narrow beam allowing for localization of treatment and specificity of effect.

Laser is an acronym for *Light Amplification by the Stimulated Emission of Radiation*, a name that refers to its method of production (Fig. 10.2).

Light of a specific wavelength passing through the gain medium is amplified by emitted photons; the surrounding mirrors then ensure that most of the light makes many passes through the gain medium, being amplified repeatedly. Part of the light that is between the mirrors (that is, within the cavity) passes through the partially transparent mirror and escapes as a beam of light.

Clinical applications show that there may be some efficacy for the treatment of soft tissue injury, chronic pain and in promoting wound healing, although many trials are, at best, ambiguous. One possible reason for this is that, whereas certain frequencies of light at certain intensities may have a positive physiological effect, the exact mechanism – which appears to be photochemical rather than related to heating effects – is still being explored, although it is now known to include changes in cell

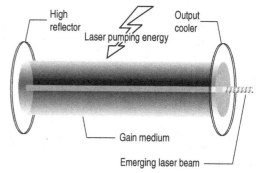

**Figure 10.2** • Laser generation. A laser consists of a highly reflective optical cavity, surrounded by a *gain medium*, which can consist of crystals doped with rare-earth elements, a variety of gases or semiconductors. There will also be a means to supply 'pumping' energy to the gain medium, either by an electric current or by light of a different wavelength. The gain medium absorbs this energy, which raises some electrons into a higher-energy state. It is the transition between this state and the lower level that gives laser its potential for being monochromatic. The cavity consists of two mirrors arranged such that light bounces back and forth, each time passing through the gain medium, allowing it to be amplified by photons from the gain material. Typically one of the two mirrors, the output coupler, is partially transparent. The output laser beam is emitted through this mirror.

membrane permeability and regulation of adenosine triphosphate and nitric oxide.

The effect of varying of wavelength, effective dose, dose-rate effects, beam penetration and pulsation are still poorly understood in the clinical setting. Laser power is typically low level, in the range of 0.001–0.5 W, although pulsed devices may go higher than this. This gives a typical beam irradiance of $10\,\mathrm{mW/cm^2}$–$5\,\mathrm{W/cm^2}$. The wavelength is typically in the range 600–1000 nm (see Table 8.1).

# Magnetic field therapy

The application of magnets to painful areas is more often than not carried out by the patient themselves as a self-help measure and many popular magazines and newspapers carry advertisements for magnetic bands, jewellery and even dog collars. It is an area that has started to be researched in some depth but the results have done little to clarify the evidence base. There seems to be a difference between static and pulsed magnets but little has been done to establish the condition-specific variables for the latter, which may be the reason behind the significant variability of research findings.

The Magneto Max machine offers the therapist a series of static toruses inside which the patient sits.

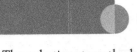

The pulsation strength, duration, polarity and intensity can all be controlled; there is some suggestion of anti-inflammatory and haematological effects and of decreased fracture healing time from this modality.

One peculiarity that is starting to emerge from meta-analysis of the trials carried out to date is that the dose–response curve, if indeed there is one, is atypical – medium strength magnetic fields (1–2T) do appear to have more effect that weak magnetic fields (<0.5T) but also more effect than higher strength fields (>3T).

No mechanism appears to have been established for the means by which pain relief is obtained, although the effect is purported to be neurological.

## TENS

Of all the electrically powered modalities, Transcutaneous Electrical Nerve Stimulation (TENS), has perhaps the widest usage, though not necessarily by therapists; most TENS applications are performed by patients on themselves either with guidance from healthcare professionals or at their own instigation – the machines are readily available for purchase by the general public.

There is a degree of controversy as to the indications for and effectiveness of TENS, and although it is frequently touted as a 'cure-all' for pain of any kind, many of the trials are of poor quality and those with sufficient power and appropriate methodology have produced results that are, at best, equivocal. As with other modalities, part of the problem is the lack of standardization in the application of the treatment; certainly, intensive, high-frequency TENS may have a greater benefit than placebo in the management of acute pain, although this effect appears to be short-term and does not include two of the commonest conditions presenting to the manual physician, low back pain and whiplash.

The idea that electrical stimulation could be used for pain control was first recorded in ancient Rome, when the court physician to the Roman emperor Claudius, Scribonius Largus, noted that his foot pain was relieved by standing on an electrical fish at the seashore. Electrostatic devices were used from the 16th through to the early 20th century; amongst others, Benjamin Franklin was a proponent of this method for pain relief in conditions ranging from headache to cancer. The most commercially successful device was the 'electric rejuvenator',

invented by Otto von Overbeck. The first modern TENS machine was patented in the USA in 1974.

Neurophysiological trials demonstrate that high- and low-frequency TENS produce their effects by activation of opioid receptors in the central nervous system, although their actions are subtly different (high-frequency TENS activates δ-opioid receptors whilst low-frequency TENS activates μ-opioid receptors). TENS has also been shown to have an inhibitory effect on central nociceptive neurons.

At lower frequencies (5–10 Hz), TENS is thought to produce muscle contractions and provide pain reduction for several hours. At high frequencies (80–100 Hz), TENS is thought to temporarily reduce pain by acting as a counterirritant stimulus.

## Interferential

As with the other modalities that we have discussed, the trials on interferential current therapy on musculoskeletal conditions produce little in the way of an evidence base for the use of this modality. Poor methodology and lack of consistency in the parameters for the machine mean that such trials as there are not amenable to meta-analysis.

Interferential works by superimposing two or sometimes three medium-frequency (3–5 kHz) alternating (sinusoidal) currents, which are generated by independent oscillatory circuits. These are programmed to deliver 'beats' between 1–200 times per second as the currents move in and out of phase with each other, creating pulses of superimposition, felt by the patient as a tingling sensation, similar to that produced in TENS (Fig. 10.3). This superimposition is identical to that seen in light, sound and other wave forms (Fig. 6.5).

Interferential is usually applied using quadripolar technique. Two pairs of electrodes – usually applied using carbon-rubber electrodes or suction cups – are placed around the site of therapy. Each pair of electrodes produces one of the two medium-frequency currents that interfere with each other, producing an effect that is, to all intents and purposes, identical to that in TENS. Unlike TENS, the electrodes can be placed posteriorly and anteriorly to generate a three-dimensional effect. The frequency range of the amplitude modulated 'beat' frequency can be low (<10 Hz) or high (>100 Hz), depending on the desired therapeutic effect.

In contrast to TENS, interferential machines also allow the operator to vary this pulsing over time.

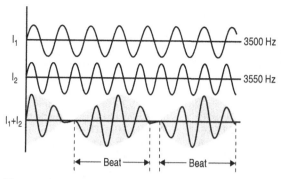

**Figure 10.3 •** Interferential currents. Two medium frequency electrical currents move in and out of phase with each other creating pulses of higher intensity, where the superimposed currents reinforce each other. These are interspersed with null areas where the currents cancel each other out.

This **sweep frequency** is superimposed on top of the beat frequency: a sweep frequency of 10 Hz superimposed on a base beat frequency of 10 Hz will result in a therapeutic dose that varies from 10 Hz to 20 Hz over the treatment period; the rate at which this frequency changes can also be controlled by the operator. The therapeutic benefit this imparts is unknown as few trials have addressed this parameter; its suggested application also varies between manufacturers, sometimes quite significantly. It does, however, seem probable that the greater variety of frequencies may stimulate a greater variety of nerve types and help prevent habituation.

As with TENS, interferential should not be applied to the neck or cranium; the most common complication is iatrogenic burns from overheating.

## Electrical muscle stimulation

The modalities that we have discussed so far have mainly been directed at symptomatic relief rather than rehabilitation; electrical currents can, however, also be applied to stimulate muscles. This can help rehabilitate and rebuild muscle damaged by trauma or neurological damage, where voluntary contraction is no longer possible.

It has been known for many years that electrical currents can cause muscle to contract (remember Galvani and the frog's legs). In combination with appropriate sensor technology and feedback control, this can be exploited to elicit functional movements, such as walking and cycling, and hence to restore certain motor functions. Depending on the degree of disability, the goal may be temporary assistance – for example, re-learning of gait following spinal cord injury – or permanent replacement of lost motor functions, a means of neurological prosthesis.

Electrical stimulation also has biomechanical benefits: it can improve the size and strength of muscles, increase the range of joint motion and enhance cardiopulmonary fitness.

Stimulation can either be applied directly to the peripheral motor nerves or, if the reflex arcs in the lower spinal cord are still intact, to the sensory nerves. The latter causes an indirect stimulation of motor nerves whilst ensuring the natural inhibition of antagonistic muscles. Typically, the pulses applied are of milliamp intensity ($\leq$ 120 mA) with a frequency of <20 Hz and a pulse width of $\leq$ 1 ms.

The major problem with electrical stimulation is that the external stimuli, which replace the missing commands from the central nervous system, tend to reverse the recruitment order of muscle fibres: motor neurons with larger diameter are activated first as they have a lower threshold; they recruit the faster and more powerful type II (white) fibres, which fatigue more quickly than the slower, but less powerful, type I (red) muscle fibres.

As well as in stroke and spinal cord victims, the technique is also widely used in rehabilitation of sports injuries (in racehorses as well as humans), particularly where weightbearing is contraindicated. Initially, the modality can prevent muscle wasting (which begins within 48 hours of immobilization) and disuse osteoporosis (contraction of Sharpey fibres helps stimulate osteoblastic activity). As the biomechanical integrity of the affected area improves, electrical stimulation can be used to re-develop muscle strength prior to exercise therapy.

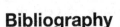 

# Bibliography

Adedoyin, R.A., Olaogun, M.O.B., Fagbeja, O.O., 2002. Effect of interferential stem cells seeded on a three-dimensional biomatrix. Lasers Med. Sci. 20 (3), 143–157.

Adedoyin, R.A., Olaogun, M.O.B., Fagbeja, O.O., 2002. Effect of interferential current stimulation in management of osteo-arthritic knee pain. Physiotherapy 88, 493–499.

Alexiades-Armenakas, M., 2007. Laser and light-based treatment of cellulite. J. Drugs Dermatol. 6 (1), 83–84.

Al-Kurdi, D., Bell-Syer, S.E.M., Flemming, K., 2008. Therapeutic ultrasound for venous leg ulcers. Cochrane Database Syst. Rev. 2008 Issue 1. Art No CD001180. doi: 10.1002/14651858.CD001180. pub2.

Allen, R., Schwarz, C. (Eds.), 1998. The Chambers dictionary. Chambers Harrap, Edinburgh.

Baba-Akbari Sari, A., Flemming, K., Cullum, N.A., et al., 2006. Therapeutic ultrasound for pressure ulcers. Cochrane Database Syst. Rev. 2006 Issue 3. Art No CD001275. doi: 10.1002/14651858.CD001275. pub2.

Bélanger, A., 2002. Interferential currents. In: Evidence-based guide to therapeutic physical agents. Lippincott Williams and Wilkins, Philadelphia, pp. 66–90.

Brosseau, L., Casimiro, L., Robinson, V., et al., 2001. Therapeutic ultrasound for treating patellofemoral pain syndrome. Cochrane Database Syst. Rev. 2001 Issue 4. Art No CD003375. doi: 10.1002/14651858. CD003375.

Brown, C.S., Ling, F.W., Wan, J.Y., et al., 2002. Efficacy of static magnetic field therapy in chronic pelvic pain: A double-blind pilot study. Am. J. Obstet. Gynecol. 187, 1581–1587.

Casimiro, L., Brosseau, L., Robinson, V., et al., 2002. Therapeutic ultrasound for the treatment of rheumatoid arthritis. Cochrane Database Syst. Rev. 2002 Issue 3. Art No CD003787. doi: 10.1002/14651858. CD003787.

Cheing, G.L., Tsui, A.Y., Lo, S.K., et al., 2003. Optimal stimulation duration of TENS in the management of osteoarthritic knee pain. J. Rehabil. Med. 35, 62–68.

Chesterton, L.S., Foster, N.E., Wright, C.C., et al., 2003. Effects of TENS frequency, intensity and stimulation site parameter manipulation on pressure pain thresholds in healthy human subjects. Pain 106, 73–80.

Chipchase, L., Williams, M., Robertson, V.J., 2007. Electrophysical agents in physiotherapy practice and education: still a good idea after all these years? WCPT 2007, Vancouver, Canada, Physiotherapy 93, S97.

Chou, R., Huffman, L.H., 2007. American Pain Society; American College of Physicians. Nonpharmacologic therapies for acute and chronic low back pain: a review of the evidence for an American Pain Society/American College of Physicians clinical practice guideline. Ann. Intern. Med. 147, 492–504.

Enwemeka, C.S., 1989. The effects of therapeutic ultrasound on tendon healing. A biomechanical study. Am. J. Phys. Med. Rehabil. 68, 283–287.

Enwemeka, C.S., 1989. Inflammation, cellularity, and fibrillogenesis in regenerating tendon: implications for tendon rehabilitation. Phys. Ther. 69, 816–825.

Enwemeka, C.S., Rodriguez, O., Mendosa, S., 1990. The biomechanical effects of low-intensity ultrasound on healing tendons. Ultrasound Med. Biol. 16, 801–807.

Fernandez, M.I., Watson, P.J., Rowbotham, D.J., 2007. Effect of pulsed magnetic field therapy on pain reported by human volunteers in a laboratory model of acute pain. Br. J. Anaesth. 99 (2), 266–269.

Garrood, J.R., 1979. Electromagnetic waves and optics. In: Physics. Intercontinental Book Productions, Maidenhead, pp. 140–176.

Haedersdal, M., Togsverd-Bo, K., Wulf, H.C., 2008. Evidence-based review of lasers, light sources and photodynamic therapy in the treatment of acne vulgaris. J. Eur. Acad. Dermatol. Venereol. 22, 267–278.

Hand, J.W., 2008. Modelling the interaction of electromagnetic fields (10 MHz–10 GHz) with the human body: methods and applications. Physics in Medical Biology 53 (16), R243–R286. Epub 2008 Jul 24.

Harden, R.N., Remble, T.A., Houle, T.T., et al., 2007. Prospective, randomized, single-blind, sham treatment-controlled study of the safety and efficacy of an electromagnetic field device for the treatment of chronic low back pain: a pilot study. Pain Practice 7 (3), 248–255.

Harvey, W., Dyson, M., Pond, J.B., et al., 1975. The stimulation of protein synthesis in human fibroblasts by therapeutic ultrasound. Rheumatol. Rehabil. 14, 237.

Hay, G.A., Hughes, D.H., 1983. Electromagnetic radiation. In: First year physics for radiographers, third ed. Ballière Tindall, Eastbourne, pp. 27–38.

Hummelsheim, H., Maier-Loth, M.L., Eickhof, C., 1997. The functional value of electrical muscle stimulation for the rehabilitation of the hand in stroke patients. Scand. J. Rehabil. Med. 29 (1), 3–10.

Hurley, D.A., Minder, P., McDonough, S.M., et al., 2000. Evidence for interferential therapy for acute low back pain. Physiotherapy 86, 36.

Hyland, G.J., 2008. Physical basis of adverse and therapeutic effects of low intensity microwave radiation. Indian J. Exp. Biol. 46 (5), 403–419.

Itoh, K., Itoh, S., Katsumi, Y., et al., 2009. A pilot study on using acupuncture and transcutaneous electrical nerve stimulation to treat chronic non-specific low back pain. Complement. Ther. Clin. Pract. 15 (1), 22–25.

Jan, M.H., Chai, H.M., Wang, C.L., et al., 2006. Effects of repetitive shortwave diathermy for reducing synovitis in patients with knee osteoarthritis: an ultrasonographic study. Phys. Ther. 86, 236–244.

Johnson, K., 1986. Physics at work: electromagnetic waves. In: GCSE physics for you. Hutchinson Education, London, p. 251.

Johnson, M.I., 1999. The mystique of interferential currents when used to manage pain. Physiotherapy 85, 294–297.

Johnson, M., Martinson, M., 2006. Efficacy of electrical nerve stimulation for chronic musculoskeletal pain: a meta-analysis of randomized controlled trials. Pain 130 (1), 157–165.

Jorge, S., Parada, C.A., Ferreira, S.H., et al. Interferential therapy produces antinociception during application in various models of inflammatory pain. Phys. Ther. 86 (6), 800–808.

Kerem, M., Yigiter, K., 2002. Effects of continuous and pulsed short-wave diathermy in low back pain. The Pain Clinic 4, 55–59.

Khoromi, S., Blackman, M.R., Kingman, A., et al., 2007. Low intensity permanent magnets in the treatment of chronic lumbar radicular ain. J. Pain Symptom Manage. 34, 434–445.

Langford, J., McCarthy, P.W., 2005. Randomised controlled clinical trial of magnet use in chronic low back pain; a pilot study. Clinical Chiropractic 8, 13–19.

Laughman, R.K., Youdas, J.W., Garrett, T.R., et al., 1983. Strength changes in the normal quadriceps femoris muscle as a result of electrical stimulation. Phys. Ther. 63, 494–499.

Liboff, A.R., 2007. Local and holistic electromagnetic therapies. Electromagn. Biol. Med. 26 (4), 315–325.

Markov, M.S., 2007. Expanding use of pulsed electromagnetic field therapies. Electromagn. Biol. Med. 26 (3), 257–274.

Maxwell, L., 1992. Therapeutic ultrasound: its effects on the cellular and molecular mechanisms of inflammation and repair. Physiotherapy 78 (6), 421–426.

McManus, F.J., Ward, A.R., Robertson, V.J., 2006. The analgesic effects of interferential therapy on two experimental pain models: cold and

mechanically induced pain. Physiotherapy 92, 95–102.

Munavalli, G.S., Weiss, R.A., 2008. Evidence for laser- and light-based treatment of acne vulgaris. Semin. Cutan. Med. Surg. 27 (3), 207–211.

National Trust, Overbeck's. Online. Available from: www.nationaltrust. org.uk 1 November 2008, 15:45 GMT.

Nicolin, V., Ponti, C., Baldini, G., et al., 2007. In vitro exposure of human chondrocytes to pulsed electromagnetic fields. Eur. J. Histochem. 51 (3), 203.

Nussbaum, E.L., 1997. Ultrasound: to heat or not to heat – that is the question. Phys. Ther. Rev. 2, 59–72.

Oosterhof, J., Samwel, H.J.A., de Boo, T.M., et al., 2008. Predicting outcome of TENS in chronic pain: a prospective, randomized, placebo controlled trial. Pain 136, 11–20.

Orringer, J.S., Kang, S., Maier, L., et al., 2007. A randomized, controlled, split-face clinical trial of 1320-nm Nd:YAG laser therapy in the treatment of acne vulgaris. J. Am. Acad. Dermatol. 56 (3), 432–438.

Ozcan, J., Ward, A.R., Robertson, V.J., 2004. A comparison of true and premodulated interferential currents. Archives of Physical Medical Rehabilitation 85, 409–415.

Poitras, S., Brosseau, L., 2008. Evidence-informed management of chronic low back pain with transcutaneous electrical nerve stimulation, interferential current, electrical muscle stimulation, ultrasound, and thermotherapy. Spine J. 8, 226–233.

Pope, G.D., Mockett, S.P., Wright, J.P., 1995. A survey of electrotherapeutic modalities: ownership and use in the NHS in England. Physiotherapy 81, 82–91.

Ramirez, A., Schwane, J.A., McFarland, C., et al., 1997. The effect of ultrasound on collagen synthesis and fibroblast proliferation in vitro. Med. Sci. Sports Exerc. 29, 326–332.

Robinson, V.A., Brosseau, L., Peterson, J., et al., 2001. Therapeutic ultrasound for osteoarthritis of the knee. Cochrane Database Syst. Rev. 2001 Issue 3. Art No CD003132. doi: 10.1002/14651858.CD003132.

Searle, R.D., Bennett, M.I., Johnson, M.I., et al., 2009. Transcutaneous electrical nerve stimulation (TENS) for cancer bone pain. J. Pain Symptom Manage. 31 (3), 424–428.

Ter Haar, G., 2008. The resurgence of therapeutic ultrasound – a 21st century phenomenon. Ultrasonics 48 (4), 233.

Ter Haar, G., Dyson, M., Oakley, E.M., 1985. The use of ultrasound by physiotherapists in Britain. Ultrasound Med. Biol. 13, 659–663.

Van der Windt, D.A.W.M., Van der Heijden, G.J.M.G., Van den Berg, S.G.M., et al., 2002. Therapeutic ultrasound for acute ankle sprains. Cochrane Database Syst. Rev. 2002 Issue 1. Art No CD001250. doi: 10.1002/14651858.CD001250.

Walker, N.A., Denegar, C.R., Preische, J., 2007. Low-intensity pulsed ultrasound and pulsed electromagnetic field in the treatment of tibial fractures: a systematic review. Journal of Athletic Training 42 (4), 530–535.

Watson, T., 2000. The role of electrotherapy in contemporary physiotherapy practice. Man. Ther. 5 (3), 132–141.

Watson, T., 2006. Electrotherapy and tissue repair. Sportex-Medicine 297–313.

Watson, T., 2006. Tissue repair: the current state of the art. Sportex-Medicine 28, 8–12.

Watson, T., 2007. Modality and dose dependency in electrotherapy. WCPT 2007, Vancouver, Canada: Physiotherapy 93 (S1), S674.

Weintraub, M.I., Cole, S.P., 2004. Pulsed magnetic field therapy in refractory neuropathic pain secondary to peripheral neuropathy: electrodiagnostic parameters – pilot study. Neurorehabil. Neural Repair 18 (1), 42–46.

Young, S.R., Dyson, M., 1990. Effect of therapeutic ultrasound on the healing of full thickness excised skin lesions. Ultrasonics 28, 175–180 (Abstract).

Young, S.R., Dyson, M., 1990. The effect of therapeutic ultrasound on angiogenesis. Ultrasound Med. Biol. 16, 261–269.

# Index

Page numbers in *italic* denote material in boxes and tables.

## A

A-scan mode ultrasonography, 229
abduction, *17*, 19
acceleration, 30, 32
  in equations of motion, 35–6
  in laws of motion, 34
acceleration–deceleration injury, 113
accessory joints, spinal, 108
accessory ribs, 108
actin, 86–7
actinides, 142
action potentials, 164
adduction, *17*, 19
adenosine triphosphate (ATP), 87
adhesive capsulitis (frozen shoulder), 107
algebra, 9–11
  clinical application, 11
alpha (α) particles, 128, 190–2
alternating current, 158–9, *159*
  drawbacks, 159–60
  rectifier, 160
    smoothed, *161*
alveolar gas exchange, 44
ammeters, 158
amperes, 6, *7*
amphiarthroses, 73
amplification, 165, *166*
amplitude modulation (AM), 182
anatomical planes, 17, *19*
anatomical position, 16–17, *17*
AND gates, 166
Angstrøms, 3
angular velocity, 31
ankle, 105
ankylosis, *111*
annulus fibrosus, 110
antalgic gait, *120*
anterior, 16, 17
antimatter, 191
aponeuroses, 86
arthralgia, 72
arthritis, 29, 72
arthrokinematics, 102–5
  circumduction, 104

roll and glide, 102, *103*
  spin, 102–4
arthropathy, 72
arthrosis, 72
atlanto-odontoid joint, *80*
atlas, 113, *114*
atmospheric pressure, 41
atomic mass numbers, 129, *212*
atomic structure, 125–50
atomic theory, 125–36
  intra-atomic forces, 131
attenuation, 196
*Australiopithecus afarensis*, 104–5
Autistic Spectrum Disorder, 33
Avogadro's constant, 130
axes, orthogonal, 19, 20
  scaling, 20
axial skeleton, 108
axis bone, 113, *114*
azimuthal quantum number, 137

## B

B-scan mode ultrasonography, 229
Bacon, Roger (Dr Miribalis), 28–9
balance, 117–18
ball and socket (spheroidal) joint, *79*, 81
Balmer spectral lines, 137
barium contrast, 212
barometers, 41
batteries (electric cells), 155
beams, 58
  bending moment, 58, 59–60
  cantilevered, 58
  non-cantilevered, 58–9
  second moment of area, 61
  *see also* shearing forces
bending moment, 58
  calculation, 59–60
  relation to beam length, 60
  sign conventions, *59*
bending moment diagrams
  cantilevered beams, *59*
  non-cantilevered beams, *60*

bending moment diagrams (*Continued*)
   self-loading characteristics, *60*
   sign conventions, 58
beta (β) particles, 192–3
biaxial joints, 101
biceps brachialis muscles
   in lever system, 52, *53*
      calculation of forces, 56–7
bicondylar joint, *79*, 83
binding energies, 194, *195*
bipedal gait, 120
bipedal stance, 116
   stability, 117
bipennate muscles, *94*
birth anomalies
   feet, 105
   suture anomalies, 75
blood pressure, 42
   classification, *43*
blood supply to muscles, 87, *88*
body mass index (BMI), 32
   and osteoarthritis, 106
body tissues
   ionizing radiation
      fetal tissue, 216
      weighting factors, *216*
   MRI $T_1/T_2$ weighting, 224
   ultrasound
      absorption, 237
      wave velocities, *236*
Bohr, N., 135, *136*
   atomic model, *128*, 135–6, *137*
   wave–particle duality, 131
bone(s)
   cancellous *vs* cortical, 62
   classification, 62
   construction, 62
   elasticity, 65
   photoelectric absorption, 211–12
   polar moment of inertia, 63
   Young's modulus, *67*
Boyle's law, 45
brachycephaly, 75
breaking point, 65
British thermal unit (BTU), 38
de Broglie wavelengths, *128*, 134, 136
Bucky, G., *217*
bulk modulus, 67
bulk stress/strain, 66

## c

calculus, 30, *31*, 33
calories, 38

cancers
   and electromagnetic radiation, 183
   and magnetic fields, 171
   from radioactive materials, 191–2
   from ultraviolet radiation, 185
candelas, 6, *7*
cantilevered beams, 58
capacitance, 162–4
capacitors, 162, 164
   discharge, *164*
carbon isotopes, 130, 131
cardiac muscle, 84
cardiology, PET in, *228*
carpal tunnel, 106
carpometacarpal joint, *82*
cartilage
   in amphiarthroses, 73
   viscoelastic properties, 67
cartilaginous joints, 76–7
   primary, 76
   secondary, 76–7
      injuries, 76, 77
cathode rays, 185
cauda equina injuries, 77
cauda equina syndrome, 110
caudal, 16, 17
cellular function and water, 147
Celsius scale, 39
centre of gravity (centre of mass)
   geometric shapes, 63–4
   humans, 63, 116–17
cephalad (cranial), 16, 17, *17*
cerebellar ataxia, *120*
'cervical ribs', 108
cervical spine, 113–15
   mobility, 113
   motion, ranges of, *113*
   whiplash-associated disorders, 113–15
   X-ray indications, *213*
characteristic photon, *194*
Charles' law, 45
circuit diagrams, 158
   symbols, *158*
circumduction, 104
claustrophobia and MRI, 224, *225*
cleft palate, 75
close-packed joint position, 105
cobalt-60, 187
Cobb–Lippman method, *108*
collagen, Young's modulus of, 67
colour perception, 193
colourblindness, 193
comparators, 166
compressive stress/strain, 66

Compton effect (scattering), 197–8, *198*, 212, *213*
computed tomography (CT), 218–20
   spiral CT, 220
conductance, 156
conductors, 156
condyloid joint (ellipsoid), *79*, 81, *82*
cones, 193
conservation of energy, 38
contact point and moment of inertia, 58
coordinates/planes, 16–24
coronal plane, *17*
   orthogonal equivalent, 20
coronoid process, 115
Coulomb's law, 131, *153*, 154
coupled motion, 109
covalent bonding, 144–5
   common types, *145*
   hydrogen, *145*
cranial *see* cephalad
creep, 66
cruciate muscles, *93*
cryotherapy, 238
cubits, 4, 5
Curie, P. & M., 187
current, 158–61
   alternating, 158
      waveform, 158–9, *159*
   direct, 158
      waveform, *159*
   flow, 158, *159*
      direction, 169, *170*
   rectifier, 160
      smoothed, *161*
   three-phase, 159

**D**

*d*-block elements, 142
Dalton's Law, 43–4
'daylight' electric bulbs, 185
de Broglie wavelengths, *128*, 134, 136
de Quervain's disease, 86
decimal system, 3
degrees of freedom, 101–2
dens of axis, 113
dentate ligaments, 107
dentate sutures, 74
deuteranomaly, 193
deuteranopia, 193
diagnostic imaging, 186, 203–33
   *see also specific modalities*
diarthroid joints, 78
diarthroses, 73

diathermy
   microwave, 238
   short-wave, 238
dichromacy, 193
differential calculus, *31*
digastric muscles, 95
diodes, *164*, 165
   back-up, *165*
direct current, 158, *159*
direct muscle action, 52, *54*, 92
displacement, 37
distal, *17*
distance ratio (DR), 50
dolichocephaly, 75
Doppler effect, 231
Doppler ultrasonography, 231
dorsal, 17
dorsiflexion, *17*, 19
Dr Miribalis (Bacon, Roger), 28–9
dynamos, 169
   increasing output, *170*

**E**

ectomorphs, 120
efficiency ($\eta$) of system, *50*
Einstein, A.
   photoelectric equation, 136
   psychological status, 33
elastic limit, 65
elasticity, 65, 66
   Hooke's law, 65, 66
   Young's modulus, 66–7
elbow, *79*, 106
electric cells (batteries), 155
electric muscle stimulation, 241
electricity, 152–68
   appliance power requirements, *174–5*
   clinical focus, 153–5, 164–5
   conductors/insulators, 156–7
   current, 158–61
   domestic/industrial, 171, *172–3*, *173–4*, *175*
   electric potential, 155
   electrodynamics, 158–61
   and magnetism, 153–4
   plugs/sockets by country, 174
   power, 161
   power transmission and health, 171
   systems, 165–8
   voltage and frequency by country, 171, *172–3*, 173
electrodynamics, 158–61
electromagnetic field therapies, 238–9
   diathermy
      microwave, 238

electromagnetic field therapies (*Continued*)
short-wave, 238
infrared therapy, 239
laser therapy, 239
ultraviolet therapy, 239
visible light therapy, 239
electromagnetic induction, 168–9
direction of fields/flow, 169, *170*
first law, 169, 170
electromagnetic radiation, 182–6, 192–8
direction of fields/flow, 180
and health, 183
propagation, *182*
wave equation, 181
electromagnetic spectrum, 182–7
electromagnetic system, *181*
electromagnetism, 153–4
electron(s)
discovery, 127
flow, measurement of, 158
photoelectric effect, 136
spin, 142, 148
electron configurations of elements, *139–42*
electron shells, 137–43
in elements, *139–42*
nomenclature, *137*
sub-levels, 137–8, 142–3
energy states, 138
nomenclature, *137*
van der Waals bonds, 148
electron shielding, 138
electronics, 161–5
capacitors, 162–4
diodes, 165
resistors, 161
thermistors, 161
electropositivity/electronegativity, 144
electrostatic forces, 153, 154–5
Coulomb's law, 131, *153*, 154
in water, 147
electroweak force, 131
elements, *126*, 127
electron configurations, *139–42*, *143*
quantum configurations, *143*
spin configurations, *143*
ellipsoid *see* condyloid joint
endomorphs, 120
energy, 37–8
clinical focus, 38
conservation of, 38
transfer, process of, 37
equations, 9–11
clinical application, 11
transformation, 11

eversion, *17*
excited state, 136
extension, *18*
as rotation, 24
external rotation, 19

**F**

facet (zygapophyseal) joints, 77
Fahrenheit scale, 39, *40*
fasciculi, 84
fast inversion recovery, 226
fast twitch (phasic) muscles, 87, 89
fat, photoelectric absorption in, 212
feet, 105
fenestration, *120*
ferromagnetism, 168
fibreoptics, 192
fibrous joints, 73, 74–5
Fleming's right hand rule, 169, *170*
flexion, 17–18
as rotation, 24
floating ribs, 113
fluorodeoxyglucose (FDG), 226
fontanelles, 74
force(s), 32
in laws of motion, 34
moment created, 53, *54–5*, 55–7
in biceps muscle, 56–7
by manipulation, 58
and work, 37
force ratio, 50
force (spring) constant., 65, 66
fractures, iatrogenic, 58
Franklin, R. *186*
free electrons, 136
frequency, 180–1
frequency modulation (FM), 182
frozen shoulder (adhesive capsulitis), 107
fulcrums, 50, *51*
in first order levers, 51
in second order levers, 51
in third order levers, 51, *52*
functional spinal units, 77, 109
furlongs, 2
fusiform muscles, *95*

**G**

gadolinium contrast, 224
gait(s), 120
assessment, 120
cycle, 120, *121*
pathological, *120*

Galileo, 29
Galvani, L. *153*
gamma (γ) rays, 186, 192–3
    diagnostic, 186
    therapeutic, 186
gas exchange, alveolar, 44
gas laws, 44–6
Gay–Lussac's law, 45
Geiger, H., *127*
    Geiger–Muller counter, *127*
ginglymus *see* hinge joint
gliding joint *see* plane joint
gomphoses *see* peg and socket joints
gravitational potential energy, 37
gravity, 36–7, *37*
    forces on astronomical bodies, *31*
    and mass, 31
ground state, 136
growth plates, 76

**H**

half-life, 131, 187, *190*
heat, 38–9
heat of vaporization, 147
heel effect, 208, *209*
    clinical implications, 208–9, 214
hemiplegic gait, *120*
Henry's Law, 44
high functioning Asperger's (HFA), 33
high-stepping gait, *120*
hinge joint (ginglymus), 79–80
hip, 106
    mobility *vs* stability, 100–1
    rotation, 101
Hooke, Robert, 29
    Hooke's law, 65
horizontal plane, *17*
human body, elemental make-up, *126*
Hund's rule, 142–3
hydrogen
    covalent bonding in, *145*
    energy levels in electron, *136*
    isotopes, *130*
hydrogen bonds, 147–8
    clinical aspects, 148
hydrogen nuclei in MRI
    flipping, *222*
    net magnetization vector, 222
hypertension
    classification, *43*
    epidemiology, 42
hypothermia, 40

**I**

I-beams, 58, 61
iatrogenic fractures, 58
ideal gas equation, 46
iliofemoral joint, *81*
imaging, diagnostic, 186, 203–33
Imperial system of measurement, 6
indirect muscle action, 52, 92
inertia, 34
    *see also* moment of inertia
inferior, 16, *17*
infrared radiation, 184
infrared therapy, 239
instantaneous axis of rotation (IAR), 64
insulators, 156–7
integral calculus, *31*
interference patterns, 133
interferential current therapy, 240–1
    complications, 241
intermolecular bonding, 147–8
internal rotation, 19
intervertebral discs
    anatomy, 110
    damage, 77
    degeneration, 111
    dysfunction, 109
    height loss, 110, 111
    herniation, *109*
        stages, *111*
    imaging, *78*
    movement, *110*
    in seated posture, 119
intervertebral joints, 77
    dislocation, 80
intra-atomic forces, 131
intramolecular bonding, 143–7
inverse square law, 37
inversion, *17*
inversion recovery (MRI), 226
inverters, 165–6
involuntary muscle *see* smooth muscle
iodine contrast, 212
ionic bonding, 144
ionizing energy, 136
ionizing radiation, 191–2
    dosage, 214–15
    injury, 191
        fetal tissue, 216
    patient exposure, 205, 207, 211–12
        chronic *vs* acute, 216
        clinical aspects, 206, 213–14
    protection, *214*
    weighting factors

ionizing radiation (*Continued*)
    body tissues, *216*
    X-rays, 215
ions, 129
isotopes, 129–31
  carbon, 130, 131
  hydrogen, *130*
  natural, *132*
  nomenclature, *132*
  radioactive, *187*

# J

joints
  classification, 72–3
    with degrees of freedom, *101*
    structural *vs* functional, 72
  close-/loose-packed position, 105
  degrees of freedom, 101–2
  extra/fewer in human body, 73, *74*
  features of specific joints, 105–16
    lower extremities, 105–6
    spine/pelvis, 107–15
    temporomandibular joint, 115–16
    upper extremities, 106–7
  human *vs* other primates, 104
  mobility *vs* stability, 73, 99–100
  movements, 99–103
    active *vs* passive, 104
    anatomical system, 17–19, *18*, *19*
    assessment, 103–4
    multifunctional transformations, 21, *22*, *23*
    normal, 103–4
    right hand rule, 24
    rotation, 20, 21, *22*, *23*
    three-dimensional, 21, *23*, 24
    translation, 20, 21, *22*, *23*

# K

Kelvin scale, 39
kelvin units, 6, 7
keyhole surgery, 192
kilograms, 7
kinematic chains, 100
  clinical aspects, 101
  open/closed loop chains, 100
kinetic energy, 38
knee, 105–6
  disorders, 106
  rotation, 106
$kV_p$, 207, 210, *213*, 215
kyphosis, 107–8

# L

lanthanides, 142
laser generation, *239*
laser therapy, 239
lateral, *17*
lateral rotation, *17*, 19
leagues, 2
leukemia and magnetic fields, 171
lever systems, 50–2, *51*
  first order, 51
  human examples, 51, 52, *53*
  muscle action, 52–3
  second/third order, 52
ligaments, 100
  association fibres, 100
  classification, 83–4
  function, 83
  injuries (sprains), 84
limbus sutures, 74
load, 50, *51*
  in first order levers, 51
  in second order levers, 51
  in third order levers, 51, *52*
logic circuits/components, 166–7
loose-packed joint position, 105
lordosis, 107
  in seated posture, 119
low back pain, 111
  treatment, 111–12
    guidelines, 112
lumbar spine, 109–12
  computed tomography, *219*
    three-dimensional, *220*
  injuries, 111
  motion, ranges of, *112*
  X-ray indications, *213*

# M

M-scan mode ultrasonography, 229
magnetic field therapy, 239–40
  dose–response curve, 240
magnetic fields and health, 171
magnetic healing, 155
magnetic resonance imaging (MRI) *181*, 221–6
  contraindications, 224
  contrast, 222–3, 224
  cost of machine, 204
  echo time (TE), 223–4
  energy absorption, 222
  fast inversion recovery, 226
  fast/turbo spin echo (FSE/TSE), 225
  free induction decay, 222

image detector, 222
intervertebral discs, *78*
inversion recovery, 226
MR signal, 222
net magnetization vector, 222
'open' scanners, 224, *225*
proton density weighting, 224
proton precession, 221–2
pulse sequences, *223*, 225, *226*
   time from inversion (TI), 226
relaxation times, 222
repetition time (TR), 222–3
short TI inversion recovery (STIR), 226
spin echo (SE), 225
$T_1/T_2$ relaxation, 222
$T_1/T_2$ weighting, *223*, 224
  in body tissues, *224*
  pulse sequences, 225, *226*
magnetic resonance (MR), 221–2
  MR signal, 222
magnetism, 142, 152, 168
  clinical focus, 153–4
  and electricity, 153–4
  magnetic fields, 154
Marsden, E., 128, 129
mAs, 205–6
mass, 31–2
mass densities and X-rays, 212
mastication, muscles of, 115, 116
Maxwell, J.C., 153, 154
measurements, 2–7
mechanical advantage (MA), 50
mechanoreceptors, 100
medial, *17*
medial plane, *17*
medial rotation, *17*, 19
Ménière's disease, 118
mercury barometers, 41
mesomorphs, 120
metatarsalgia, 105
metre–kilogram–second system *see* MKS system of
    measurement
metres, 6, 7
microcephaly, 75
microwave diathermy, 238
microwave ovens, *183*
microwaves, 183
miles, *5*
MKS system of measurement, 6
mobile phones and health, 183
moles, 6, *7*, 130
moment, bending *see* bending moment
moment of area, second *see* second moment of area
moment of force, 63

moment of inertia, 53, 55–7
  calculation, 53, *54–5*, 55–7
   in biceps muscle, 56–7
  created by manipulation, 58
  polar, 62–3
momentum, 31
  and force, 32
  in laws of motion, 34
moons, *37*
motor end plates, 86
motor units, 86
movements of joints *see* joints, movement
MRI *see* magnetic resonance imaging
multi-pennate muscles, *94*
muscle tone, 87
muscle(s), *88*
  action, 52–3, 92
   direct *vs* indirect, 52, 92
   line of action, 53
   viscoelastic properties, 67
  classification, 84–97
   according to blood supply, *88*
  contraction, 86–7
   aerobic *vs* anaerobic, 87
  crossing other structures, 101
  essential fixators, 92
  extra/fewer in human body, 89
  in joints, 100
  nerve supply, 86
  origin/insertion, 90
  prime movers, 92
  relaxation, 87
  structure, *85*
  synergism/antagonism, 92
  variants, 100
  vascular supply, 87
musculoskeletal ultrasonography, 229–30
myelin, 164
myocytes, 84
myoglobin, 87
myosin, 86–7

**N**

NAND gates, 167
natural philosophy, 27–48
  clinical focus, 29–30
Neanderthals, 104
nerve entrapment
  disc herniation, *109*
  elbow, 106
  wrist, 106
nerve transmission, 164–5

nerves
    supply to muscles, 86
    supply to shoulder, 107
neurology, PET in, *228*
neurons
    as capacitors, 164
    polarization, 164
    wave propagation, 164–5
neuropsychology, PET in, *228*
neutrons, 130
Newton, Isaac, 33, *34*
    equations of motion, 35–6
    law of gravitation, 36
    laws of motion
        first/second, 34
        third, 34–5
Nobel Prizes, *186*
noble gases, 142
nodes of Ranvier, 164, 165
non-cantilevered beams, 58–9
NOT gates, 167
nuclear magnetic resonance (NMR) *221*
nucleons, 130, 131
nucleus pulposus, 110
numbers, 2–3
numerical units, 4–6

## O

obesity, 32
    and osteoarthritis, 106
    sleeping posture, 119
    and X-rays, 206
obstetric ultrasonography, 229–30
    clinical aspects, 230
odontoid process of axis, 113
Ohm's law, 156, *157*
oncology, PET in, *228*
operational amplifiers (OP-AMP), 165, 166
OR gates, 167
origin, 19
orthogonal planes, 19, 20
orthogonal position, 19
orthogonal system, 19–24
osteoarthritis, 106
osteoporosis, 106
otolith organs, 117
ozone/ozone layer, 185

## P

*p*-block elements, 142
Pacinian corpuscles, 100

pain
    low back pain, 111–12
    whiplash-associated, 113
pair production, 198
palmar, *17*
palmaris longus anomalies, 89–90, 97
Palmer, D., 155
parsecs, 2
partial pressures, 43–4
    clinical focus, 44
    in pulmonary–cardiovascular system, 44, *45*
passive infrared (PIR) technology, 184
patella, 62
    as pulley, 52, *54*, 92
Pauli exclusion principle, 138, 144
peg and socket joints (gomphoses), 75
pennate muscles, *94*
'perched facet' syndrome, 80
periodic table, *126*, 130
    and electron shells, 138, 142
*pes planus* (flat feet), 105
PET *see* positron emission tomography
pharmacology, PET in, *228*
phasic muscles *see* fast twitch muscles
photodisintegration, 198
photoelectric effect, 136, 196–7
    X-ray absorption, *197*, 211–12
photons, 134, 180
    waveform, 180
pivot joint (trochoid), *79*, 80–1
plagiocephaly, 75
Planck's constant, 134
plane (gliding) joint, *79*, 80
    degrees of freedom, 101–2
plane sutures, 75
plantar, *17*
plantar pressure receptors, 117
plantarflexion, *17*, 19
plantigrade stance, 116
plasticity, 65
'plum-pudding' atomic model, 127, *128*
Poisson's ratio, 67
polar moment of inertia, 62–3
polarity, 146
polonium, 187, *188–9*, 189
polydactyly, 105
positron (proton) emission tomography (PET), *181*,
        226–7
    clinical applications, *228*
    cranium, *227*
positrons, *191*
posterior, 17
posture, 116–20
    analyzer, *118*

anatomical markers, 118
anteroposterior, 118, *119*
balance, 117–18
evaluation, 118, *119*
recumbent, 119
seated, 118–19
potential energy, 37
power, electrical, 161
pressure, 40–4
atmospheric, 41
blood, 42
clinical focus, 41, 42–3
standard temperature and pressure (STP), 41
units, commonly used, *42*
*see also* partial pressures
pressure receptors, plantar, 117
pronation, *17*
properties of materials, 65–6
protanomaly, 193
protanopia, 193
proton emission tomography (PET) *see* positron emission
    tomography
protons, 153–4
flipping, *222*
net magnetization vector, 222
precession, 221–2
proximal, *17*
psoas minor anomalies, 89
psychiatry, PET in, *228*
pubic symphysis, 77
pulleys, 52
pyrexia, 40
Pythagorus' theorem., 12, *13*
solving vectors, *16*

## Q

Q-angle, 106
quadriceps muscles, 52, *54*
quadrilateral muscles, *93*
quantum mechanics, 133–5, *136*, 137–8
chemical bonding, 143–4, 148
de Quervain's disease, 86

## R

RADAR, 183
radial muscles, *95*
radial tunnel, 106
radiation *see* ionizing radiation
radiation pressure, 134
radio tracers, 186

radio waves, 182
encoding signal, 182
station identification, 182
radioactive half-life, 131, 187, *190*
radioactive isotopes, 187, *188–9*
radioactive sources, 187, *188–9*, 189
radioactivity, 187–92
natural exposure, 192
radiation types, 190–2
radiocarpal joint, *82*
radiolucency/radio-opacity, 211, 212
radionucleotides, 187, *188–9*
radiotherapy, 186
radium, 187, *188–9*, 189
injury, 191–2
Rankine scale, 39
raphés, 86
rear impact whiplash, 114–15
recumbent posture, 119
red muscle, 89
reflection, 192–3
laws of, *193*
refraction, 193–4
laws of, *194*
refractory period, 164
resistance, electrical, 156
resistors, 161, *162*
retrolisthesis, 112
rheumatism, 29
ribs
false ribs, 113
floating, 113
fractures, 113
true ribs, 112–13
rods, 193
roentgens, 209
roll and glide joint movements, 102, *103*
Röntgen, W., 185, *186*
rostral, *17*
rotation, 20
external, 19
internal, 19
lateral, *17*, 19
medial, *17*, 19
orthogonal system, 21, *22*, *23*
positive *vs* negative, 24
right hand rule, 24
*see also* instantaneous axis of rotation
the Royal Society, 29, 33
Ruffini end organs, 100
Rutherford, E.
alpha particles, 128–9, *190*
atomic model, 127–9, *128*, 131
beta particles, *190*

# S

s-block elements, 142
sacroiliac joint, 109
sacroiliac joint syndrome, 119
saddle joint (sellaris), 79, 81, 82
sagittal plane, 17
scalars see vectors/scalars
scattering
  classical (coherent), 197
  Compton (modified), 197–8, 198, 212, 213
schindylesis, 75
sciatica, 29–30
'Scientific Method', 28
scientific notation, 3–4, 5
  prefixes, 7, 9
scissor gait, 120
scoliosis, 108
seasonal affective disorder (SAD), 184–5, 239
seated posture, 118–19
  ideal, 119
second moment of area, 61–2
seconds, 6, 7
sellaris see saddle joint
semicircular canals, 117
semiconductors, 157
sensory ataxia, 120
serrate sutures, 74
Sharpey fibres, 86
shear force diagrams, 58
  cantilevered beams, 59
  non-cantilevered beams, 60
  self-loading characteristics, 60
  sign conventions, 58, 59
shear modulus, 63, 67
shear stress/strain, 66
shearing forces, 58
  calculation, 59–60
  relation to beam length, 60
short TI inversion recovery (STIR), 226
short-wave diathermy, 238
shoulder
  arthrokinematics, 102, 103, 107
  joint features, 107
  mobility vs stability, 100–1
  rotation, 101
SI units, 6–7, 7
  base units, 7
  derived, 8–9
  names/symbols, 8–9
  prefixes, 7, 9
skeletal muscle, 84–97
  architecture, 92, 93–6
  contraction, 86–7

  aerobic vs anaerobic, 87
  nerve supply, 86
  nomenclature, 89–90, 91
  variants, 87, 88, 89–90
    features, 89
  vascular supply, 87, 88
skin cancer, 185
sleeping posture see recumbent posture
'slipped disc', 77
slow twitch (tonic) muscles, 87, 89
smooth muscle, 84
sodium channels, 164
sodium chloride
  hydrogen bonds, 147
  ionic bonding in, 144
somatotypes, 120
  sleeping posture, ideal, 119
sound waves, range of, 236
space charge, 204
space charge effect, 205
specific heat, 147
spectral lines, visible, 137
spheroidal joint see ball and socket joint
sphygmomanometers, 42, 43
spin echo (SE), 225
spin joint movements, 102–4, 107
spinal units, functional, 77, 109
spinal X-rays, 213
spine
  compressive resistance, 107
  curves, normal, 107
  degrees of freedom, 109
  dislocated, 80
  injuries, 113–15
  joint features, 107–13
  transitional segments, 108
spiral CT, 220
spiral muscles, 96
spondylolisthesis, 112
spondylosis, 112
sprains, 84
spring (force) constant., 65, 66
squamous sutures, 75
standard temperature and pressure (STP), 41
standing wave modes, 135
stenosing tenosynovitis, 86
step-up/-down transducers, 169, 170–1, 171
strain, 66
strap muscles, 93
stress, 66
striated muscle, 84
suboccipital muscles, 113
superconductors, 156
superficial, 17

superior, 16
supination, 17
surge protection, 161
sutures, 73, 74
  closure anomalies, 75
  false sutures, 74–5
  true sutures, 74
symphyses, 76
synarthrosis, 73
synchondroses, 76
syndactyly, 105
syndesmoses, 75, *76*
synostoses, 74
synovial joints, 73, 77–83
  classification, 78–9
    structural, 83
  degrees of freedom, 101
  mobility, 78
synovial sheaths, 86
synovium, *77*
Système International D'unités *see* SI units
systems, electrical, 165–8

**T**

talipes equinovarus, 105
telegraphy, *153*
television, 182
temperature, 38, 39–40
  body, 40
  standard temperature and pressure (STP), 41
temporomandibular disorder (TMD), 115
temporomandibular joint (TMJ), 115–16
10 day rule, 216
tendons, 86
  damage, 86
  surgical repair, 97
tenosynovitis, stenosing, 86
TENS (transcutaneous electrical nerve stimulation), 240
tensile stress/strain, 66
therapeutic modalities, 235–43
thermionic emission, 204–5
  profile for tungsten, *204*
thermistors, 161, 205
Thompson, J. J.
  atomic model, 127, *128*
  Thompson prizes, *127*
thoracic outlet compression syndrome, 108
thoracic spine, 112–13
  motion, ranges of, *112*
  X-ray indications, *213*
thorium-232 series, *189*
three-dimensional movement, 21, *23*, 24

threshold frequencies, 136
tonic muscles *see* slow twitch muscles
tonic neck reflexes, 117
torque, 63
transcutaneous electrical nerve stimulation (TENS), 240
transducers, 165
transformers, 169–71
transistors, 165
transition metals, 142
transition values, 194, *195*
transitional spinal segments, 108
translation, 20
  orthogonal system, 21, *22*, *23*
transverse plane, *17*
  orthogonal equivalent, 20
triangular muscles, *96*
triaxial joints, 101
tricipital muscles, *96*
trigonocephaly, 75
trigonometry, 12–15
trochoid *see* pivot joint
truth tables, 166, *167*, *168*
tungsten electrons, *195*
  X-ray emission spectrum, *196*
tunnel of Guyon, 106

**U**

ultrasonography
  advantages, *229*
  coupling medium, 236
  diagnostic, 227–31
  Doppler, 231
  musculoskeletal, 229–30
  obstetric, 229–30
    clinical aspects, 230
  therapeutic, 235–8
    complications, 237
    drug uptake, 238
    energy absorption, 237
    healing/scarring, 237
    non-thermal effects, 237–8
    thermal effects, 237
  ultrasound, 235–6
    beam power/intensity, 236
    wave production, 236
    wave velocities in tissues, *236*
ultraviolet radiation, 184–5
  protection from, 185
  therapeutic, 184, 239
ultraviolet therapy, 184, 239
uniaxial joints, 101
unified field theory, 153

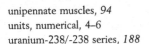 

unipennate muscles, *94*
units, numerical, 4–6
uranium-238/-238 series, *188*

## V

van der Waals bonds, 148
variable resistors, *161*
vectors/scalars, 7, 9
   addition of vectors, 16
   resolving vectors, 15–16
velocity, 30–1
   angular, 31
   in equations of motion, 35–6
   in laws of motion, 34
velocity ratio, 50
ventral, 16, *17*
vertebrae
   instantaneous axis of rotation, 64
   in transitional segments, 108
vestibular system, 117
viscoelasticity, 65–6
visible light, 184, 192–4
   reflection, 192–3
   refraction, 193–4
visible light therapy, 239
visual imaging, *181*
visual system and balance, 117
vitamin D production, *184*
Volta, A., *153*
voltage, 155

## W

waddling gait, *120*
water
   clinical aspects, 147
   density, 146
   electrostatic forces, 147
   heat of vaporization, 147
   molecule, 146–7
      electron shells, 146
   polarity, 146
   properties, 145–6
   as solvent, 146, 147
   specific heat, 147
wave equation, 181
wave–particle duality, 131, 180
wave theory, 133
wavelength, 180
weak nuclear force, 131
weight, 31
   clinical focus, 32
weights/measures, 2–7

whiplash-associated disorders, 113–15
   ramping force, 115
   rear impact whiplash, 114–15
   speed of incident, 115
'white coat syndrome, 42
white muscle, 89
work/energy, 37–8
   clinical focus, 38
work functions, 136, 205
wrist, 106

## X

X-ray(s), 185–6
   absorbed dose, 215
   absorption, *197*, 211–12
      differential, 211
   attenuation, 196–8, 210
   clinical indicators, *213*
   collimation, 208, 212
   contrast agents, 212
   diagnostic, 186
   effective dose, 215
   first radiograph, 185, *186*
   heel effect, 208, *209*
      clinical implications, 208–9, 214
   image production, 216–18
   imaging, *181*
   intensity, 209–10
   interaction with matter, 196–8
   $LD_{50}$, 216
   motion artifact, 214
   pair production, 198
   patient exposure, 205, 207, 211–12
      chronic *vs* acute, 216
      clinical aspects, 206, 213–14
   patient positioning, 206
   penetrability, 210–11
   photodisintegration, 198
   production, 194, *195*, 196, 207–9
      quality/quantity, 209–11
   radiation dosage, 214–15
   radiation weighting factor, 215
   radiolucency/radio-opacity, 211
   scattering
      classical (coherent), 197
      Compton (modified), 197–8, *198*, 212, *213*
   shielding, *214*
   ten day rule, 216
   therapeutic, 186
   tissue weighting factors, *216*
   *see also* computed tomography
X-ray diffraction, *186*

X-ray machines, 204–18
  autotransformer, 207
  Buckies, 216
  cathode, 206
  collimator, 208
  cost, 203–4
  dental, 208
  electron energy, 206–7
  electron production, 205–6
  filament, 205
  filament current, 205
  filtration, *211*
    compensating, 211
    inherent, 211
    and patient exposure, *214*
  full wave rectification, 207
  grids, 216, *217*
  half-value layer (HVL), 210
  image production, 216–18
  image receptor, 217–18
  intensifying screens, 217, *218*
  kilovolts peak (kV$_p$), 207, 210
    and absorption/transmission, *213*
  line compensator, 207
  quality/quantity of rays, 209–11
    factors affecting, *211*
  source-image distance (SID), 210, 214
  targets, 206, 207, 208, *209*
  thermionic emission, 204–5
  thermionic filament, 205
  thermionic tube, *207*
  tube current, 205–6
  X-ray circuit, 207, *208*
  X-ray tube, 206, *207*
  *see also* X-rays, production
X-ray profiles, *196*

**Y**

yield point, 65
Young, T., 134
  Young's fringes, 133
  Young's modulus, 66–7
    values for materials, *67*

**Z**

zygapophyseal (facet) joints, 77

Printed in the United States
By Bookmasters